T0293748

Mental Health Issues
of Child Maltreatment

Contemporary Strategies

Volume 2: Interventions &
Intersectional Considerations & Applications

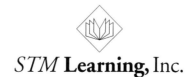

STM **Learning,** Inc.

Leading Publisher of Scientific, Technical, and Medical Educational Resources
Saint Louis
www.stmlearning.com

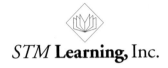

STM **Learning,** Inc.

We've partnered with Copyright Clearance Center to make it easy for you to request permissions to reuse content from STM Learning, Inc.

With copyright.com, you can quickly and easily secure the permissions you want.

Simply follow these steps to get started:

— Visit **copyright.com** and enter the title, ISBN, or ISSN number of the publication you'd like to reuse and hit "Go."
— After finding the title you'd like, choose "Pay-Per-Use Options."
— Enter the publication year of the content you'd like to reuse.
— Scroll down the list to find the type of reuse you want to request.
— Select the corresponding bubble and click "Price & Order."
— Fill out any required information and follow the prompts to acquire the proper permissions to reuse the content that you'd like.

For questions about using the service on **copyright.com**, please contact:

Copyright Clearance Center
222 Rosewood Drive
Danvers, MA 01923
Phone: +1-(978) 750-8400
Fax: +1-(978) 750-4470

Additional requests can be sent directly to **info@copyright.com**.

About Copyright Clearance Center

*Copyright Clearance Center (CCC), the rights licensing expert, is a global rights broker for the world's most sought-after books, journals, blogs, movies, and more. Founded in 1978 as a not-for-profit organization, CCC provides smart solutions that simplify the access and licensing of content that lets businesses and academic institutions quickly get permission to share copyright-protected materials, while compensating publishers and creators for the use of their works. We make copyright work. For more information, visit **www.copyright.com**.*

Mental Health Issues
of Child Maltreatment

Contemporary Strategies

Volume 2: Interventions &
Intersectional Considerations & Applications

Paul Thomas Clements, PhD, RN, ANEF, DF-IAFN, DF-AFN
Clinical Professor
Center for Excellence in Forensic Nursing
Texas A&M University
College Station, TX
President-Elect
Academy of Forensic Nursing

David T. Solomon, PhD, HSP-P
Associate Professor/ Director of Health Services Psychology
PsyD Program
Department of Psychology
Western Carolina University
Cullowhee, NC

Beth I. Barol, PhD, LSW, BCB, NADD-CC
Associate Dean (Retired)
Widener University Center for Social Work Education
Consultant (National and International)
Institute Director
Pennsylvania Capacity Building Institute
Ridley Park, PA

Ciera E. Schoonover, PhD, MSW, MPH, HSP
Assistant Professor
Department of Psychology
Middle Tennessee State University
Murfreesboro, TN

Soraya Seedat, PhD, MBChB, FC Psych (SA), MMed Psych, MPhil Applied Ethics (Bioethics)
Distinguished Professor and Executive Head
Department of Psychiatry
Stellenbosch University
Cape Town, South Africa

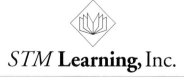

STM **Learning,** Inc.

Leading Publisher of Scientific, Technical, and Medical Educational Resources
Saint Louis
www.stmlearning.com

Publishers: Glenn E. Whaley and Marianne V. Whaley
Managing Editor: Samantha Brown
Graphic Design Director: Glenn E. Whaley
Graphic Designer: Connie H. C. Wang
Curriculum Developer: Samantha Brown
Associate Editors: Miya Russell, Tammy Arnow, Gracie York
Copy Editors: Miya Russell, Katie Slaten
Proofreaders: Katie Slaten, Tammy Arnow, Gracie York

Copyright ©2024 STM Learning, Inc.

All rights reserved. No part of this publication may be reproduced, stored in a retrieval system, or transmitted in any form or by any means, electronic, mechanical, photocopying, recording, or otherwise, without prior written permission from the publisher.

Printed in the United States of America.

Publisher:
STM Learning, Inc.
Saint Louis, Missouri 63033
Phone: (314) 434-2424
http://www.stmlearning.com orders@stmlearning.com

Print ISBN: 978-1-953119-26-1
eBook ISBN: 978-1-953119-27-8

Library of Congress Cataloging-in-Publication Data

Names: Clements, Paul T. (Paul Thomas), 1962- editor. | Solomon, David T.,
    editor. | Schoonover, Ciera, editor. | Barol, Beth I., editor. | Seedat,
    Soraya, 1966- editor.
Title: Mental health issues of child maltreatment : contemporary strategies
    / [edited by] Paul Thomas Clements, David T. Solomon, Ciera Schoonover,
    Beth I. Barol, Soraya Seedat.
Description: Saint Louis : STM Learning, Inc., [2023]- | Includes
    bibliographical references. | Contents: v. 1. Presentations & assessment
    | Summary: "A contemporary overview of strategies to identify and assess
    mental health issues arising from child maltreatment"-- Provided by
    publisher.
Identifiers: LCCN 2023046741 | ISBN 9781953119209 (v. 1 ; paperback) | ISBN
    9781953119216 (v. 1 ; ebook)
Subjects: MESH: Child Abuse--psychology | Stress Disorders,
    Traumatic--diagnosis | Adverse Childhood Experiences | Child
Classification: LCC RC569.5.C55 | NLM WS 350.8.A2 | DDC
    616.85/82230019--dc23/eng/20231113
LC record available at https://lccn.loc.gov/2023046741

CONTRIBUTORS

Eileen M. Alexy, PhD, RN, APN, PMHCNS-BC
Professor
Department of Nursing
The College of New Jersey
Ewing, NJ

Patrick C. Barton, MA
Doctoral Student
Department of Psychology
Western Carolina University
Cullowhee, NC

Andrea Blaskan, BSN, BA (Psychology)
Registered Nurse
Emergency Department
HCA
Las Vegas, NV

Beth I. Barol, PhD, LSW, BCB, NADD-CC
Associate Dean (Retired)
Widener University Center for Social Work Education
Consultant (National and International)
Institute Director
Pennsylvania Capacity Building Institute
Ridley Park, PA

Irene Brodd, PhD, LT, MSC, USN, Navy Medical Readiness and Training Command (NMRTC), Portsmouth

Sarah H. Buffie, MSW, LSW
Founder/Director/Lead Trainer/Consultant
Soul Bird Consulting
Cincinnati, OH

Paul Thomas Clements, PhD, RN, ANEF, DF-IAFN, DF-AFN
Clinical Professor
Center for Excellence in Forensic Nursing
Texas A&M University
College Station, TX
President-Elect
Academy of Forensic Nursing

Kelly Cummings, PhD, RN, 200 RYT, Caritas Coach®

Savannah Dettman, MA, LCMHCA
Psychotherapist
Asheville, NC

Ann C. Eckardt, PsyD, ABPP
Associate Research Scientist/Director of Military Research and Community-Based Prevention Science
Family Translational Research Group
New York University
New York, NY

Mitzy D. Flores, PhDc, MSN, RN, AHN-BC, CHSE, COI, Caritas Coach©, Introspective Hypnosis Practitioner
Visiting Professor/ Academic and Clinical Nurse Educator
School of Nursing
University of South Florida
Tampa, FL

Cathy L. Grist, PhD
Professor
Department of Human Services
Western Carolina University
Cullowhee, NC

Anna Johnson, MA

Adrienne N. Kennedy, DSW
Founder/ CEO
Pioneering Connections, LLC
Columbus, OH

Eva Klain, JD

Linda K. Knauss, PhD, ABPP
Professor
Institute for Graduate Clinical Psychology
Widener University
Chester, PA

Christopher A. Mallett, PhD, Esq, LISW-S
Professor
School of Social Work
Cleveland State University
Cleveland, OH

Kaleigh Mancha, MS, LMFT, Certified Full Spectrum Doula
Licensed Marriage & Family Therapist/ Co-Founder
Heart & Sol Collective
Las Vegas, NV

Ash Moomaw, MA
Department of Counseling Psychology
Ball State University
Muncie, IN

Matthew A. Myrick, PhD, LSW
Assistant Professor
Widener University
Chester, PA

Yewande Oshodi, MBBS, MPH, FMCPsych, Mphil, Cert CA Psych
Associate Professor of Psychiatry
Psychiatry Department
College of Medicine University of Lagos
Consultant Child and Adolescent Psychiatrist
Psychiatry Department
Lagos University Teaching Hospital (LUTH)
Lagos, Nigeria

C. Danae Riggs
Certified Trauma Consultant/Resilience Worker
Soul Bird Consulting
Certified Trauma Consultant/Resilience Worker
Humans Being Human Consulting
Cincinnati, OH

Adjoa D. Robinson, PhD, MSW

Ciera E. Schoonover, PhD, MSW, MPH, HSP
Assistant Professor
Department of Psychology
Middle Tennessee State University
Murfreesboro, TN

Soraya Seedat, PhD, MBChB, FC Psych (SA), MMed Psych, MPhil Applied Ethics (Bioethics)
Distinguished Professor/Executive Head
Department of Psychiatry
Stellenbosch University
Cape Town, South Africa

Anna Segura, PhD
Assistant Research Scientist
Family Translational Research Group
New York University
New York, NY

Amy M. Smith Slep, PhD
Professor
Family Translational Research Group
New York University
New York, NY

David T. Solomon, PhD, HSP-P
Associate Professor/ Director of Health Services Psychology
PsyD Program
Department of Psychology
Western Carolina University
Cullowhee, NC

Caelan Soma, PsyD, LP, LMSW
Chief Clinical Officer
Starr Commonwealth
Albion, MI

Eileen F. Starr, PhD, LCSW

Alicia Summers, PhD
Director
Data Savvy Consulting, LLC
Reno, NV

Sandra Swart, MBChB, MMed (Psych)
Consultant Psychiatrist
Cape Town, South Africa

Lisa Ann Tauai, RD, MBA, CWP
Healthcare to Health Dietitian
99th Operations Medical Readiness Squadron
United States Air Force
Nellis Air Force Base, NV

Nancy Thaler, MHOS
Co-Director
National Capacity Building Institute
National Association of State Directors of Developmental Disabilities Services
Alexandria, VA

Cathi Tillman, MSW, ACSW, LSW, Certificate: Harvard Program in Refugee Trauma
Executive Director
La Puerta Abierta, Inc
Philidelphia, PA

Rebecca Vlam, MSS, LCSW
Clinical Assistant Professor
The Center for Social Work Education
Widener University
Chester, PA

Madelyne Williams, BS

Jeannette B. Wyatt, PhD, LCSW
Associate Professor
Center for Social Work Education
Widener University
Chester, PA

FOREWORD

In 1988, I was a newly minted prosecutor working in a rural county of approximately 13 000 people. As is often the case with new prosecutors, I was assigned to handle the less glamorous cases that rarely catch the public's eye—child protection cases, juvenile justice cases, and criminal cases involving interpersonal violence in which children were witnesses to the cruelties adults inflict on one another.

If truth be told, none of us back then knew what we were doing—not the judges, prosecutors, defense attorneys, child protection workers, law enforcement officers, medical or mental health professionals. This was approximately a decade before the publication of "Adverse Childhood Experience"[1] research and terms such as "poly-victimization"[2] and "trauma-informed practice"[3] were not yet in our vocabulary.

We were not far removed from high-profile daycare cases in which well-intentioned professionals unaware of child development, linguistics, and other factors that need to be considered when interviewing young children, made errors which resulted in the overturning of convictions. The collection of evidence was also very different back then. Cell phones, the internet, laptops, and other technology were not widely used.

We have come a long way since then. Today, there are over 950 Children's Advocacy Centers serving nearly every community in the United States. We now implement forensic interview training programs to thousands of frontline interviewers as well as other members of the medical community.[4] The growth of the internet and cell phone usage made it easier to locate and sexually abuse children, but it also created an online footprint that makes it easier to prosecute those who prey on children. Although still in its infancy, there is even movement to develop spiritual care workers or specially trained chaplains who can respond to the spiritual impact of child abuse.[5]

Perhaps the most exciting development in recent decades is the idea that the past need not be prologue and that, working together, we can significantly reduce child abuse.

There is a simple reason for the decline in child abuse: we have dramatically improved the education of teachers, doctors, nurses, child protection workers, criminal justice professionals and medical and mental health providers to prevent abuse and, when it cannot be prevented, to respond with excellence.

This is why the publication of *Mental Health Issues of Child Maltreatment* is so important. In these pages, frontline professionals of today and tomorrow will find concrete, research-supported responses to nearly every aspect of child maltreatment. Perhaps best viewed as a toolkit, this invaluable resource will guide these professionals to even greater heights of responding to child maltreatment in a trauma-informed manner.

Although the complete eradication of child abuse may not be within our grasp anytime soon, it is clear we are making great strides, and the best is yet to come. To that end, *Mental Health Issues of Child Maltreatment* is a welcome addition to the child protection canon.

Victor I. Vieth, JD[6]
Director, Center for Faith & Child Protection

REFERENCES

1. Vincent Felitti & Robert F. Anda, *The Relationship of Adverse Childhood Experiences to Adult Medical Disease, Psychiatric Disorders and Sexual Behavior: Implications for Healthcare,* in Ruthe A. Lanius, eric Vermeten & Clare Pain (EDS) The Impact of Early Life Trauma on Health and Disease: The Hidden Epidemic 77 (Cambridge Medicine 2010).

2. Heather A. Turner, David Finkelhor, and Richard Ormrod, *Poly-Victimization in a National Sample of Children and Youth,* 38(3) American Journal of Preventive Medicine 323 (2010), David Finkelhor, Richard K. Omrod, Heather A. Turner, *Poly-victimization: A Neglected Component in Child Victimization,* 31 Journal of Child Abuse & Neglect 7 (2007).

3. SAMHSA's Concept of Trauma and Guidance for a Trauma-Informed Approach. HHS Publication No. (SMA) 14-4884. Rockville, MD: Substance Abuse and Mental Health Services Administration, 2014.

4. Rita Farrell and Victor Vieth, *ChildFirst® forensic interview training program,* 32(2) APSAC Advisor 56-63 (2020); Kathleeen Coulborn Faller, *Forty Years of Forensic Interviewing of Children Suspected of Sexual Abuse, 1974-2014: Historical Benchmarks,* 4 Social Sciences 34, 49 (2015).

5. Victor I. Vieth, Mark D. Everson, Viola Vaughan-Eden, Suzanna Tiapula, Shauna Galloway-Williams, Carrie Nettles, *Keeping Faith: The Potential Role of a Chaplain to Address the Spiritual Needs of Maltreated Children and Advise Child Abuse Multi-Discplinary Teams,* 14(2) Liberty University Law Review 351 (2020).

6. Chief Program Officer for Education & Research, Zero Abuse Project. Mr. Vieth is a former child abuse prosecutor who received national attention for his work to address child abuse in rural communities. He went on to direct the National Center for Prosecution of Child Abuse. He is the recipient of the Victim Rights Legend Award from the United States Department of Justice, the Lifetime Achievement Award from the Institute on Violence, Abuse & Trauma (IVAT), and the Change Maker Award from the Academy on Violence & Abuse.

PREFACE

As the first volume of this book highlights, child maltreatment can have long-lasting negative effects on survivors. This includes a high incidence of psychological distress throughout childhood and into adulthood, including higher rates of post-traumatic stress disorder (PTSD),[1] depression,[2] anxiety,[3] delinquent behavior,[4] non-suicidal self-injury,[2] and suicide attempts.[5] Compounding the issue is the high comorbidity between types of child maltreatment[6] (ie, when a child has experienced one type of child maltreatment, it is more likely that they have experienced others as well). Although the problem is immense, it is heartening that there are a number of options at the hands of communities and clinicians that can potentially prevent child maltreatment and assuage its negative impact when it does occur. For example, heightened awareness toward the importance of earlier screening and identification of child maltreatment, the significant expansion of mandatory reporting laws across the nation to include a broader array of child care providers (including volunteers at camps and youth centers, members of the clergy, athletic staff, and even photographic processors),[7] and an enhanced understanding of the impact of adverse childhood experiences (ACES)[8] and the need for subsequent therapeutic mitigation, all provide hope for preventing an overwhelming derailment of on-time intrapsychic growth and development for maltreated children.

Increasing access to information also increases access to misinformation. For example, although popular social media site TikTok® has been suggested as a powerful tool for disseminating mental health information,[9] a 2023 study of the most viewed videos related to autism spectrum disorder on TikTok® found that only 27% of them could be classified as accurate.[1] Professionals are likewise not immune from the influence of misinformation. In the journal *Research on Social Work Practice,* Cox & Codd[7] outline a pressing issue: despite the existence of multiple evidence-supported treatments for trauma and anxiety symptoms, many trauma survivors do not receive such treatments. They highlight that many clinicians are more familiar with pop-psychology books promoting treatments with little-to-no empirical basis than they are with research-backed work. In fact, the majority of clients seeking help for anxiety in community settings receive supportive therapies,[8] which tend to be less effective than cognitive-behavioral or other evidence-based treatments.[10,11] Receiving ineffective interventions can lead to a person experiencing additional suffering because they are not given the opportunity to lessen or eliminate their symptoms through more effective interventions.[12] Worse, some unsupported treatments may cause further harm to maltreatment and trauma survivors than if no intervention is administered at all. For example, both critical incident stress debriefing and attachment therapy have been found to be harmful to recipients compared to no treatment at all, yet they continue to be administered in some settings.

Dissemination of accurate information regarding effective intervention is integral to curtailing the negative effects of child maltreatment and bettering the lives of survivors. In direct response to these ongoing inaccuracies, misperceptions, and misuses of approaches (even if well-intentioned), this volume encourages the translation of the latest evidence into sound clinical practice, including efforts related to prevention, intervention, and building resilience. This volume also increases its utility through its use of an intersectional viewpoint to focus on specific considerations and applications of effective prevention and intervention strategies when working with a variety of populations.

As with the first volume, *Mental Health Issues of Child Maltreatment: Contemporary Strategies, Volume 2* is not limited to a particular discipline or part of the globe. It is both a book for the professional in need of a quick, yet evidence-based, resource check and a source for the student who is just learning about the scope of child maltreatment. Specifically, in direct response to the overarching and overwhelming needs of this vulnerable population of at-risk children, *Mental Health Issues of Child Maltreatment* intends to do the following:

— **Define the problem** of child maltreatment conceptually and numerically, using statistics that describe the state of maltreatment and the characteristics of those most affected by it

— **Identify causes and risk factors** that appear to affect susceptibility to maltreatment, such as factors that increase a child's risk of abuse or obstacles to delivering effective child protection services

— **Design interventions** that are trauma-informed, sensitive, and developmentally targeted for children and their caregivers

— **Disseminate information** about the evidence and effectiveness of these interventions to increase the profile for their usage in clinical practice

— **Educate students and future professionals** in psychology, medicine, nursing, social work, and creative arts therapies to mitigate the effects of child maltreatment for future generations.

It is with these thoughts and intentions that we, both individually and collectively, are hopeful that the following chapters will provide support and guidance to you, the reader, in your efforts toward providing trauma-informed care to children seeking mental health care during a time or times of need. The world, indeed, can be a complex and often traumatic place for children to navigate. We are optimistic that the information contained within this book can provide direction during the journey.

Paul Thomas Clements, PhD, RN, ANEF, DF-IAFN, DF-AFN

David T. Solomon, PhD, HSP-P

Beth I. Barol, PhD, LSW, BCB, NADD-CC

Ciera E. Schoonover, PhD, MSW, MPH, HSP

Soraya Seedat, PhD, MBChB, FC Psych (SA), MMed Psych, MPhil Applied Ethics (Bioethics)

REFERENCES

1. Shenk CE, O'Donnell KJ, Pokhvisneva I, et al. Epigenetic age acceleration and risk for posttraumatic stress disorder following exposure to substantiated child maltreatment. *J Clin Child and Adolesc Psychol.* 2022;51(5):651-661. doi:10.1080/15374416.2020.1864738

2. Yan R, Ding W, Wang D, et al. Longitudinal relationship between child maltreatment, bullying victimization, depression, and nonsuicidal self injury among left behind children in China: 2 year follow up. *J Clin Psychol.* 2023;79(12):2899-2917. doi:10.1002/jclp.23585

3. Liu J, Deng J, Zhang H, Tang X. The relationship between child maltreatment and social anxiety: A meta-analysis. *J Affective Disord.* 2023;329:157-167. doi:10.1016/j.jad.2023.02.081

4. Gauthier-Duchesne A, Hébert M, Blais M. Child sexual abuse, self-esteem, and delinquent behaviors during adolescence: The moderating role of gender. *J Interperson Violence.* 2022;37(15-16):NP12725-NP12744. doi:10.1177/08862605211001466

5. Ernst M, Brähler E, Kampling H, et al. Is the end in the beginning? Child maltreatment increases the risk of non-suicidal self-injury and suicide attempts through impaired personality functioning. *Child Abuse Negl.* 2022;133:1-13. doi:10.1016/j.chiabu.2022.105870

6. Matsumoto M, Piersiak HA, Letterie MC, Humphreys KL. Population-based estimates of associations between child maltreatment types: A meta-analysis. *Trauma Violence Abuse.* 2023;24(2):487-496. doi:10.1177/15248380211030502

7. Cox KS, Codd RT. Advocates of research-supported treatments for PTSD are losing in lots of ways: What are we going to do about it? *Res Soc Work Pract.* 2023;34(4). doi:10.1177/10497315231206754

8. Wolitzky-Taylor K, Zimmermann M, Arch JJ, De Guzman E, Lagomasino I. Has evidence-based psychosocial treatment for anxiety disorders permeated usual care in community mental health settings? *Behav Res Therapy.* 2015;72:9-17. doi:10.1016/j.brat.2015.06.010

9. Chochol MD, Gandhi K, Elmaghraby R, Croarkin PE. Harnessing youth engagement with mental health TikTok and its potential as a public health tool. *J Am Acad Child Adolesc Psychiatry.* 2023;62(7):710-712. doi:10.1016/j.jaac.2022.11.015

10. Nordh M, Wahlund T, Jolstedt M, et al. Therapist-guided internet-delivered cognitive behavioral therapy vs internet-delivered supportive therapy for children and adolescents with social anxiety disorder: A randomized clinical trial. *JAMA Psychiatry.* 2021;78(7):705-713. doi:10.1001/jamapsychiatry.2021.0469

11. Norman SB, Capone C, Panza KE, et al. A clinical trial comparing trauma informed guilt reduction therapy (TrIGR), a brief intervention for trauma related guilt, to supportive care therapy. *Depress Anxiety.* 2022;39(4):262-273. doi:10.1002/da.23244

12. Kalokairinou L, Choi R, Nagappan A, Wexler A. Opportunity cost or opportunity lost: An empirical assessment of ethical concerns and attitudes of EEG neurofeedback users. *Neuroethics.* 2022;15:1-13. doi:10.1007/s12152-022-09506-x

13. Aragon-Guevara D, Castle G, Sheridan E, Vivanti G. The reach and accuracy of information on autism on tiktok. *J Autism Dev Disord.* August 2023. doi:10.1007/s10803-023-06084-6

Our Mission

To become the world leader in publishing and

information services on child abuse,

maltreatment, diseases, and domestic violence.

We seek to heighten awareness of these issues

and provide relevant information to

professionals and consumers.

REVIEWS

The authors have expertly woven together a comprehensive exploration of children who have encountered Adverse Childhood Experiences that is both informative and engaging. This book is an indispensable resource for anyone in the field of child maltreatment, offering a wealth of knowledge, practical guidance, and insightful perspectives.

The authors' deep understanding of forensic issues is evident throughout the book, making it a trusted companion for professionals, students, and anyone interested in the subject. The content is well-structured and covers a wide range of essential topics, from evidence collection and documentation to legal considerations and the emotional aspects of patient care.

One of the book's notable strengths is its commitment to staying current with the latest advancements and best practices in forensic mental health. It not only provides a solid foundation but also incorporates up-to-date information and case studies, ensuring that readers are well prepared to meet the challenges of this dynamic field.

What sets Mental Health Issues of Child Maltreatment *apart is its compassionate approach. The authors pay special attention to the emotional and psychological needs of patients, which is a critical aspect of our work. This focus on holistic care makes it an invaluable resource for anyone striving to excel in the field of child maltreatment.*

Overall, the authors have crafted a must-read book that combines expertise with empathy, making it an indispensable reference for mental health professionals and an enlightening read for anyone interested in this essential field of health care. I wholeheartedly recommend Mental Health Issues of Child Maltreatment *to all those committed to providing the highest standard of care and justice.*

Ann Wolbert Burgess
Professor
William Connell School of Nursing
Boston College
Chestnut Hill, MA

Mental Health Issues of Child Maltreatment *is a long overdue comprehensive resource that should be required reading for all mental health professionals, child welfare workers, court personnel and administrators—in fact, all who come into contact with survivors of child maltreatment. The text addresses the biological and neurological manifestations and consequences of child maltreatment, providing an up-to-date review of the state-of-the-art of our understanding of the sequelae of trauma. The text goes on to provide a thorough review of the challenges of accurate assessment and offers the reader a number of innovative strategies for effective interventions. Finally, the reader is presented with the challenges and strategies for extending our understanding in these areas through research. In summary, this text is an important contribution to capturing what we currently know about child maltreatment and trauma and how to intervene appropriately and effectively.*

Paula Silver, PhD
Educator and Administrator
Retired Dean
School of Human Services
Widener University
Chester, PA

This two-volume book offers a fresh perspective of childhood trauma for multidisciplinary professionals. It both questions past methods and offers successful approaches to thinking about, assessing, and treating children. The book has thoughtful, practical, and clinically relevant material for thinking about children who are now adults. Children are our future, and this book promotes means to prevent childhood maltreatment and promote their wellbeing. It honors what a whole person and whole family may need. The books highlight that children do not know what to ask for when they have had adverse childhood experiences. They do not have the resources to work on understanding and influencing what has happened to them. It is clearly up to clinical practitioners to recognize and treat the whole person, a whole family, and overarching systems.

I highly recommend this two-volume book, as it is comprehensive, clear, and compassionate in assessing and treating these often "invisible victims."

Ginny Focht-New, PhD, PMH-CNS,
BCB, NADD-CC, BCN

Contents in Brief

Contents in Detail

Mental Health Issues
of Child Maltreatment

Contemporary Strategies

*Volume 2: Interventions &
Intersectional Considerations & Applications*

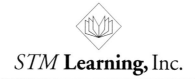

STM Learning, Inc.

Leading Publisher of Scientific, Technical, and Medical Educational Resources
Saint Louis
www.stmlearning.com

Section

I

INTERVENTIONS

INTRODUCTION TO EVIDENCE-SUPPORTED TREATMENTS FOR CHILD MALTREATMENT

David T. Solomon, PhD, HSP-P
Cathy L. Grist, PhD
Anna Johnson, MA

OBJECTIVES

After reading this chapter, the reader will be able to:

1. *Articulate the rationale for the use of evidence-supported treatments over novel, untested treatments.*

2. *Evaluate the evidence for child maltreatment (CM) interventions.*

3. *Describe the important components of implementing of evidence-supported treatments.*

BACKGROUND AND SIGNIFICANCE

Although definitions of CM vary, types of maltreatment include physical, emotional, and sexual abuse, and physical and emotional neglect. These acts of maltreatment affect children worldwide. One meta-analysis, published in 2015, found that the global incident rates of CM in the general population were estimated at 22.6% for physical abuse, 36.3% for emotional abuse, 16.3% for physical neglect, 18.4% for emotional neglect, and between 7.6% of boys and 18% of girls for sexual abuse.[1] These prevalence estimates indicate that between 7 and 36 out of 100 children will experience some form of maltreatment during childhood.[1] Additionally, a 2010 World Health Organization retrospective survey across 21 countries found that of those who had experienced CM, almost 40% had experienced multiple instances.[2]

Experiences of maltreatment during childhood can have short-term and long-term effects, including but not limited to: an increased risk for mood disorders, eating disorders, and other mental illnesses,[3,4] substance use,[5,6] suicide risk,[7] homelessness, and adult incarceration.[8] For example, a recent study found that individuals with mental health diagnoses were more likely to report a history of CM than those with no diagnoses, and CM history was related to an earlier age for the onset of mood disorders as well as more severe symptoms.[3]

Based on the high prevalence of CM and its multiple potential negative sequelae, effective interventions and preventions related to CM are crucial. Children who have experienced maltreatment deserve effective intervention to reduce the resulting distress of a difficult life experience that they had no control over. Effective intervention can potentially save them from years of emotional hardship and unfulfilled potential. The most reliable way to meet these goals is through the utilization of evidence-supported treatments (ESTs) that have been objectively shown to result in meaningful improvements for individuals impacted by CM. The work done to research ESTs eliminates many of the potential "unknowns" that are still present with novel, untested treatments, which may, for many reasons that will be discussed, appear to be effective when they are not.

CONTROVERSY RELATED TO EVIDENCE-SUPPORTED TREATMENTS

Although this introduction focuses broadly on ESTs, and many of the chapters throughout this section focus on specific ESTs, it should be noted that ESTs comprise just 1 piece of an overarching concept called evidence-based practice (EBP). EBP involves the integration of research evidence on which treatments, and which components of treatments, are effective in improving relevant clinical outcomes, a therapist's or counselor's clinical expertise, and the values and preferences of the client.[9] For example, parent-child interaction therapy (PCIT; see **Chapter 5: Promoting Healthy Parent-Child Interactions**) has been shown to be effective in reducing future instances of parental use of physical abuse with their children[10] and decreasing child externalizing behaviors.[11,12] Although PCIT is a manualized treatment in which most sessions will involve the therapist coaching caregivers through interactions with their children, the therapist uses clinical judgement and expertise to determine the focus of each coaching session and the methods utilized in order to meet the family's specific goals. The therapist must make quick, in-the-moment decisions based on an expert understanding of the theoretical underpinnings of the treatment. This is further demonstrated by the fact that, in some situations, the interactions that the therapist is coaching the caregiver through may be intense (eg, if the caregiver is having to put the child in time-out); therefore, the therapist also needs the interpersonal skills to reduce caregiver distress and to calmly talk them through the interaction. These relate to therapist-specific skills and expertise that are integral to the process. However, while clinical expertise is extremely valuable to effective implementation of treatment, there are several reasons why it should not be used in isolation from, or take precedence over, sound clinical research for the selection of specific treatments.

Still, some clinicians have been resistant to utilizing ESTs. For example, in the late 1990s, Myers & Thyer[13] sparked a small debate when they suggested that social work clients should have a right to effective, empirically validated treatments. Witkin[14] responded that "Myers and Thyer's article is less about 'rights' than it is about tightening the grip of empiricism on social work practice research education." It is clear that Witkin viewed the concept of empiricism with some antagonism. Years later, in 2013, Lilienfeld and colleagues[9] commented on a similar resistance to ESTs in the field of clinical psychology, and it is clear that there are disagreements about the need for EBPs in other disciplines as well.[15] Furthermore, a review of survey research found that in most studies, clinicians rated empirical evidence as less important than their own clinical experiences while making treatment decisions, indicating that there is possible indifference towards clinical research within the field.[9] For example, a large survey of licensed clinical social workers found that most had used at least 1 EST as well as at least 1 novel, unsupported treatment in their practice.[16] Even as of the early 2020s, several qualitative studies indicated that some clinicians still either lack knowledge about evidence-based practices or are reluctant to use ESTs due to beliefs that they do not meet the needs of their client populations or could negatively impact therapist-client relationships.[17,18]

Why do some clinicians avoid or ignore ESTs and research evidence? One possibility is that these professionals have little faith in research in general. This attitude may be intensified when the research does not support a person's current clinical practice. The scientific impotence discounting hypothesis, inspired by cognitive dissidence theory, suggests that when individuals are exposed to scientific evidence that disconfirms their current beliefs, they tend to rationalize the disconfirming evidence by asserting that the given topic under investigation cannot be accurately assessed using extant scientific methods. Indeed, a series of studies by Munro,[19] found that when participants read research abstracts with results contrary to their current beliefs, they were more likely to say that science was not able to examine that topic. Strikingly, they were also more likely to say that science was not able to examine several other unrelated topics. These findings suggest that when individuals are exposed to research that contradicts their beliefs, they are not only more likely to discount that research, but also to discount all research more generally.

Additionally, some clinicians feel that it is not necessary to utilize ESTs because all treatments are roughly equivalent in their effectiveness. The supposed axiom that all treatments are equally as effective is also known as the dodo verdict (harkening to the dodo bird's proclamation in *Alice's Adventures in Wonderland* that all the participants in a race were winners). Certainly, it would be heartening to have a plethora of effective treatments for a variety of mental and emotional struggles. This concept, however, first originated in the 1930s,[20] and while research does support that non-therapy specific factors, such as therapeutic alliance, do account for some proportion of the outcomes of therapy,[21] it is no longer accurate to say that the majority of the evidence indicates that every treatment modality is equally as effective for every type of psychopathology.[22] It is also likely that some forms of psychological distress are more treatable by a wider array of therapeutic modalities than others. Take, for example, post-traumatic stress disorder (PTSD) and borderline personality disorder, which are 2 diagnoses that are linked to a history of CM;[23-25] both of these diagnoses show clear responsiveness to a relatively small set of treatments.[26,27] However, even when multiple effective treatments exist, some treatments are still more effective than others.

Finally, some clinicians may feel that research evidence is not important because they can determine the effectiveness of their work with their clients. It is nearly impossible, though, to determine that because a client has improved *during* therapy, it means that they have improved *because of* therapy. This understanding may make treatment seem more effective than it actually is. When a client shows improvement during therapy, there are a host of competing explanations for their improvement, such as the placebo effect, natural recovery, and multiple treatments co-occurring (eg, a client may be in individual therapy, join a support group, and start taking medication all during the same period).[9] Additionally, while clinical expertise is required for good clinical decision making, clinicians need to be aware that they are subject to the same cognitive biases that can impact any person's judgement, such as confirmation bias.[28] For example, because clinicians assume the therapy they are providing is helpful, they may "see" improvement that is not actually occurring or come up with alternative explanations when improvement is not occurring. However, the majority of all the potential threats to making valid inferences about the effectiveness of a treatment with individual clients can be accounted for through sound research design (eg, by using randomized control trials), thereby allowing for much firmer statements about the effectiveness of a treatment to be made.

USE OF EVIDENCE-SUPPORTED TREATMENTS: A LOGICAL AND ETHICAL RATIONALE

Despite disagreement in the field, the authors of this chapter argue that the use of ESTs can help clinicians engage in effective and ethical practices. Most professional ethical codes indicate that clinicians should avoid harm to their clients, while others specify that services should also benefit clients. For example, the first principle of the American Psychological Association's ethical code[29] is Beneficence and Nonmaleficence, meaning that psychologists "strive to benefit those with whom they work and take care to do no harm." Furthermore, the American Counseling Association's code of ethics[30] indicates that "[c]ounselors have a responsibility to the public to engage in counseling practices that are based on rigorous research methodologies."

As has already been pointed out, it is difficult to determine if a treatment is effective during work with individual clients. The problem, then, is that when a treatment modality has not been researched, it is possible that it either does not significantly decrease distress or increase wellbeing or may even cause harm to clients. Lilienfeld[31] described a set of criteria for determining potentially harmful psychological treatments. First, research must indicate that the treatment results in some harm, physical or psychological, to the client or people associated with the client. Such harm could be an exacerbation of symptoms or even the stifling of natural recovery (ie, clients would have gotten better faster on their own without the treatment). The harm must also be long-term as opposed to a temporary increase in symptoms. This is important because therapy can often be emotionally tough for clients who are often asked to confront difficult issues, which can be distressing. This may be particularly true of treatments for trauma such as CM. For example, trauma-focused cognitive behavioral therapy (TF-CBT, see **Chapter 4: Trauma-Focused Cognitive Behavioral Therapy**) is an evidence-supported treatment originally designed as a treatment for child sexual abuse but later expanded for other traumas. TF-CBT requires frank and difficult discussion of traumatic experiences with both child clients and their caregivers, and the latter portion of the treatment involves the child creating a trauma narrative that they will later share with their caregiver, which may cause distress. However, TF-CBT is shown by meta-analysis to reduce PTSD symptoms, despite the temporary distress during treatment.[32] The final criterion proposed by Lilienfeld[31] is that the negative effects of the treatment must have been established by more than 1 independent research team. This final criterion mirrors similar standards for deeming a treatment effective, but it also prevents a treatment from being labeled as harmful due to some random error in the research results, poor research design, or a biased research team.

However, Mercer[33] suggested an alternate set of criteria for categorizing potentially harmful treatments for children focusing on CM, such as physical harm or emotional abuse occurring due to the treatment. She noted that children are a vulnerable population who have less autonomy over decisions made about their psychological treatment. She also pointed out that many aversive events, such as the deaths of children during therapy, are extremely serious and often occur outside of research studies. For these reasons, requiring potential harm to be uncovered by multiple research teams is not appropriate, and indeed in some cases, anecdotal evidence may be sufficient.

Despite differences in their classification systems, both Mercer[33] and Lilienfeld[31] categorize attachment therapy as a potentially harmful treatment. Attachment therapy is aimed at children with trauma and maltreatment histories, many of whom are in foster care. Harmful techniques used in attachment therapy include forced holding or having the caregiver lie on top of the child, forcing children to drink excessive amounts of water, and rebirthing techniques where the child is wrapped in a blanket or carpet and required to struggle their way out, often while pressure is being applied to them, symbolizing being reborn. These methods have resulted in water poisoning and suffocation deaths in several children.[34] Additionally, attachment therapists may rub lotion on or otherwise touch the children regardless of whether the child consents; having an unrelated adult touch a child with extensive abuse history against their will is potentially emotionally harmful.

While it may seem like harmful treatments would be easy to identify (thus arguably lessening the requirement for novel treatments to be researched), this is not always the case. One reason for this is that treatments can be potentially harmful even if the rationale for a treatment seems entirely cogent or is otherwise based on sound theory. Even attachment therapy is based, in part, on a well-supported attachment theory that has been more successfully applied to other treatments that are evidence-supported.[34] Critical incident stress debriefing (CISD) is another treatment that was identified by Lilienfeld[31] as a potentially harmful treatment. CISD is group PTSD prevention for individuals who have experienced some shared trauma (eg, groups of first responders) and is usually administered in 1 several-hour session within a few days after the trauma. It makes logical sense that responding early, providing psychoeducation about PTSD, and normalizing trauma reactions would be beneficial; however, a review of the research found that CISD, at best, has negligible effectiveness and, at worst, increases the likelihood of participants developing PTSD.[31] Interestingly, 1 study found that most individuals who received CISD stated that they were satisfied with the treatment, even though (unbeknownst to the participants) they were actually more likely to develop PTSD symptoms than those who did not receive CISD,[35] which further highlights the difficulty of determining if treatment is effective, even for the clients receiving the treatment.

Even when a treatment does not cause harm per se, a treatment that is merely ineffective (or substantially less effective than alternative treatments) is still ethically problematic. The primary reason for this is that clients are spending money on an ineffective intervention and wasting valuable time that could be used for a more effective service; this is what is termed as opportunity cost.[36] Stated more plainly, providing an ineffective treatment, when effective alternatives exist, unduly prolongs the suffering of clients, which should be considered unacceptable in any helping profession. This problem is further compounded if a client or family, after having received ineffective treatment, does not pursue further, potentially helpful treatments because they have come to believe that therapy in general is ineffective.

Are all novel, untested treatments ineffective or harmful? Most likely not. It is important to continue to develop new treatments and work on improving existing ones. However, the development of a new treatment is only the first step towards the widespread ethical use of that treatment with clients. As this chapter highlights, research is necessary to establish the effectiveness and efficacy of any treatment. Untested treatments might be effective, but they might also be ineffective or harmful. When a treatment is untested, no matter how much it *seems* like it would be beneficial, its efficacy remains speculation.

It should be noted that there are various reasons that could make a particular treatment, even an EST, contraindicated, or that might otherwise make another treatment more appropriate for a given client. However, when clinicians choose to avoid particular treatments for reasons that are not, in reality, related to probable outcomes, they could be subjecting clients to opportunity cost. For example, 1 survey of 182 exposure therapy trained therapists found that the participants' reasons for excluding clients from exposure therapy (eg, a belief that the client was emotionally frail) were not supported by the literature for predicting poor therapeutic outcomes and that some attributes of the therapist (eg, anxiety tolerance) were also predictive of the likelihood of excluding clients from exposure therapy.[37] This is problematic, given that a large meta-analysis of 65 studies found that exposure therapy resulted in large decreases in PTSD symptoms and was more effective than treatments that were not trauma-focused.[38] An additional meta-analysis also found that the amount of trauma-focus a treatment had did not predict treatment dropout,[39] which makes it unlikely that a substantial number of clients cannot tolerate discussing their trauma. This information indicates that when clinicians falsely believe a client cannot emotionally deal with a treatment that directly discusses and confronts the trauma, they may be unduly extending that client's distress through provision of ineffective or less effective services.

When the preponderance of the research favors the effectiveness of one treatment over another, the research evidence should be the deciding factor over the clinician's personal judgement, unless there is a strong objective reason, such as the client having previously not responded favorably to that treatment.[9] Even in cases when a client declines a certain treatment modality (even after a discussion of the rationale and possible benefits of that modality), the possible alternative treatments should likewise be ESTs.

SELECTING AND IMPLEMENTING EVIDENCE-SUPPORTED TREATMENTS

The authors of this chapter recommend 3 considerations for matching a client with a potential EST. First, the client's specific pattern of symptoms and difficulties, as determined through the assessment process, should be translated into specific and measurable treatment goals. Second, the clinician should consider which ESTs have been shown, using the highest rigor of scientific methods, to be effective for the client's symptoms of focus. Finally, if multiple ESTs of similar rigor exist, consider *how* effective (ie, in terms of effect sizes) each one has been in research studies.

It is important to consider that there are multiple possible outcomes following CM, ranging from little to no lasting distress to more severe reactions. When a survivor of maltreatment does exhibit symptoms following their CM experience, the types of symptoms vary. Additionally, when an EST is examined, it is usually tested for its effectiveness on specific outcomes and symptoms. For this reason, the selection of an appropriate EST should be based on clinical assessment and the specific symptoms experienced by the client. For example, if a 6-year-old child has experienced physical abuse and is exhibiting behavioral difficulties but very few PTSD-specific symptoms, TF-CBT (which focuses more on PTSD symptoms) may be less appropriate than other ESTs that focus more on externalizing problems or harsh physical parenting.

How does one determine if a treatment has sufficient evidence for its use for a given outcome? While a full discussion of evaluating research is beyond the scope of this chapter, randomized controlled trials, which utilize a control group, and meta-analyses tend to provide the strongest levels of evidence. The American Psychological Association's guidelines for determining ESTs indicates that for a treatment to be probably efficacious or well-established, the treatment must be shown to be superior to a waitlist or control group in 2 or more randomized trials or more numerous properly conducted single-case designs.[40] A helpful resource for determining ESTs is the California Evidence-Based Clearinghouse (CEBC) for Child Welfare,[41] which maintains a registry rating treatments relevant to child welfare on a scale from 5 (concerning) to 1 (well-supported) based on the strength of the treatments' research base. The rating system considers factors such as the number of randomized controlled trials conducted related to the treatment, how long the research projects followed-up with participants to ensure long-lasting results, and the quality of the outcome measures used in those studies. Furthermore, treatments may have multiple ratings for various potential outcomes. The authors of this chapter recommend selecting treatments identified as having a rating of 2 (supported) or 1 (well-supported) when available. The CEBC can be accessed and searched online at https://www.cebc4cw.org/

In addition to matching the appropriate treatment with the appropriate goals of treatment, it should be noted that some treatments are, on average, more effective than others and lead to greater improvement in symptoms. Effect sizes are often used as an indicator by researchers to determine the optimal efficacy of intervention techniques and programs, and they are standardized in such a way that they are directly comparable to each other. While there are a number of different effect sizes depending on the design of a study and types of analyses conducted, a commonly-used effect size in clinical research is Cohen's d, which is a straightforward method of quantifying the mean difference between 2 groups and is a true measure of the clinical significance of the difference.[42] Specifically, it looks at how many standard deviations apart the average score for the group receiving the treatment were from the control which did not receive the treatment. Larger values of Cohen's d indicate more effective treatments. Typically, the effect size is interpreted as significant at a small magnitude of .2 (56% probability that the intervention is effective), significant at a medium magnitude of .5 (64% probability that the intervention is effective), and significant at a large magnitude of .8 (71% probability that the intervention is effective).[42] Because effect sizes often vary somewhat from study to study, meta-analyses, which, among other things, combine the effect sizes of multiple studies to determine an average effect size, can be useful in determining how effective a treatment is overall across studies. Some meta-analyses will also compare the average effect sizes for multiple treatments. For example, assume that both Treatment A and Treatment B are effective at reducing PTSD symptoms in children. If meta-analysis finds that Treatment A has an average effect size of .5 and Treatment B has an average effect size of .8, it indicates that Treatment B tends to be more effective at reducing PTSD in children, meaning children tend to improve *more* after receiving treatment B. While there are a number of factors involved in comparing treatments, when comparing treatments with similar attributes that may be similarly appropriate for a given client, the authors of this chapter recommend considering those with the strongest (largest) effect sizes.

In a large meta-analysis of CM interventions conducted by van der Put et al,[43] 121 studies were examined for the effectiveness of different components of interventions, and 352 effect sizes were obtained. A small effect size was found for both preventative and therapeutic interventions. Large effect sizes were found for preventative interventions which were short in duration and interventions that focused on increasing self-confidence in the client. There was also an increase in effect size as follow-up duration increased. With regards to therapeutic interventions, larger effect sizes were found for those interventions that focused on parenting skills and social and emotional support. Again, it should be noted that this meta-analysis focused on a very specific outcome or aim of treatment: preventing future instances of CM. Other types or components of treatments may be more or less effective for different types of outcomes that may be the goals of therapy (eg, reducing PTSD or other symptoms in children who have experienced CM).

Once an EST has been selected, it is important to review how the treatment is implemented. Appropriate implementation can be as important as any specific component included in the implementation. There are 3 considerations that are important guidelines when implementing an EST. First is fidelity, which is when an EST is used as it was intended and performed as designed without excluding important components of the treatment. Secondly is sustainment, which is when the EST is implemented with fidelity for long enough to determine if there are effective changes. The third component is scale. Scale occurs when an EST is implemented with fidelity but on a smaller scale, which makes establishing evidence of effectiveness difficult. For example, a pilot study is conducted on an EST, but the research is only implemented in 1 community center in the state. The study may be too small to see an impact on a larger group of individuals, such as members of an entire state or region. When considering choosing an EST, in order for implementation to be meaningful, all 3 components should be considered.[44]

KEY POINTS
1. The multiple long-term negative effects of CM necessitate effective interventions for maltreatment survivors.

2. The use of evidence-supported treatments is the surest way to provide effective and ethical treatment in the aftermath of CM.

3. The selection of an appropriate evidence-supported treatment should be based on the specific symptoms of the client and the effectiveness of each given treatment against those symptoms.

REFERENCES
1. Stoltenborgh M, Bakermans KMJ, Alink LRA, van IJzendoorn MH. The prevalence of child maltreatment across the globe: review of a series of meta-analyses. *Child Abus Rev.* 2015;24(1):37-50. doi:10.1002/car.2353

2. Kessler RC, McLaughlin KA, Green JG, et al. Childhood adversities and adult psychopathology in the WHO World Mental Health Surveys. *Br J Psychiatry.* 2010;197(5):378-385. doi:10.1192/bjp.bp.110.080499

3. Struck N, Krug A, Yuksel D, et al. Childhood maltreatment and adult mental disorders—the prevalence of different types of maltreatment and associations with age of onset and severity of symptoms. *Psychiatry Res.* 2020;293. doi:10.1016/j.psychres.2020.113398

4. Afifi TO, Sareen J, Fortier J, et al. Child maltreatment and eating disorders among men and women in adulthood: results from a nationally representative United States sample. *Int J Eat Disord.* 2017;50(11):1281-1296. doi:10.1002/eat.22783

5. Cicchetti D, Handley ED. Child maltreatment and the development of substance use and disorder. *Neurobiol Stress.* 2019;10. doi:10.1016/j.ynstr.2018.100144

6. Santo T Jr, Campbell G, Gisev N, et al. Prevalence of childhood maltreatment among people with opioid use disorder: a systematic review and meta-analysis. *Drug Alcohol Depend.* 2021;219. doi:10.1016/j.drugalcdep.2020.108459

7. Hoertel N, Franco S, Wall MM, et al. Childhood maltreatment and risk of suicide attempt: a nationally representative study. *J Clin Psychiatry.* 2015;76(7):916-923. doi:10.4088/JCP.14m09420

8. Edalati H, Nicholls TL. Childhood maltreatment and the risk for criminal justice involvement and victimization among homeless individuals: a systematic review. *Trauma Violence Abuse.* 2019;20(3):315-330. doi:10.1177/1524838017708783

9. Lilienfeld SO, Ritschel LA, Lynn SJ, Cautin RL, Latzman RD. Why many clinical psychologists are resistant to evidence-based practice: root causes and constructive remedies. *Clin Psychol Rev.* 2013;33(7):883-900. doi:10.1016/j.cpr.2012.09.008

10. Kennedy SC, Kim JS, Tripodi SJ, Brown SM, Gowdy G. Does parent–child interaction therapy reduce future physical abuse? A meta-analysis. *Res Soc Work Pract.* 2016;26(2):147-156. doi:10.1177/1049731514543024

11. Thomas R, Abell B, Webb HJ, Avdagic E, Zimmer-Gembeck MJ. Parent-child interaction therapy: a meta-analysis. *Pediatrics.* 2017;140(3):1-2. doi:10.1542/peds.2017-0352

12. Ward MA, Theule J, Cheung K. Parent–child interaction therapy for child disruptive behavior disorders: a meta-analysis. *Child Youth Care Forum.* 2016;45(5):675-690. doi:10.1007/s10566-016-9350-5

13. Myers LL, Thyer BA. Should social work clients have the right to effective treatment? *Soc Work.* 1997;42(3):288-298. doi:10.1093/sw/42.3.28

14. Witkin SL. The right to effective treatment and the effective treatment of rights: rhetorical empiricism and the politics of research. *Soc Work.* 1998;43(1):75-80. doi:10.1093/sw/43.1.75

15. Thyer BA, Pignotti MG. *Science and Pseudoscience in Social Work Practice.* Springer Publishing Company, LLC; 2015.

16. Pignotti M, Thyer BA. Novel unsupported and empirically supported therapies: patterns of usage among licensed clinical social workers. *Behav Cogn Psychother.* 2012;40(3):331-349. doi:10.1017/S135246581100052X

17. Bergmark M, Sundberg LR, Markström U, Rosenberg D. Evidence-based methods in rural areas—knowledge and national guideline utilization in mental health service development. *J Evid Based Soc Work.* 2022;19(2):161-184.

18. Finne J. Attitudes toward and utilization of evidence-based practice among Norwegian social workers. *J Evid Based Soc Work.* 2020;17(2):149-162.

19. Munro GD. The scientific impotence excuse: discounting belief-threatening scientific abstracts. *J Appl Soc Psychol.* 2010;40(3):579-600. doi:10.1111/j.1559-1816.2010.00588.x

20. Rosenzweig S. Some implicit common factors in diverse methods of psychotherapy. *J Psychother Integr.* 2002;12(1):5-9. doi:10.1037/1053-0479.12.1.5

21. Priebe S, Conneely M, McCabe R, Bird V. What can clinicians do to improve outcomes across psychiatric treatments: a conceptual review of non-specific components. *Epidemiol Psychiatr Sci.* 2020;29. doi:10.1017/S2045796019000428

22. Lilienfeld SO. The Dodo bird verdict: status in 2014. *Behav Ther.* 2014;37(4):91-95.

23. Frost R, Hyland P, Shevlin M, Murphy J. Distinguishing Complex PTSD from Borderline Personality Disorder among individuals with a history of sexual trauma: a latent class analysis. *Eur J Trauma Dissociation.* 2020;4(1). doi:10.1016/j.ejtd.2018.08.004

24. McRae EM, Stoppelbein L, O'Kelley SE, Fite PK, Smith SB. Pathways from child maltreatment to proactive and reactive aggression: the role of posttraumatic stress symptom clusters. *Psychol Trauma.* 2022;14(3):357-366. doi:10.1037/tra0001051

25. Tschoeke S, Bichescu-Burian D, Steinert T, Flammer E. History of childhood trauma and association with borderline and dissociative features. *J Nerv Ment Dis.* 2021;209(2):137-143. doi:10.1097/NMD.0000000000001270

26. Stoffers-Winterling JM, Storebø OJ, Kongerslev MT, et al. Psychotherapies for borderline personality disorder: a focused systematic review and meta-analysis. *Br J Psychiatry.* 2022:1-15. doi:10.1192/bjp.2021.204

27. Watkins LE, Sprang KR, Rothbaum BO. Treating PTSD: a review of evidence-based psychotherapy interventions. *Front Behav Neurosci.* 2018;12. doi:10.3389/fnbeh.2018.00258

28. Garb HN, Boyle PA. Understanding why some clinicians use pseudoscientific methods. In: Lilienfeld SO, Lynn SJ, Lohr JM, eds. *Science and Pseudoscience in Clinical Psychology.* 2nd ed. The Guilford Press; 2015:19-41.

29. Ethical principles of psychologists and code of conduct. American Psychological Association. Updated January 1, 2017. http://www.apa.org/ethics/code/index.aspx

30. ACA Code of Ethics. American Counseling Association. 2014. http://www.counseling.org/docs/ethics/2014-aca-code-of-ethics.pdf

31. Lilienfeld SO. Psychological treatments that cause harm. *Perspect Psychol Sci.* 2007;2(1):53-70. doi:10.1111/j.1745-6916.2007.00029.x

32. Lewey JH, Smith CL, Burcham B, Saunders NL, Elfallal D, O'Toole SK. Comparing the effectiveness of EMDR and TF-CBT for children and adolescents: a meta-analysis. *J Child Adolesc Trauma.* 2018;11(4):457-472. doi:10.1007/s40653-018-0212-1

33. Mercer J. Evidence of potentially harmful psychological treatments for children and adolescents. *Child Adolesc Social Work J.* 2017;34(2):107-125. doi:10.1007/s10560-016-0480-2

34. Chaffin M, Hanson R, Saunders BE, et al. Report of the APSAC Task Force on attachment therapy, reactive attachment disorder, and attachment problems. *Child Maltreat.* 2006;11(1):76-89. doi:10.1177/1077559505283699

35. Carlier IVE, Voerman AE, Gersons BPR. The influence of occupational debriefing on post-traumatic stress symptomatology in traumatized police officers. *Br J Med Psychol.* 2000;73(1):87-98. doi:10.1348/000711200160327

36. Lilienfeld SO, Lynn SJ, Lohr JM. Science and pseudoscience in clinical psychology: initial thoughts, reflections, and considerations. In: Lilienfeld SO, Lynn SJ, Lohr JM, eds. *Science and Pseudoscience in Clinical Psychology.* 2nd ed. The Guilford Press; 2015:1-16.

37. Meyer JM, Farrell NR, Kemp JJ, Blakey SM, Deacon BJ. Why do clinicians exclude anxious clients from exposure therapy? *Behav Res Ther.* 2014;54:49-53. doi:10.1016/j.brat.2014.01.004

38. McLean CP, Levy HC, Miller ML, Tolin DF. Exposure therapy for PTSD: a meta-analysis. *Clin Psychol Rev.* 2022;91:1-10. doi:10.1016/j.cpr.2021.102115

39. Imel ZE, Laska K, Jakupcak M, Simpson TL. Meta-analysis of dropout in treatments for posttraumatic stress disorder. *J Consult Clin Psychol.* 2013;81(3):394-404. doi:10.1037/a0031474.supp

40. American Psychological Association Presidential Task Force on Evidence-Based Practice. Evidence-based practice in psychology. *Am Psychol.* 2006;61(4):271-285.

41. California Evidence-Based Clearinghouse for Child Welfare. CEBC. 2022. https://www.cebc4cw.org

42. Coe R. It's the effect size, stupid: what effect size is and why it is important. Paper presented at: Annual Conference of the British Educational Research Association; September 12-14, 2002; University of Exeter, England.

43. van der Put CE, Assink M, Gubbels J, Boekhout van Solinge NF. Identifying effective components of child maltreatment interventions: a meta-analysis. *Clin Child Fam Psychol Rev.* 2018; 21(2):171-202. doi:10.1007/s10567-017-0250-5

44. Walsh C, Rolls Reutz J, Williams R. Selecting and implementing evidence-based practices: a guide for child and family serving systems. California Evidence-Based Clearinghouse for Child Welfare. 2015. https://www.nj.gov/dcf/about/divisions/dcsc/ImplementationGuide-Apr2015-onlineprint.pdf

Chapter 2

TELEHEALTH: *PROMOTING TARGETED AND SAFE ASSESSMENT AND INTERVENTION*

Paul Thomas Clements, PhD, RN, ANEF, DF-IAFN, DF-AFN
Andrea Blaskan, BSN, BA (Psychology)

OBJECTIVES

After reading this chapter, the reader will be able to:

1. Describe the evolution and ongoing expansion of telehealth in health care.

2. Examine the role of telehealth as a method of assessment and intervention for suspected and confirmed cases of child maltreatment.

3. Identify foundational facets for sensitive, targeted, and safe assessment and intervention when using a telehealth platform for clinical evaluation in suspected or confirmed cases of child maltreatment.

BACKGROUND AND SIGNIFICANCE

EARLY BEGINNINGS

The Health Resources Services Administration[1] defines telehealth as the use of electronic information and telecommunications technologies to support long-distance clinical health care, patient and professional health-related education, and public health and health administration services. Furthermore, telehealth can be defined as the transmission of health data and medical care via electronic communications.[2] Telehealth's roots trace back to the 19th century with the inception of telecommunications technology, such as the telephone and radio, which established the ability for information to be transmitted quickly over long distances. The application of such technology in medicine became of significant interest in the 20th century following several experiments focused on its application in the health care setting. In 1959, physicians at the University of Nebraska created a 2-way interactive television system to transmit data from neurological examinations to medical students across the university's campus.[3-4] Five years later, the same team of physicians established the earliest recorded use of hospital-based telemedicine by way of video conferencing with closed-circuit television links in order to conduct therapy sessions and psychiatric consultations between the Nebraska Psychiatric Institute and Norfolk State Hospital.[4]

In the 1970s, the National Aeronautics and Space Administration (NASA) embarked on a large-scale telemedicine project called Space Technology Applied to Rural Papago Advanced Health Care (STARPAHC), in which the feasibility of providing medical care to Papago Indians through telecommunications was tested on the Papago Indian Reservation in Arizona.[5] Following the success of STARPAHC, the intent of telehealth shifted to focus on delivering accessible health care to underserved populations in rural areas. With the rapid advancement of technology in the 21st century and increased reliance on electronic communication during COVID-19, telehealth has continued to evolve in its ability to grant remote health care services to the general population.

APPLICATION TO HEALTH CARE

Telehealth, across all aspects of health care, has become an important and ever-growing aspect of patient care delivery. Notable advantages to telehealth include its ease of access in obtaining medical care and consultations at an individual's own convenience, as well as its ability to extend health care to individuals in remote locations with little to no access to medical resources and personnel. As a result of its accessibility, follow-up care between the patient and provider can be more easily managed, which is an advantage that is considerably relevant in cases when consistent evaluation and treatment are imperative for patient improvement.[6]

As a health care delivery medium, telehealth can be divided into 4 modes of transmission[7]: live-video conferencing, asynchronous video, remote patient monitoring, and mobile health. Live-video conferencing is the most well known form, where both the patient and provider can communicate via a live, 2-way video. In the scope of pediatrics, clinicians typically favor live-video conferencing to conduct consultations, in part due to the real-time ability to interact with and assess patients, as well as convenience for both the provider and patient. In contrast, asynchronous video, also known as "store-and-forward" transmission, involves the electronic delivery of patient health data between clinicians for further patient evaluation and treatment. Remote patient monitoring is a form of patient data collection in which a health care professional is able to continuously track a patient's status, either through direct video monitoring or review of electronically transmitted diagnostic tests.[8] The most recently developed mode of telehealth is mobile health, whereby individuals are able to seek and obtain medical care as well as track aspects of their health and wellness through mobile applications. These applications are designed to store health data, track medical progress, and connect individuals with a medical professional in a matter of seconds.[9]

Telehealth has been recognized as a cost-effective means of providing health care services related to increased care efficiency and a reduction in hospital readmission rates resulting from patient diagnosis and treatment through teleconsultation.[10] However, there are limitations to the use of telehealth, including a health care professional's diminished ability to perform thorough physical and mental health examinations on patients. This limitation can lead to an increase in the number of incorrect or incomplete diagnoses and prescribed treatment courses for patients, thus putting patient safety at risk.[11]

Turning the focus to child maltreatment, protection of patient privacy and confidentiality across electronic platforms is of special concern. Though programs through which telehealth operate are often encrypted and in accordance with Health Insurance Portability and Accountability Act (HIPAA) regulations, internet-hosted platforms still run the risk of data breaches by cyberhackers.[12] Additionally, related to privacy concerns with telehealth, ensuring that a patient is alone and in a safe environment for a consultation, especially in cases of suspected abuse, is difficult. The abuser may overhear conversations or position themselves outside of the camera's view, preventing providers from guaranteeing the patient's safety and privacy. This situation also puts the patient at risk for coercion, nonverbal threats, and other forms of intimidation,[13] underscoring the importance of identification and utilization of strategies uniquely tailored to telehealth in cases of suspected or actual child maltreatment.

ASSESSMENT AND INTERVENTION

The COVID-19 public health crisis and subsequent social distancing measures both contributed to an increased risk for survivors of intimate partner violence (IPV) and their children, including making it harder to stay connected to support networks like emergency rooms, psychiatric crisis centers, and even domestic violence, which can be an ongoing source of stress. These circumstances increased stress and forcibly increased proximity to the person causing harm.[14] Once in-person appointments became available again, with the increasing focus on the interface and impact of Social Determinants of Health (SDHs) on access to mental health care and the ongoing risk for increasing violence,[15,16] many agencies have continued to shift to telehealth (in some settings, referred to as *telemental health*[17]) to provide virtual support to patients, including those who may be experiencing abuse or exploitation. Providers and agencies are working to establish or build upon their existing policies and practices designed to achieve safe and effective telehealth for survivors of IPV while simultaneously promoting the survivors' health and wellbeing.[18] Furthermore, COVID-19 substantially increased telehealth use across many health care service disciplines. One survey[19] of 3500 family physicians and pediatricians indicates that only 12% of primary care physicians worked in a practice that used telehealth in 2016, while more than 90% offered telehealth after the first 2 months of COVID-19.

When many patients rely on telehealth for connection to and support from their health care team, providers should educate all patients during telehealth appointments about IPV resources. If IPV is disclosed in a telehealth context, clinicians should tailor support to their patient's circumstances (ie, the child or a non-offending parent). Sources of support can include a social worker within the clinical care team, online support services, local community-based organizations that specialize in IPV, or support groups with text/chat options. In addition to providing such resources to all patients, an in-person health care visit may be needed due to the correlation between IPV and physical ailments. With telehealth-based clinical care continuing beyond COVID-19, universal IPV training, regardless of the health care delivery modality, should be considered to teach clinicians how to recognize, support, and refer persons experiencing IPV. If the person agrees to a referral for support, provide it and ask if it is okay to follow up with them, using a question that can be answered with "yes" or "no."[13]

It is important to note that there have not been any large, randomized trials evaluating the accuracy of identifying IPV in telehealth formats. However, there have been studies documenting the acceptability and feasibility of trauma-informed, digitally-delivered interventions focused on preventing violence to increase safety and decision making of persons in abusive relationships and linking them to online support.[20] Thus, telehealth has posed new challenges to child maltreatment screening and support. To help facilitate access to and use of screening questions and resource lists, it is recommended that *smart phrases* be created in the electronic health record.[12]

Overall, as of 2023, the findings on telehealth are encouraging, as they demonstrate that perceived barriers or peculiarities resulting from this medium of service delivery do not necessarily come at the expense of efficacious outcomes. In fact, clients have demonstrated rather dramatic symptom improvement, thereby demonstrating that this treatment modality may effectively meet the needs of rural populations who would otherwise be unlikely to receive services at all.[7,12,18]

Because the experience of violence and trauma can affect both physical and mental health, it is important to support clinicians in screening, identifying, and responding to child maltreatment, including within the context of telehealth encounters.[21] Often, clinicians do not want to ask about child maltreatment because of logistical concerns (eg, ensuring patient privacy and safety) or because they may not know how to respond to an affirmative answer. During COVID-19, telehealth communications with health care providers may conceivably have been the only external points of contact available to some children experiencing maltreatment. For example, rural survivors of sexual abuse and physical violence experience considerable difficulties accessing mental health services, so telehealth could give them an opportunity to disclose and seek treatment.[21] Regardless of the modality of screening, the same basic approach remains: to first recognize that violence and abuse could be occurring, and proceed with caution so that the child experiencing maltreatment is approached in a person-centered way, prioritizing access and privacy.

For children who are living with the offending parent, confidentiality is not just a professional standard but is critically important for their safety. Participating in at-home telehealth therapy decreases clients' privacy and confidentiality and enables further power and control behaviors in the home. **Table 2-1** provides guidance and strategies to preemptively prepare for safe and effective telehealth assessments during cases of suspected childhood maltreatment.

Table 2-1. "CUES" Strategy for Safe and Effective Telehealth Assessments for Violence, Abuse, and Human Trafficking[18]	
TIME	APPROACH
Before the Visit	— Prepare a "script," integrating information into the visit about IPV and available survivor support resources for people to share with their family and friends. — Understand that telehealth visits may not be a safe time for discussing IPV, since others may be in the room or listening in. — Connect with local domestic violence advocacy agencies and hotlines to understand what services they offer.
During the Visit	— Offer normalizing information about relationships, health, and stress during COVID-19. One method for this is the "CUES" intervention for IPV, which can be used within telehealth visits: **C:** Prioritize **confidentiality** by ensuring it is safe for the patient to speak over the phone/video and letting them know that their health information will be kept safe (disclosing any reporting requirements). Ask: "Are you somewhere where you can speak freely?" **UE:** Offer **universal education** to all patients about how stress can affect relationships which, in turn, can affect health. Relay that there are supportive resources available. Share with the client: "Before we get started, I want to say that I know COVID-19 has made things harder for everyone. Because people are stressed, we're sharing ideas about helping yourself and the people you care about. For example, we may experience more stress now in our relationships, including increased fighting or harm, and that can affect our health. There is free, confidential help available if you know someone who is being hurt in their relationship. Would it be okay if I sent some resources for you to share? I will also send information on support around parenting, access to food, and stress. How are things going right now for you?" Providers can also offer universal education to patients that normalize financial struggles to pay for necessary things like food and shelter and where to go for support if they need it. **E: Empower** patients to share these resources with friends and family. Research has shown that being able to support and encourage others is a form of empowerment that can also be healing. Say: "You can also share these resources with friends or family if you think it may help them, too." **S:** Provide **support** if patients disclose experiences of IPV or other needs and offer validating messages, information to support health, a warm referral to a domestic violence advocacy program, and a crisis text line.

(continued)

Table 2-1. "CUES" Strategy for Safe and Effective Telehealth Assessments for Violence, Abuse, and Human Trafficking[18] *(continued)*

TIME	APPROACH
During the Visit	Say: "Thank you for sharing this with me. I am so sorry this is happening. What you are telling me makes me worry about your safety and health. A lot of my patients experience things like this, and there are people who can help. I can connect you today if that interests you, even right now if you like, and I can stay on the line with you."
	Providers may also be able to brainstorm with patients who are experiencing violence or exploitation about ways in which to stay connected when someone is controlling their access to health care and support networks.
	Say: "I'd like to think about your health, too, and hear if your partner or someone else is interfering in any way with your plans to help your child stay healthy, for example by messing with your medicines, taking away hand sanitizer, preventing you from seeking help, or keeping you from connecting with friends and family."

While telehealth care poses new challenges, health care professionals should still assess patients as they would if they were seeing them in person. In addition to standard patient assessment procedures, the strategies in **Table 2-2** may be helpful. There has been a rise in the use of nonverbal gestures to alert clinicians to abuse as a result of an increase in IPV due to self-isolation measures stemming from COVID-19. In particular, the *Signal for Help*, introduced by the Canadian Women's Foundation in 2020,[22] has been identified as a universal signal of abuse by more than 40 organizations across Canada and the United States. The signal is designed as a single continuous

Table 2-2. Recognizing Child Abuse and Neglect in Telehealth Care[23-27]

DESCRIPTION OF THEORY

— Observe and consider family/child interactions.

— Does the child seem fearful of the caregiver? Does the caregiver speak for the child directly without allowing the child the opportunity to share?

— Observe any nonverbal cues that may be indicative of potential abuse and neglect. Does the child demonstrate expressions of pain even in the absence of any visible marks or bruises? Does the child seem shut down? Do members of the home engage in traumatic play?

— Pay attention to the background. Are there any safety hazards, either physical or environmental? Can yelling or screaming be overheard? How does the child appear in the environment?

— Be mindful of who may be listening in the background. Ask probing questions such as: What does a day look like at home for you right now? What's your favorite part about being at home? What is the hardest? Avoid yes and no questions if possible.

— Continue to assess suspicious injury or illness the same way you would in an office or clinic. Request photos of the injury via a secure message to analyze and compare the appearance of the injury to how the parent reports it occurred.

— When discussing a suspicious mark with a child, make every effort to ensure the child is alone and can answer questions safely and confidentially.

— Listen to patient responses, both verbal and nonverbal (ie, body language). Are patients or their parents or caregivers deflecting or avoiding responses to particular questions? Are parents or caregivers interrupting?

(continued)

Table 2-2. Recognizing Child Abuse and Neglect in Telehealth Care[23-27] *(continued)*

DESCRIPTION OF THEORY

— Listen to how caregivers describe their interactions with their children. For example, a parent may say, "they are so ill-behaved, next time they act out I'm going to…."

— Ensure minor patients know how to reach out securely and confidentially should they need specific support, counsel, or medical treatment that may be sensitive.

— Create a safety plan and identify a safe word that a patient can use to signal the presence of someone else whom they fear speaking in front of.

— Encourage patients to use self-care strategies for both mental and physical health. Provide some stress-relieving stretches, breathing techniques, or physical activities for both children and parents.

— Encourage ending the phone or video call, if necessary, during the intake with the understanding that there are absolutely no consequences to doing so. Informing clients that there will be no consequences to a shortened or missed session is especially relevant for clients who are court-ordered to receive treatment related to domestic violence.

hand movement marked by holding one's hand up with the thumb tucked inside the palm, then folding the remaining fingers down to entrap the thumb (see **Figure 2-1**).[23]

Gestures such as the Signal for Help can allow providers to recognize cases of abuse while also maintaining patient safety compared to using designated phrases, which may alert a perpetrator in close proximity to the patient during the telehealth appointment.

Figure 2-1. The Signal for Help, created by The Canadian Women's Foundation is a nonverbal hand signal that provides a way to discreetly communicate when someone needs help

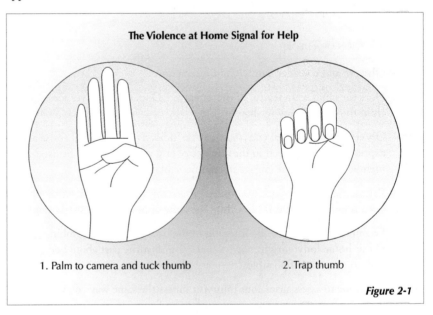

The Violence at Home Signal for Help

1. Palm to camera and tuck thumb   2. Trap thumb

Figure 2-1

CASE STUDY

Case Study 2-1

Nathan was a 9-year-old male with a history of ADHD, recently referred for mental health assessment after multiple suspensions from his local elementary school. He was on a mandatory homeschool Individual Curriculum Plan until getting re-evaluated by the multidisciplinary team, including by the mental health division. His suspension resulted from verbally disruptive behavior in the classroom, including rude and inappropriate comments to the teachers, frequently containing expletives. When Nathan was approached for de-escalation efforts, he repeatedly stated, "Don't touch me! You are not allowed to touch me! It's illegal if you touch me. You could go to jail if you touch me!" This behavior required Nathan to be physically escorted from the classroom. His parents, particularly his father, were calling the principal's office with hostile comments, saying that it was illegal for school personnel to touch Nathan and that it was a form of "child molestation." Nathan's father had been unemployed since losing his job during COVID-19, when the factory he worked at closed. His mother was unemployed and an undocumented immigrant from Mexico.

— What care goals can you identify that a telehealth model could target for Nathan, his mother, and his father?

— What challenges might be faced in coordinating care via telehealth?

— What risk factors and warning signs should you be aware of/watch for during the telehealth visit?

— What SDHs should be addressed with both Nathan and his parents?

— How will you measure the success of telehealth with Nathan and his parents?

KEY POINTS

1. Telehealth continues to evolve and expand as an option for conducting assessment and planning for intervention in cases of suspected or actual child maltreatment.

2. Child trauma treatment offered via telehealth can increase access to treatment for children and families in remote communities, reduce travel costs for families (eg, transportation, time off work), increase clinical capacity for the agency, and increase likelihood of treatment attendance.

3. In the post-pandemic era, the most significant benefit of telehealth services is the ability to provide child trauma treatment services to facilitate Social Determinant of Health needs and enhance access to services.

REFERENCES

1. Frequently asked questions. Office of the National Coordinator for Health Information Technology. 2023. https://www.healthit.gov/faq/what-telehealth-how-telehealth-different-telemedicine

2. NEJM Catalyst. What is telehealth? Innovations in care delivery. *N Engl J Med Catal.* 2018. doi:10.1056/CAT.18.0268

3. Kichloo A, Albosta M, Dettloff K, et al. Telemedicine, the current COVID-19 pandemic and the future: a narrative review and perspectives moving forward in the USA. *Fam Med Community Health.* 2020;8(3). doi:10.113610.1136/fmch-2020-000530

4. Doarn CR. Telemedicine and psychiatry - a natural match. *MHealth.* 2018;4:60. doi:10.21037/mhealth.2018.12.04

5. Freiburger G, Holcomb M, Piper D. The STARPAHC collection: part of an archive of the history of telemedicine. *J Telemed Telecare.* 2007;13(5):221-223. doi:10.1258/135763307781458949

6. Gajarawala SN, Pelkowski JN. Telehealth benefits and barriers. *J Nurse Pract.* 2021;17(2):218-221. doi:10.1016/j.nurpra.2020.09.013

7. What is telehealth? Key components of telehealth. The National Telehealth Policy Resource Center. 2022. https://www.cchpca.org/what-is-telehealth/

8. Mechanic OJ, Persaud Y, Kimball AB. Telehealth systems. StatPearls Publishing. Updated September 12, 2022. https://www.ncbi.nlm.nih.gov/books/NBK459384/

9. Vaghefi I, Tulu B. The continued use of mobile health apps: insights from a longitudinal study. *JMIR Mhealth Uhealth.* 2019;7(8):12983. doi:10.2196/12983.

10. Rutledge CM, Kott K, Schweickert PA, Poston R, Fowler C, Haney TS. Telehealth and eHealth in nurse practitioner training: current perspectives. *Adv Med Educ Pract.* 2017;26(8):399-409. doi:10.2147/AMEP.S116071

11. Khoong EC. Policy considerations to ensure telemedicine equity. *Health Affairs.* 2022;42(5):643-646. doi:10.1377/hlthaff.2022.00300

12. Jalali MS, Landman A, Gordon WJ. Telemedicine, privacy, and information security in the age of COVID-19. *J Am Med Inform Assoc.* 2020;28(3):1-2. doi:10.1093/jamia/ocaa310

13. Simon MA. Responding to intimate partner violence during telehealth clinical encounters. *JAMA.* 2021;325(22):2307-2308. doi:10.1001/jama.2021.1071

14. How COVID-19 may increase domestic violence and child abuse. American Psychological Association. 2020. https://www.apa.org/topics/covid-19/domestic-violence-child-abuse

15. Hunter AA, Flores G. Social determinants of health and child maltreatment: a systematic review. *Pediatr Res.* 2021;89(2):269-274. doi:10.1038/s41390-020-01175-x

16. Social determinants of health. US Department of Health and Human Services. 2023. https://health.gov/healthypeople/priority-areas/social-determinants-health

17. Racine N, Hartwick C, Collin-Vézina D, Madigan S. Telemental health for child trauma treatment during and post-COVID-19: limitations and considerations. *Child Abuse Negl.* 2020;110:104698. doi:10.1016/j.chiabu.2020.104698

18. Telehealth, COVID-19, intimate partner violence, and human trafficking: increasing safety for people surviving abuse. A guide for community health centers and partnering domestic violence advocacy programs. Futures Without Violence. https://www.futureswithoutviolence.org/wp-content/uploads/Telehealth-COVID-19-IPV-and-HT_Guide.pdf

19. North S. Telemedicine in the time of COVID and beyond. *J Adolesc Health.* 2020;67(2):145-146. doi:10.1016/j.jadohealth.2020.05.024

20. Emezue C. Digital or digitally delivered responses to domestic and intimate partner violence during COVID-19. *JMIR Public Health Surveill.* 2020; 6(3):e19831. doi:10.2196/19831

21. Gray MJ, Hassija CM. Provision of evidence-based therapies to rural survivors of domestic violence and sexual assault via telehealth: treatment outcomes and clinical training benefits. *Train Educ Prof Psychol.* 2015;9(3):235-241. doi:10.1037/tep0000083

22. Become a signal for help responder. Canadian Women's Foundation. 2023. https://canadianwomen.org/signal-for-help/

23. Henry TA. Tips to help you ID intimate partner violence via telehealth. American Medical Association (AMA). 2021. https://www.ama-assn.org/delivering-care/public-health/tips-help-you-id-intimate-partner-violence-telehealth

24. Kaukinen C. When stay-at-home orders leave victims unsafe at home: exploring the risk and consequences of intimate partner violence during the COVID-19 pandemic. *Am J Crim Just.* 2020;45(4):668-679. doi:10.1007/s12103-020-09533-5

25. Ahuja L. Telehealth therapy concerns for clients engaging in treatment for domestic violence. Society for the Advancement of Psychotherapy. 2021. https://societyforpsychotherapy.org/telehealth-therapy-concerns-for-clients-engaging-in-treatment-for-domestic-violence/

26. Recognizing child abuse and neglect in telehealth care. North Central Missouri Children's Advocacy Center. Accessed December 22, 2020. https://www.nc-mochildren.org/ncmcac/2020/12/recognizing-child-abuse-and-neglect-in-tele-health-care.html

27. Jones AM, Shealy KM, Reid-Quinones K, Moreland AD, Davidson TM, Lopez CM. Guidelines for establishing a telemental health program to provide evidence-based therapy for trauma-exposed children and families. *Psychol Serv.* 2014;11(4):398-409. doi:10.1037/a0034963

Psychopharmacological Interventions for Childhood Maltreatment

Soraya Seedat, PhD, MBChB, FC Psych (SA), MMed Psych, MPhil Applied
    Ethics (Bioethics)
Yewande Oshodi, MBBS, MPH, FMCPsych, Mphil, Cert CA Psych
Sandra Swart, MBChB, MMed (Psych)

Objectives

After reading this chapter, the reader will be able to:

1. *Understand the role of psychopharmacology in the management of maltreated children and adolescents using a developmentally-informed biopsychosocial approach and trauma-informed principles.*

2. *Identify key considerations and principles for choosing pharmacotherapy as a treatment modality.*

3. *Be familiar with the common medication options for maltreated children and adolescents.*

Background and Significance

Child maltreatment includes physical, sexual, and emotional (psychological) abuse, as well as physical and emotional neglect. It is estimated globally that 1 billion children aged 2 to 17 years have experienced past-year physical, sexual, or emotional violence or neglect, or multiple types of abuse and neglect, yet there exists a silent burden of child maltreatment, both in high-income and low- and middle-income economies.[1] Exposure to adversity in childhood and adolescence is associated with an increased risk of several long-term mental and physical health sequelae.[2,3] These long-term outcomes are mediated by the severity, timing, and duration of adverse childhood experiences (ACEs). ACEs often co-occur, as do the mental, physical, and health consequences of ACEs, with a dose-response relationship between ACEs and negative health outcomes and a substantial impact on disability and economic costs.[3,4] For example, it has been estimated that a 10% reduction in the prevalence of ACEs in North America and Europe would result in annual savings of 3 000 000 disability-adjusted life years (DALYs) or $105 billion.[4]

Addressing childhood maltreatment necessitates a trauma-informed approach and consideration of a broad range of interventions, including psychotherapy and pharmacotherapy to address presenting mental health conditions. An in-depth understanding of the mental health sequelae in maltreated children and adolescents, along with an understanding of psychopharmacologic treatment options, will aid health care providers in approaching the management of this population more holistically.

Psychotherapeutic and pharmacotherapeutic treatment options are not mutually exclusive and should preferably be used in combination. Mental disorders such as post-traumatic stress disorder (PTSD), major depressive disorder (MDD), anxiety disorders, and attention deficit hyperactivity disorder (ADHD), which are overrepresented in children with histories of child maltreatment, may require medication intervention. Rational prescribing of pharmacotherapy (ie, medication) is essential in this population, considering that maltreated children and adolescents tend to be prescribed more psychotropic medications than non-maltreated peers receiving psychiatric care, and over-prescription must be guarded against. There continues to be much controversy and debate surrounding the prescription of antidepressants and other psychotropic medications for children and adolescents. Notably, there is no evidence that selective serotonin reuptake inhibitors (SSRIs), which are the most widely prescribed class of antidepressants in adolescents, have deleterious effects on developing brains.[5]

All medications carry side effects that must be outweighed by the clinical benefits of prescribing them. There is also no evidence to indicate that psychotherapy is safer than pharmacotherapy. It is also relevant to note that adverse events have generally been poorly documented across psychotherapy trials in children and adults.

Before the initiation of pharmacotherapy, assessment of the child should be conducted by a clinician trained and experienced in the assessment of children exposed to maltreatment. A comprehensive assessment of the nature of the maltreatment and the child's psychiatric, medical, family, social, and academic attainment history is key in determining the intervention needs of the child and family.

In clinical settings, the varied presentation of psychiatric disorders in children and adolescents exposed to maltreatment (both at clinical threshold and subthreshold levels) has implications for prescribing pharmacotherapy. Pharmacotherapy is effective and safe when judiciously prescribed and can be used alongside psychotherapeutic treatment in the management of mental disorders secondary to child maltreatment.[6]

Importantly, comprehensive, holistic, and individualized care for maltreated children and adolescents, informed by a multidisciplinary team, is required. Child and adolescent survivors of maltreatment presenting to psychiatric care are a unique population. Individually tailored interventions need to address the child's clinical presentation and must include parental involvement, cooperation (eg, adherence to the child's treatment plan), supervision, and support.

RATIONAL PRESCRIBING

Children who have experienced childhood maltreatment may be at higher risk of internalizing and externalizing problems, discrete mental disorders as classified in the *Diagnostic and Statistical Manual of Mental Disorders, 5th edition* (DSM-5), and other long-term sequelae.[2,3] While the exact causal relationship is still unknown, genetic and environmental factors should be taken into consideration. These disorders include mood and anxiety disorders, suicidality, self-harming behaviors, offending behaviors, delinquency, impulsivity, disruptive behaviors, ADHD, oppositional defiant disorder (ODD), and substance use disorders (SUD), among others. These problems and disorders often co-occur. For example, PTSD may co-occur with panic disorder, obsessive-compulsive disorder (OCD), and generalized anxiety disorder (GAD), as well as with ADHD, ODD, SUD, and depression. It is also important to consider the presence of disordered patterns of attachment, particularly in maltreated children, as severe attachment disorders themselves may mimic other psychiatric disorders and influence treatment response and outcome.[7]

Maltreated children are traditionally "research orphans,"[8] and the evidence base on the management of psychiatric disorders in this group is sparse. Whilst psychotherapeutic treatments such as cognitive behavior therapy (CBT) are considered first-line interventions in maltreated children and adolescents with mood, anxiety, and trauma- and stressor-related disorders,[9] pharmacotherapy, particularly SSRIs, may have an important role in the management of these debilitating disorders. Pharmacotherapy should preferably be prescribed in combination with a psychotherapeutic intervention.

FACTORS TO CONSIDER IN THE DIAGNOSIS AND MANAGEMENT OF A MALTREATED CHILD OR ADOLESCENT

Several factors need to be considered when deciding on the use (or not) of pharmacotherapy for maltreated children and adolescents. These are outlined below:

CHILDHOOD MALTREATMENT OR BEHAVIORAL PROBLEMS?

Sometimes, there is a clear history of maltreatment or one suspects it in a child or adolescent presenting for care with severe agitation, self-harming behavior, or nightmares, among other behaviors. The behavioral manifestations consequent to childhood maltreatment can vary from child to child and are dependent on several other factors, such as protective factors (eg, social or parental support), developmental age, and the chronicity of maltreatment.[10,11]

The presence of emotional and behavioral disturbances in some instances may be sufficient to meet DSM-5 diagnostic criteria for a specific disorder; in others the presentation of symptoms may be subthreshold or unclear but still require pharmacological intervention. For example, medications may be prescribed for brief periods and with close monitoring in order to help a child regulate experiences of physiologic hyperarousal, such as nightmares, sleep difficulties, and high anxiety. Thus, medication treatment may be necessary even in suspected cases of maltreatment. However, even when medication is helpful in reducing stress responses in children and adolescents, it should be considered an adjunct to, rather than a substitute for, psychotherapy.

IS A PSYCHIATRIC DISORDER PRESENT?

Generally, children may respond adaptively or maladaptively depending on the quality of early life experiences and relationships with caregivers, temperamental styles, genetic vulnerability, and interaction with their environment.[12,13] If we think of each child as an individual with a genetic blueprint (resilience, vulnerability, genes of inheritance), molded by inherent temperamental characteristics and influenced by the early experiences of caregiving, we can consider that a response to a certain stressor (eg, childhood maltreatment) will depend on the experience of, and environmental support to, that stressful event, and therefore the development of a disorder will depend on a set of complex interactions among these sets of factors.

A disorder may be present within the child, but the degree of distress and dysfunction may differ according to the individual child and their developmental stage. In addition, it is important to consider the extent of functional impairments (eg, family and social relationships, academic performance) and the strengths of the child (eg, emotion regulation, resilience) in various contexts.[14]

Variations in early attachment patterns (ie, secure, insecure, or disorganized) with the primary caregiver may be seen as a potential predictor of variations in the response a child may display to stressful life situations and social adversity.[12] Temperament refers to the style of behavior that is inherent in a child and is dynamically influenced by their environment. If there is a discrepancy between a child's temperament or capacity and the demands or expectations of the child's environment (eg, attunement of the parent or social or cultural expectations), then maladaptive or dysfunctional adaptations are potentiated.

A child may function adaptively within a particular domain while struggling in another. The child's overall functioning (impairments and strengths) will also contribute to the presentation of a psychiatric disorder.[7] It is important to emphasize that the key is a careful and correct diagnosis with a treatment plan that is tailored to the child in question.

EVALUATION AND TREATMENT OF MALTREATED CHILDREN/ADOLESCENTS WITH PSYCHIATRIC SYMPTOMS

In the assessment of a child or adolescent who presents with psychiatric symptoms after maltreatment, the following should be taken into account before making a diagnosis: the child's age during the maltreatment or other traumatic experiences; the frequency, severity, and multiplicity of ACEs; the home environment; prior medical conditions; and existing neurodevelopmental disorders or neurocognitive delays. The functioning of the child prior to the maltreatment is also important.[15]

DEFINING THE PSYCHIATRIC DISORDER

A psychiatric disorder in a child can be defined as "a condition characterized by distress and dysfunction in the child, which is persistent in time, pervasive across each domain of experience and severe in degree, but not limited to social deviance or disadvantage alone."[16] Categorizing potential disorders according to the DSM-5[17] or the *International Statistical Classification of Diseases and Related Health Problems, 11th edition* (ICD 11)[18] is useful when considering multifactorial contributions to childhood disorders.

The diagnosis of a psychiatric disorder in childhood also depends on the developmental stage of the child, as a disorder may present with different symptomatic and clinical manifestations depending on the stage. In assessing a child who has been maltreated or exposed to violence, it is useful to assess the child's response to adversity by considering what would be appropriate for that stage of a child's emotional and psychosocial development. According to Erikson,[19,20] each stage of maturation is tied to a key psychosocial life crisis or challenge that an individual needs to negotiate. Attention to developmental stages in childhood assists the clinician in differentiating "normal" versus pathological responses or behaviors to adverse situations.

Diagnosis of psychiatric disorders should only be made after screening and evaluation by a trained professional.

In treating a maltreated child or adolescent with a psychiatric disorder, any decision to prescribe pharmacotherapy in combination with psychotherapy will depend on the degree of dysfunction of that child in their environment and the difficulties (that may present at the outset or arise over time) in treating the psychiatric disorder(s) with initial psychotherapy alone.

The use of pharmacotherapy in a child requires the consideration of a variety of factors. A useful way of organizing these contributory factors is to construct an etiological formulation, which should include the information in **Table 3-1**.

Table 3-1. Factors to Consider when Constructing an Etiological Formulation	
Predisposing factors	Genetic vulnerability, prenatal and perinatal trauma, exposures (including toxins, viral exposure, early hypoxic compromise during labor and delivery, and nuchal chord during delivery), developmental delays, medical conditions, attachment styles, temperament, and maternal mental illness.
Precipitating factors	Vulnerability versus resilience, ongoing trauma, environmental factors (eg, psychosocial, cultural, or societal stressors), parental factors (eg, mental illness, attunement), developmental stage of the child, and intellectual or school difficulties.

(continued)

Table 3-1. Factors to Consider when Constructing an Etiological Formulation *(continued)*

Perpetuating factors	Ongoing trauma, poor support, psychological or environmental (including school and cultural) stressors, and substance abuse.
Protective factors	Psychosocial support, early intervention, and resiliency factors.

PROVIDING PSYCHOEDUCATION

In younger children, medication adherence and response (efficacy or side effects) are often dependent on parent/caregiver reporting. It may be useful to have educative discussions with parents/caregivers as well as the child regarding medication myths and stigma associated with medication use to help dispel misinformation prior to initiating medication. The caregiver and child need to understand the nature of the medication, the importance of adherence, and what to expect from the side effect profile.[21]

PHARMACOTHERAPY TREATMENT GUIDELINES: PRINCIPLES OF PRESCRIBING

When deciding on pharmacotherapy, it is helpful to consider a child's developmental age as this often determines the clinical presentation of the disorder and impacts on the choice of treatment modality. See **Figure 3-1** for additional factors to consider.

Figure 3-1. Evaluating a child or adolescent for pharmacological intervention

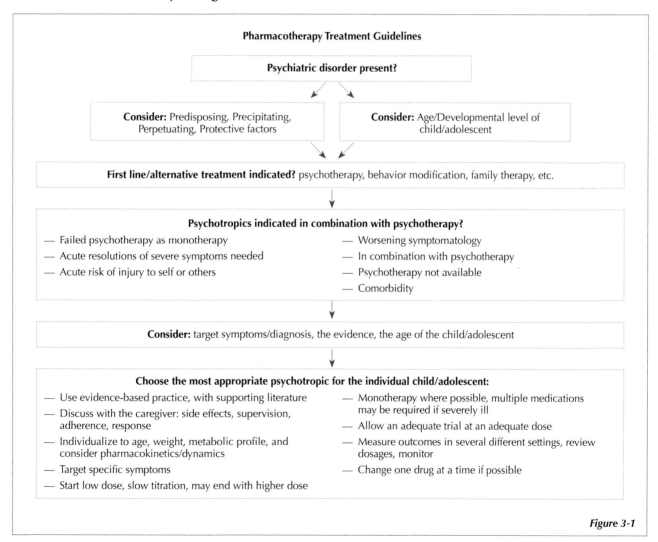

Figure 3-1

Medication should be considered in the following cases where[22]:

— Psychotherapy as monotherapy has failed.

— Acute resolution of severe symptoms is needed.

— There is an acute risk of injury to self or others.

— There is worsening symptomatology.

— It is in combination with psychotherapy.

— Psychotherapy is not available (eg, lack of trained personnel, the cost is prohibitive).

— There are comorbid conditions present that require concurrent treatment.

The following principles are relevant when prescribing psychotropic medications to children and adolescents[23]:

— Use evidence-based practice, supported by the literature.

— Discuss supervision of medication, adherence, response, and side effects with the caregiver(s).

— Individualize to age, weight, and metabolic profile.

— Target specific symptoms and measure progress over time.

— Start with a low dose, titrate up slowly, but be prepared to aim for higher doses depending on response and tolerability.

— Promote awareness of potential side effects of the medication(s) prescribed and continuously monitor for these side effects over time.

— Use monotherapy where possible; however, multiple medications may be needed.

— Allow an adequate trial at an adequate dose for each medication prescribed, provided that the medication is tolerated.

— Measure outcomes in several different settings, review dosage, and monitor the response and side effects.

— Change one drug at a time, if possible.

— Do not prescribe medications indefinitely, treat optimally, and taper off medication when needed.

— Appropriate biologic testing is an important principle before the commencement of psychopharmacological agents (eg, height and weight for stimulants; height, weight, and lipid testing for antipsychotics).[24-26]

— The affordability and availability of medication.

The following factors should be considered if there is a poor response to treatment[27]:

— That a wrong diagnosis may have been made.

— That a comorbid medical or psychiatric disorder is present that has not been recognized or adequately treated.

— That the type of psychotherapy or pharmacotherapy used was not appropriate.

— That the dose or duration of treatment was inadequate.

— That the child may be non-adherent to treatment.

— That there may be medication side effects that need attention.

— That there may be ongoing exposure to negative life events.

— That ethnic or cultural factors may be at play.

Children have larger hepatic capacity, increased glomerular filtration in the kidneys, and reduced amounts of fat tissue. Therefore, psychotropic medications, such as stimulants, antipsychotics, tricyclic drugs, and lithium are more rapidly eliminated in children, and fewer drugs are stored in fat tissue. The half-life of medications may be shorter in children due to their quicker elimination. This may contribute to differential response rates and the need for different doses.[28]

PSYCHOTROPIC MEDICATIONS COMMONLY USED IN CHILDREN AND ADOLESCENTS

SSRIs

SSRIs are currently the most commonly used class of antidepressants in children and adolescents. There is evidence for their efficacy and safety for MDD and strong evidence for their efficacy for anxiety disorders and OCD in those younger than the age of 18.[29] There is no evidence to indicate superiority of one SSRI agent over another.[29-31]

It is estimated that 4 to 6 children need to be treated with an SSRI in order to find 1 who will improve on an SSRI who would otherwise not improve on placebo (this number is known as the ***number needed to treat***).

Side effects may include increased behavioral activation and suicidality (usually early in treatment), insomnia, headaches, restlessness, sweating, gastrointestinal disturbances (eg, nausea, diarrhea), and sexual dysfunction.[24] Younger children compared to older children are more susceptible to the activation effects of SSRIs. Weight gain and sedation are unusual side effects.[30] Severe agitation or activation should alert the clinician to a possible underlying bipolar disorder diagnosis.[27] Treatment is often introduced with the lowest tolerated daily dose (usually given in the morning) and may be slowly increased, depending on the indication, response, and tolerability to dose increments.

MOOD STABILIZERS

Sodium Valproate

Sodium Valproate can be classified as an anticonvulsant, mood stabilizer, or voltage-sensitive sodium channel modulator.[30] Valproate is indicated for the treatment of bipolar disorder and epilepsy. It is sometimes prescribed off-label for the management of mood dysregulation. Valproate should generally not be used in children younger than 10 years old, unless it is prescribed by an expert when alternative options have been examined.[30] Side effects include sedation, dizziness, gastrointestinal disturbances, weight gain, and hair loss. Valproate is teratogenic so its prescription in adolescent females should be done with great caution. There is a significant increased hepatotoxicity risk if used in children younger than 2 years of age.[23,30]

Valproate is prescribed at a dose of 10-60 mg/kg/day in 2 divided doses for the controlled released preparation, depending on indication and severity of symptoms. Slow down-titration is needed when discontinuing valproate.[30]

Lithium

Lithium (Li) is a very well known and widely researched antimanic agent with good evidence for efficacy and safety. The FDA has approved it for children aged 12 years to 17 years. It has been found to be safe and efficacious in studies in children aged 7 years to 17 years with a good treatment response in adolescent bipolar disorder, childhood aggression and disruptiveness, behavioral disorders associated with mental retardation, and developmental disorders.[32,33] It has a very narrow safe therapeutic safety window and can be toxic at certain levels and, as such, must be monitored closely by a qualified child and adolescent psychiatrist. Its use in children who have experienced maltreatment is aimed at treating comorbid conditions or in stabilizing mood. Primary indication for use is mania in bipolar mood disorder. Lithium's side effects include fine tremor, polyuria, polydipsia, ankle edema, weight gain, metallic taste in mouth, gastrointestinal irritation, leukocytosis, and worsening of acne and psoriasis.

Treatment can be initiated at 250 to 300 mg twice daily and up-titrated weekly by 250 to 300 mg until a therapeutic dosage of 0.8 mmol/l to 1.2 mmol/l is reached in acute mania. The lithium dose for children should be 30 mg/kg. Discontinuation should be slow with close monitoring as abrupt discontinuation can precipitate a manic episode. Monitoring of lithium levels and kidney function must be done regularly, initially every 5 days until blood levels are reached. Thyroid function, parathyroid function, calcium and magnesium, fasting blood glucose, and lipogram should also be monitored.

ANTIPSYCHOTICS

Risperidone

Risperidone is a second-generation/atypical antipsychotic and serotonin-dopamine antagonist.[30] Paliperidone is an active metabolite of risperidone and is available in tablet form and as a monthly injection. Indications for their use include schizophrenia, other psychotic disorders, acute mania/mixed mania, and irritability in autism spectrum disorders.[30]

Side effects include dizziness, hypotension, sedation, and extrapyramidal side effects (usually at higher dosages).[30] Body mass index (BMI) must be recorded prior to initiating oral treatment with risperidone at 0.25 mg to 0.5 mg daily or twice a day depending on the child or adolescent's age. Duration of treatment with Risperidone or with Paliperidone will vary depending on the indication for use.

Monitoring of BMI and metabolic profile (blood pressure, fasting glucose, and lipogram) are required during treatment, especially in high-risk cases.[30]

Aripiprazole

Aripiprazole is an atypical antipsychotic agent that is referred to as a second-generation antipsychotic; it has even been described by some as a third-generation antipsychotic.[34] It is FDA approved for use in children and adolescents aged 6 years to 17 years for the treatment of irritability associated with autism spectrum disorder. Other indications for use include schizophrenia, other psychotic disorders, and mania. Side effects include extrapyramidal side effects, drowsiness, gastrointestinal symptoms, and metabolic syndrome. Other reported common side effects include dizziness, light-headedness, drowsiness, nausea, vomiting, tiredness, excess saliva/drooling, blurred vision, weight gain, constipation, headache, and trouble sleeping.

The target dose for adolescents is 10 mg/day. Subsequent dose increases should be administered in 2 to 5 mg increments. Sudden stoppage of Aripiprazole could result in the "Aripiprazole discontinuation syndrome," characterized by anxiety and restlessness. Discontinuation should therefore not be abrupt, but rather, Aripiprazole should be tapered off gradually.

Other Second-Generation Antipsychotics

Olanzapine and Quetiapine are also used in the treatment of schizophrenia, schizoaffective disorder, and bipolar mood disorder. Side effects include risk of metabolic syndrome, but both drugs have less tendency to increase prolactin. Dizziness and somnolence with postural hypotension can occur with both. Olanzapine additionally causes tremor, constipation, akathisia, and dry mouth. Those who take Olanzapine are also more prone to weight gain due to increased appetite.

Clozapine is indicated after optimal treatment with two consecutive antipsychotics has failed. It can cause blood abnormalities (eg, agranulocytosis) and a white cell count should be done weekly for 18 weeks. Other side effects are constipation, ECG changes, dizziness, sedation, muscle weakness, hypersalivation, hypotension, and seizures.

BENZODIAZEPINES

Benzodiazepines should not be used routinely in the treatment of anxiety disorders in children/adolescents.[35] Benzodiazepines are classified as anticonvulsants and anxiolytics.[30]

Indications include anxiety disorders, seizures, acute agitation, and catatonia.[30]

Sedation, dizziness, slurred speech, confusion, memory impairment, paradoxical disinhibition/hyper-excitability, dependence, and withdrawal are among the myriad of side effects associated with benzodiazepine use.[23,30]

Treatment initiation and discontinuation: The lowest possible dose should be used for the shortest possible time period. If tolerance and dependence develop, substitution with diazepam and gradual down-titration are recommended.[23]

TRICYCLIC ANTIDEPRESSANTS (TCAS)

TCAs are serotonin and noradrenaline reuptake inhibitors.[30] They enhance serotonin and noradrenaline neurotransmission by blocking the serotonin and noradrenalin reuptake pump. TCAs also have actions at a variety of other receptors. TCAs, while efficacious, have significant side effects and should be used with caution. TCAs should not be prescribed for children and adolescents with depression.

STIMULANTS

Methylphenidate is a central nervous stimulant and a controlled drug.[23]

It enhances the actions of dopamine and noradrenaline in various brain regions by blocking dopamine and noradrenaline reuptake and facilitating their release. This enhances attention, concentration, executive function, and wakefulness and improves hyperactivity, tiredness, and depression.[30] It is a first-line drug for ADHD with a large evidence base to support its use in ADHD.[23]

Side effects include anorexia, deceleration of growth, insomnia, headaches, nervousness, irritability, overstimulation, and exacerbation of tics.[23,30]

Treatment should be initiated by a child and adolescent specialist and can be continued by a primary care physician once the child is stabilized on an adequate dosage of methylphenidate.[30] Stimulants have high abuse potential; adolescents should be monitored for drug diversion, especially if there is a history of drug abuse.[23]

Medications like dextroamphetamine/amphetamine salts or lisdexamfetamine dimesylate (LDX) should be prescribed in consultation with a specialist, and if side effects of methylphenidate cannot be tolerated.

NON-STIMULANTS

Atomoxetine is a selective noradrenaline reuptake inhibitor.[30] It is a suitable first-line alternative for ADHD in children older than 6 years. Atomoxetine should be considered if there is a poor response to stimulants, if medications cannot be given during the day (ie, at school), if stimulant diversion is problematic, or if there are dopaminergic side effects on conventional stimulants such as anxiety, stereotypies, and tics.[23] Sedation, fatigue, decreased appetite, and increased blood pressure and heart rate are some of the side effects associated with atomoxetine.

OTHER MEDICATIONS

These medications should be prescribed in consultation with a specialist, as the evidence base for their use in children and adolescents is limited (**Table 3-2**).

Table 3-2. Other Medications and Their Uses	
Antihistamines (eg, hydroxyzine)	— Ongoing trauma, poor support, psychological or environmental (including school and cultural) stressors, and substance abuse.
Clonidine *Note: Clonidine's approved indication is for hypertension. Its CNS uses are second, third-line or experimental.*	— Third-line medication for ADHD. — Off-label use in difficult-to-treat anxiety disorders (eg, PTSD, social anxiety disorder).
Propranolol	— Social phobia (performance anxiety). — Lithium-induced postural tremor. — Control of aggressive behavior. — Neuroleptic-induced akathisia.
Buspirone *Note: Studies in children aged 6 years to 17 years with GAD have not shown significant decrease in anxiety symptoms.*	— Anxiety disorders: for example, generalized anxiety disorder. — Short-term treatment of anxiety symptoms.

MEDICATION TREATMENT OPTIONS FOR COMMON PSYCHIATRIC DISORDERS IN CHILDREN AND ADOLESCENTS

MOOD DISORDERS

Psychotherapy and other psychosocial interventions (eg, self-help materials, sleep hygiene, exercise) should be provided for all age groups. Antidepressants have a modest effect size in pediatric MDD which is lower than that seen in adult studies of MDD.[36]

Severity Considerations
— **Mild depression:** Watchful waiting, psychoeducation, supportive treatment, case management.[27,37]

— **Moderate depression:** Psychotherapy, such as CBT, interpersonal therapy (IPT), or family therapy.[27,37]

— **Moderate to severe depression:** The combination of fluoxetine and CBT is cost-effective and of superior efficacy than CBT or fluoxetine alone in adolescents with moderate-severe depression. The addition of CBT has a protective effect against suicidality. Treatment should be for at least 6 to 9 months to reduce the risk of relapse. [27,37-39]

PTSD

A comprehensive approach should include consideration of the severity of PTSD symptoms as well as the degree of functional impairment. Individual trauma-focused cognitive behavioral therapy (TF-CBT) is regarded as first-line treatment and parents should preferably be included in the treatment plan.[22,40] There is also good evidence for the efficacy of group TF-CBT, Eye Movement Desensitization and Reprocessing (EMDR), Cognitive Processing Therapy (CPT), and Behavioral Therapy.[41]

Severity Considerations
— **Mild PTSD:** TF-CBT is considered a first-line treatment for mild PTSD.[22,40]

— **Moderate-Severe PTSD:** TF-CBT is considered the first-line treatment for moderate to severe PTSD.[22] Medications should not be routinely prescribed.[40] Combine TF-CBT with an SSRI if acute symptom resolution is needed, comorbidity that necessitates pharmacotherapy, poor response to psychotherapy, or if a potentially better outcome with combination treatment is anticipated.[23]

ANXIETY AND RELATED DISORDERS

CBT is usually the first-line treatment for children and adolescents with anxiety disorders. Medications may be considered if CBT is not suitable, if CBT fails, or if the anxiety is severe. The combination of CBT and medication (eg, Sertraline) are significantly superior to either Sertraline or CBT monotherapy for childhood anxiety disorders in a randomized controlled trial.[23,42] Start the medication at a low dose, inform caregivers about the risk of suicidality, and monitor for behavioral activation and suicidality (suicidal ideation and attempts). Allow an adequate trial at an adequate dose when assessing clinical response. Benzodiazepines should not be routinely used, and if used, only for a short period to manage acute anxiety.[23,35]

ADHD AND OPPOSITIONAL DEFIANT DISORDER

Parental management training, psychosocial interventions, and psychotherapy should be considered first. If medication is considered for ADHD, this must be done under specialist guidance. Psychosocial interventions should be considered first in school-going children and adolescents. If medication is indicated, it should be specialist-initiated after a comprehensive assessment. Methylphenidate is a first-line medication, while Atomoxetine is an alternative first-line.[23]

MOOD DYSREGULATION, IMPULSIVITY, AND SELF-HARMING BEHAVIORS

Pharmacological interventions for behaviors characterized by mood dysregulation, impulsivity, distress intolerance, and self-harming present several challenges in that there are often multiple risk factors for these behaviors that present as a consequence of childhood maltreatment. In addition, the clinical picture may be clouded by co-existing psychiatric disorders, complex psychosocial dynamics, and acute versus the chronic risk of suicide. Pharmacotherapy is not recommended as a first-line intervention in these cases. Rather, it is recommended that individual risk screening for comorbid psychiatric disorders be done with treatment individualized to the disorder. Some specific behaviors may not form part of the constellation of symptoms that are core to the presenting psychiatric disorder(s) per se; however, salient symptoms need to be targeted initially by age-appropriate behavior modifications, cognitive restructuring, dialectical behavioral therapy, and individual and group psychotherapy to reduce distress, enhance safety, and promote therapeutic alliances. If pharmacotherapy is required to assist with impulsivity or self-directed aggression, a specialist in the field should be consulted before initiating medication.

CONCLUSION

Children and adolescents exposed to childhood maltreatment have an increased risk of developing various psychiatric disorders. In general, psychosocial interventions and psychotherapy are the mainstay of treatment, especially in a very young child and where the psychiatric disorder is of mild severity. However, psychopharmacology has an important role to play in the management of certain disorders, particularly where the response to psychotherapy has been suboptimal and has failed, or simply as an adjunct to treatment where comorbid psychiatric disorders are present. Medications should be prescribed after careful consideration and with caution after a comprehensive assessment of the presentation and circumstances of the individual patient.

CASE STUDY

Case Study 3-1

Ann was a social worker and enjoyed caring for the teenagers she supported in her community. She received a complaint from Karla, a 13-year-old girl who she was coordinating the care of and who was recently referred to see a psychiatrist after an attempted suicide. Karla said she recently started experiencing trouble sleeping, feelings of anxiety, and uncontrollable tremors. As a non-prescribing care provider, Ann faced a dilemma on how to make sense of these complaints and how best to help Karla.

Discussion

The dilemma faced by Ann is fairly common, especially in settings where there is either no trained specialist to provide medication management, or there are long waiting lists to consult with a doctor. At other times, a patient may simply find it easier to access a non-prescribing clinician to ask for help.

Generally, non-prescribing clinicians, like Ann, cannot provide medication advice or prescribe any medications. However, they have a very important role in helping to facilitate access to appropriate care.

An important first principle is to recognize the limits of one's scope of practice, while also being aware of medications and their possible side effects. Second, a good understanding of the resources within the community for medication prescription and management is also necessary. Third, trauma-related inquiry, as much as possible, should be collaborative and involve the parent or legal guardian. Fourth, trauma-informed principles of care (namely, safety, trustworthiness, collaboration, choice, and empowerment) should always form the cornerstone of management.

A few further questions that could be asked by Ann include confirming the timing and nature of onset of these complaints, exploring if any medications are being used and what they are, and having some knowledge of the temporal relationship of symptoms to medication usage. All these can help Ann to establish if the complaints might be linked to a new medication that has been initiated.

Important next steps would include reassuring the patient and at the same time encouraging her to schedule an appointment with her doctor, and where possible, to assist in scheduling an earlier appointment. Assistance with arranging a telephonic consultation may also be considered in settings that permit virtual consultations.

Caution must be exercised when clients want to adjust the dosage of medications themselves or where they make requests for a non-prescribing clinician to adjust medications for them. It is also important to avoid the temptation to ask a client to stop all medications immediately as this could result in adverse reactions.

KEY POINTS

1. A biopsychosocial approach to care is imperative, as medication alone will not equip a maltreated child with new coping skills or restore a child's sense of safety.

2. Safe and effective medications are available for maltreated children and adolescents who present with psychopathology. SSRIs are the most effective medications currently for MDD, anxiety disorders, and OCD. Prescribing SSRIs requires clinical judgment and ensuring that the benefits outweigh the risks.

3. The prescribing clinician must obtain informed consent from the parent or legal guardian and assent from the child, and the values of the child and family must be upheld in treatment decisions. Informed consent entails discussion of target symptoms, the likely benefits of medication, the potential side effects, and the risks of not taking the medication in question. Informed consent and assent are ongoing processes and these discussions should always be documented.

4. Education about medication side effects and exploring other modalities of care, with patient and caregiver, is key to improving adherence.

5. Interventional treatments for severe and refractory pediatric MDD, such as electroconvulsive therapy, transcranial magnetic stimulation, and ketamine, have not yet been widely investigated in this age group and there is insufficient evidence to recommend their use.

REFERENCES

1. Hillis S, Mercy J, Amobi A, Kress H. Global prevalence of past-year violence against children: a systematic review and minimum estimates. *Pediatrics.* 2016;137(3):e20154079. doi:10.1542/peds.2015-4079

2. Dvir Y, Ford JD, Hill M, Frazier JA. Childhood maltreatment, emotional dysregulation, and psychiatric comorbidities. *Harv Rev Psychiatry.* 2014;22(3):149-61. doi:10.1097/HRP.0000000000000014

3. Hughes K, Bellis MA, Hardcastle KA, et al. The effect of multiple adverse childhood experiences on health: a systematic review and meta-analysis. *Lancet Public Health.* 2017;2(8):e356-e366. doi:10.1016/S2468-2667(17)30118-4

4. Bellis MA, Hughes K, Ford K, Ramos Rodriguez G, Sethi D, Passmore J. Life course health consequences and associated annual costs of adverse childhood experiences across Europe and North America: a systematic review and meta-analysis. *Lancet Public Health.* 2019;4(10):e517-e528. doi:10.1016/S2468-2667 (19)30145-8

5. Cousins L, Goodyer IM. Antidepressants and the adolescent brain. *J Psychopharmacol.* 2015;29(5):545-555. doi:10.1177/0269881115573542

6. Shenk CE, Keeshin B, Bensman HE, Olson AE, Allen B. Behavioral and pharmacological interventions for the prevention and treatment of psychiatric disorders with children exposed to maltreatment. *Pharmacol Biochem Behav.* 2021;211: 173298. doi:10.1016/j.pbb.2021.173298

7. Chaffin M, Hanson R, Saunders BE, et al. Report of the APSAC Task Force on attachment therapy, reactive attachment disorder, and attachment problems. *Child Maltreat.* 2006;11(1):76-89. doi:10.1177/1077559505283699

8. Spetie L, Arnold E. Ethical issues in child pharmacology research and practice: emphasis on pre-schoolers. *Psychopharmacol.* 2007;191(1):15-26. doi:10.1007/ s00213-006-0685-8

9. Putnam FW. Ten-year research update review: child sexual abuse. *J Am Acad Child Adolesc Psychiatry.* 2002;42(3):269-278. doi:10.1097/00004583-200303000-00006

10. Consequences of child abuse and neglect. In: Petersen AC, Joseph J, Feit M, eds. *New Directions in Child Abuse and Neglect Research.* National Academies Press (US); 2014:111-174.

11. Sege RD, Amaya-Jackson L, American Academy of Pediatrics Committee on Child Abuse and Neglect, Council on Foster Care, Adoption, and Kinship Care, American Academy of Child and Adolescent Psychiatry Committee on Child Maltreatment and Violence, National Center for Child Traumatic Stress. Clinical considerations related to the behavioral manifestations of child maltreatment. *Pediatrics.* 2017;139(4):e20170100. doi:10.1542/peds.2017-0100

12. Bowlby J. *Attachment.* Hogarth Press; 1969.

13. Thomas A, Chess S, Birch H. *Temperament and Behavior Disorders in Children.* New York University Press; 1968.

14. Prosser LA, Corso PS. Measuring health-related quality of life for child maltreatment: a systematic literature review. *Health Qual Life Outcomes.* 2007;5:42. doi:10.1186/1477-7525-5-42

15. Rutter M, Bishop D, Pine D, et al. *Rutter's Child and Adolescent Psychiatry.* 5th ed. Blackwell Publishing Ltd; 2008.

16. Lask B, Taylor S, Nunn KP. *Practical Child Psychiatry: The Clinician's Guide*. BMJ Books; 2003.

17. American Psychiatric Association. *Diagnostic and Statistical Manual of Mental Disorders (DSM-5)*. 5th ed. American Psychiatric Association Press; 2013.

18. World Health Organization. *International Statistical Classification of Diseases and Related Health Problems, Tenth Revision*. World Health Organization; 2004.

19. Erikson EH. *Childhood and Society*. Norton; 1963.

20. Erikson EH. *Identity, Youth and Crisis*. Norton; 1968.

21. Pescosolido BA, Perry BL, Martin JK, Mcleod JD, Jensen PS. Stigmatizing attitudes and beliefs about treatment and psychiatric medications for children with mental illness. *Psychiatr Serv*. 2007;58(5):613-618. doi:10.1176/ps.2007.58.5.613

22. Cohen JA, Bukstein O, Walter H, et al. Practice parameter for the assessment and treatment of children and adolescents with posttraumatic stress disorder. *J Am Acad Child Adolesc Psychiatry*. 2010;49(4):414-427.

23. Taylor D, Paton C, Kapur S. *The Maudsley Prescribing Guidelines*. 10th ed. Informa Healthcare; 2009.

24. Walkup J; Work Group on Quality Issues. Practice parameter on the use of psychotropic medication in children and adolescents. *J Am Acad Child Adolesc Psychiatry*. 2009;48(9):961-973. doi:10.1097/CHI.0b013e3181ae0a08

25. American Academy of Child and Adolescent Psychiatry. Practice parameter for the assessment and treatment of children and adolescents with attention-deficit/hyperactivity disorder. *J Am Acad Child Adolesc Psychiatry*. 2007;46:894Y921.

26. Bryden KE, Carrey NJ, Kutcher SP. Update and recommendations for the use of antipsychotics in early-onset psychoses. *J Child Adolesc Psychopharmacol*. 2001;11:113Y130. doi:10.1089/104454601750284027

27. Birmaher B, Brent D; AACAP Work Group on Quality Issues, et al. Practice parameter for the assessment and treatment of children and adolescents with depressive disorders. *J Am Acad Child Adolesc Psychiatry*. 2007;46(11):1503-1526. doi:10.1097/chi.0b013e318145ae1c

28. Sadock JS, Sadock VA. *Kaplan & Sadock's Synopsis of Psychiatry Behavioral Sciences/ Clinical Psychiatry*. 12th ed. Lippincott Williams & Wilkins; 2021:1319.

29. Dwyer JB, Bloch MH. Antidepressants for pediatric patients. *Curr Psychiatr*. 2019;18(9):26-42F.

30. Stahl SM. *Stahl's Essential Psychopharmacology: The Prescriber's Guide*. 7th ed. Cambridge University Press; 2020.

31. Hetrick SE, McKenzie JE, Bailey AP, et al. New generation antidepressants for depression in children and adolescents: a network meta-analysis. *Cochrane Database Syst Rev*. 2021;5(5):CD013674. doi:10.1002/14651858.CD013674.pub2

32. Amerio A, Ossola P, Scagnelli F, et al. Safety and efficacy of lithium in children and adolescents: a systematic review in bipolar illness. *Eur Psychiatry*. 2018;54:85-97. doi:10.1016/j.eurpsy.2018.07.012

33. Solmi M, Fornaro M, Ostinelli EG, et al. Safety of 80 antidepressants, antipsychotics, anti-attention-deficit/hyperactivity medications and mood stabilizers in children and adolescents with psychiatric disorders: a large scale systematic meta-

review of 78 adverse effects. *World Psychiatry*. 2020;19(2):214-232. doi:10.1002/wps.20765

34. Mailman RB, Murthy V. Third generation antipsychotic drugs: partial agonism or receptor functional selectivity? *Curr Pharm Des*. 2010;16(5):488-501. doi:10.2174/138161210790361461

35. Ipser JC, Stein DJ, Hawkridge S, Hoppe L. Pharmacotherapy for anxiety disorders in children and adolescents [review]. *Evid-Based Child Health: Cochrane Rev J*. 2010;5(2):555-628. doi:10.1002/ebch.541

36. Feeney A, Hock RS, Fava M, Hernández Ortiz JM, Iovieno N, Papakostas GI. Antidepressants in children and adolescents with major depressive disorder and the influence of placebo response: a meta-analysis. *J Affect Disord*. 2022;305:55-64. doi:10.1016/j.jad.2022.02.074

37. Depression in children and young people: identification and management in primary, community, and secondary care. National Institute for Clinical Excellence. Published 2005. Updated 2019. Accessed Aug 12 2023. https://www.nice.org.uk/guidance/ng134

38. March J, Silva S, Petrycki S, et al. Fluoxetine, cognitive-behavioral therapy, and their combination for adolescents with depression: treatment for adolescents with depression study (TADS) randomized controlled trial. *JAMA*. 2004;292(7):807-820. doi:10.1001/jama.292.7.807

39. March JS, Vitiello B. Clinical messages from the treatment for adolescents with depression study (TADS). *Am J Psychiatry*. 2009;166:1118-1123. doi:10.1176/appi.ajp.2009.08101606

40. Post-traumatic stress disorder (PTSD): the management of PTSD in adults and children in primary and secondary care. National Institute for Clinical Excellence. Published 2005. Updated 2018. Accessed August 14, 2023. https://www.nice.org.uk/guidance/ng116

41. Xiang Y, Cipriani A, Teng T, et al. Comparative efficacy and acceptability of psychotherapies for post-traumatic stress disorder in children and adolescents: a systematic review and network meta-analysis. *Evid Based Ment Health*. 2021;24(4):153-160. doi:10.1136/ebmental-2021-300346

42. Walkup JT, Albano AM, Piacentini J, et al. Cognitive behavioral therapy, sertraline, or a combination in childhood anxiety. *N Engl J Med*. 2008;359:2753-2766. doi:10.1056/NEJMoa0804633

Chapter 4

Trauma-Focused Cognitive Behavioral Therapy

Ciera E. Schoonover, PhD, MSW, MPH, HSP

Irene Brodd, PhD, LT, MSC, USN, Navy Medical Readiness and Training
    Command (NMRTC), Portsmouth

Madelyne Williams, BS

The views expressed in this chapter are those of the authors and do not
necessarily reflect the official policy or position of the Department of the
Navy, Department of Defense, or the United States Government.

Irene Brodd, PhD is a military service member. This work was prepared
as part of her official duties. Title 17 U.S.C. 105 provides that "Copyright
protection under this title is not available for any work of the United States
Government." Title 17 U.S.C. 101 defines a United States Government
work as a work prepared by a military service member or employee of the
United States Government as part of that person's official duties.

Objectives

After reading this chapter, the reader will be able to:

1. *Understand the scope and prevalence of child maltreatment along with the various domains of trauma impact on children and adolescents.*

2. *Identify the core components of trauma-focused interventions with the strongest empirical basis for children and adolescents.*

3. *Recognize the multiple domains of trauma impact and ways in which Trauma-Focused Cognitive Behavioral Therapy (TF-CBT) effectively improves symptoms of post-traumatic stress disorder (PTSD) and other internalizing and externalizing problems associated with trauma exposure.*

4. *Describe the skills and trauma-specific components of TF-CBT (eg, PRACTICE) and demonstrate precursory knowledge of how to apply those components in clinical practice.*

5. *Discuss the scope of TF-CBT as it applies to various contexts and diverse populations.*

Background and Significance

Early childhood is a critical period of development, marked by tremendous growth and change. It is also the time when children are at highest risk for maltreatment.[1] In the United States, approximately 618 000 children were victims of abuse and neglect in 2020.[1] Approximately 76.1% were victims of neglect, 16% experienced physical abuse, 9% were subjected to sexual abuse, and 0.2% were reported to have been trafficked.[1] Children from birth to age 6 are at the greatest risk for maltreatment and exposure to domestic violence.[1] While staggering, the statistics are thought to be an underestimate of true rates, as maltreatment is suspected to be grossly underreported. Given that nearly every state in the United States experienced some form of restrictions in response to COVID-19, the nation's largest group of child maltreatment reporters (ie, educators) had limited opportunities to observe and report suspected maltreatment, begging the question: *how accurate are our current statistics on child maltreatment?*

In addition to maltreatment, children may experience a wide range of potentially traumatic events that include exposure to domestic violence, death of a caregiver, serious accidents or injuries, natural disasters, community violence, and many others. The scope of traumatic experiences can vary widely, but ultimately, it is the individual's perception of the event or experience that tends to influence subsequent symptomatology. While this chapter focuses on the implementation of trauma-focused interventions as an intervention for child maltreatment, it should be noted that the interventions reviewed may be tailored as treatments for traumatic stress responses secondary to other adverse or traumatic experiences as well.

MENTAL HEALTH CONCERNS AFTER TRAUMA EXPOSURE

A portion of children who are exposed to maltreatment or other traumatic events develop difficulties in a variety of domains, including cognitive, behavioral, or emotional wellbeing.[2] These difficulties can become clinically significant, evolving into more severe mental health concerns, such as PTSD, depressive disorders, anxiety disorders, or externalizing behavior problems. There is thought to be somewhat of a dose-response relationship to trauma exposure, in which chronic exposure can lead to more severe impairment.[2] Complex trauma is a concept that has increasingly been used to describe the experience of recurring or chronic trauma exposure, such as repeated physical or emotional abuse or pervasive environmental neglect.[3]

Maltreated children are at greater risk for the following: externalizing behavior problems (eg, conduct problems, delinquency, high-risk sexual behaviors), mental health disorders (eg, anxiety, depressive or eating disorders), drug use, and suicide attempts.[4-7] In fact, children and adolescents who experience maltreatment have a 2.5 times greater risk for developing mental health problems than those in the general population.[8] The acute and chronic stress associated with the experience of abuse can also have adverse physiological and health impacts, such as heart disease, obesity, high blood pressure, and high cholesterol.[6]

TRAUMA TREATMENTS ACROSS CHILDHOOD

Trauma-focused interventions are designed to address the problems associated with traumatic events that children experience or witness. That is, trauma-focused treatments are intended for children who have primary presenting concerns related to trauma symptoms (eg, PTSD, cognitive distortions, shame, depressed mood). With trauma-focused interventions, children may be supported to overcome trauma-specific problems such as avoidance, shame, sadness, or fear. While externalizing behavior concerns are typically not a core focus of trauma-focused interventions, many include behavior management components to improve behavioral dysregulation associated with trauma exposure.

Child, caregiver, and environmental factors should be considered when deciding on an intervention for a child presenting with difficulties after a traumatic experience. Child factors include the child's age, developmental level, language ability, and type and duration of symptoms.[9] Caregiver factors may also play a role in decision making, such as the offending status of the caregiver (TF-CBT is not designed to be used with offending caregivers),[10] the caregiver's availability to engage in treatment, and the caregiver's level of impairment or functioning.[9] Finally, environmental factors must be considered, such as custodial status and availability of a caregiver to participate.

Three commonly referred interventions for childhood trauma are Child Parent-Psychotherapy (CPP), Parent-Child Interaction Therapy (PCIT), and TF-CBT. CPP is appropriate for children younger than 6 years old and is not dependent on the child's verbal expression or language abilities. In CPP, therapists help parents put the trauma narrative into words and support their children in recovery after traumatic experiences.[11] PCIT is a strong evidence-based intervention for children 2 to 7 years old and their caregivers[12] (as further discussed in Chapter 5: Promoting Healthy Parent-Child Interactions). PCIT has shown to be effective for children who have experienced trauma[13]; however, it does not directly address trauma in the child; rather, it addresses the externalizing behavior problems and focuses on improving the caregiver-child relationship.[14] Directly targeting PTSD symptoms, TF-CBT is appropriate for children 3 to 18 years old with speech and language abilities. TF-CBT involves individual child, caregiver-only, and caregiver-child therapy sessions wherein participants learn affect regulation strategies, practice cognitive coping skills, and process experienced trauma.[2]

Although there are many interventions that have been deemed efficacious in treating trauma symptoms across childhood, many interventions with the strongest evidence base consist of a set of common elements. For example, many evidence-based child interventions require involvement and active participation by a caregiver.[15] Notably, trauma-focused interventions with the strongest evidence base include components that emphasize psychoeducation on trauma and the trauma response, skill building (including exposure exercises), affect identification and regulation, parent-management strategies, and future safety planning.

TRAUMA-FOCUSED COGNITIVE BEHAVIORAL THERAPY

The National Child Traumatic Stress Network (NCTSN), an online source for families and providers that aims to improve access to services for traumatized children and families, lists 38 different trauma treatments, including TF-CBT.[16] TF-CBT is a pioneering intervention in treating childhood symptoms of trauma. With one of the strongest, longest, and most consistent evidence bases of trauma interventions, the California Evidence-Based Clearinghouse for Child Welfare[17] recognizes TF-CBT as "well-supported by research evidence" as a trauma treatment. Given TF-CBT's compelling evidence base, it will be presented as a model intervention for treating traumatic stress in early childhood and adolescence.

CONCEPTUAL MODEL

Trauma exposure can impact a variety of domains and levels of functioning. If left untreated, trauma symptoms can have negative effects on physical, emotional, cognitive, behavioral, and social development. Given that these areas of functioning all serve to impact one another, further negative developmental cascades can result from dysfunction in one domain, exacerbating maladaptive functioning. TF-CBT's theoretical underpinnings are in cognitive-behavioral, attachment, and family therapy, making it a well-rounded and ecologically valid strategy for addressing the impact of childhood trauma to reduce its negative impacts.[2] The crux of TF-CBT is that it addresses the impact of childhood trauma across all domains of functioning, thus reducing the impact and likelihood of further disrupted development.

OVERVIEW AND DESCRIPTION OF THE TF-CBT MODEL

A short-term, time-limited intervention (typically lasting 8 to 15 sessions), TF-CBT is based on elements common in cognitive behavioral therapy (CBT). CBT begins with an assessment to gather history and information about patient concerns, including symptoms and presenting problems. In the case of TF-CBT, the assessment includes all of those components in addition to gathering information about the traumatic event(s) the child has experienced. Therapists may gather information through a number of ways, using a multi-method and multi-source approach. An initial step in the assessment process typically involves a clinical interview(s) with the caregiver and child. Additional collateral interviews may be conducted as appropriate. Children may present with comorbid concerns of internalizing (eg, mood, anxiety), externalizing (eg, oppositional or disruptive behaviors), and other problems (eg, attention concerns or sleep disturbances). Standardized questionnaires to identify primary concerning symptoms may help inform treatment planning.

Common elements in TF-CBT and standard CBT treatments include session structure (eg, proposed duration of treatment, setting an agenda), psychoeducation, and out-of-session practice with review of practice during sessions. In TF-CBT, the acronym PRACTICE (**Table 15-1**) is used to summarize the components of TF-CBT that address concerns subsequent to a traumatic experience. The PRACTICE components have been evaluated in research in this order, therefore, researchers note that "the efficacy of the TF-CBT model is known only in relation to applying the components and treatment phases in this manner."[2] The components build upon one another, such that children and caregivers learn and consolidate early skills to develop skills taught later in treatment. TF-CBT is conceptualized as consisting of 3 phases: (1) stabilization and skill building, (2) trauma narration and processing, and (3) consolidation and closure.

Table 15-1. PRACTICE Model Components[2]

P	Psychoeducation; Parenting skills
R	Relaxation
A	Affective expression and modulation
C	Cognitive coping and processing skills
T	Trauma narration and processing
I	In vivo exposure and mastery of trauma reminders
C	Conjoint caregiver-child sessions
E	Enhancing safety and safety planning

PSYCHOEDUCATION AND PARENTING SKILLS

Psychoeducation provides information to children and their caregiver(s) about treatment. In TF-CBT, psychoeducation starts during the assessment phase, is emphasized in the first phase, and is ongoing over the course of treatment. Providing psychoeducation accomplishes many essential goals when addressing presenting traumatic response concerns. Specific to TF-CBT, one of these goals is to normalize caregivers' and children's responses to the traumatic experience(s). Therapists do this by offering information about typical psychological and physiological responses. This also instills hope and is moralizing for caregivers and children who have experienced a traumatic experience by letting them know that they are not alone in their experience(s). In providing psychoeducation, therapists discuss diagnoses, symptoms, and available treatments. This discussion of symptoms begins to address trauma reminders and helps children/adolescents and caregivers gain an understanding of the connections between events and responses so they can develop adaptive responses to trauma reminders.

In TF-CBT, therapists offer caregivers support around effective parenting practices with children and adolescents. Support takes the form of providing caregivers normative information about children's symptoms and reactions after traumatic experiences and ways to respond to and reduce problem behaviors (eg, tantrums, defiance, agression). Therapists teach caregivers effective parenting skills, which include reinforcing their children's positive and prosocial behaviors through parental attention and behavior charts and reducing problem behaviors through selective or differential attention and consistent and predictable discipline, such as time-out from positive reinforcement. For parents of adolescents, therapists engage adolescents with their parents to develop family rules and consequences when rules are broken.

RELAXATION SKILLS

Therapists instruct children and caregivers in relaxation skills that address the physiological symptoms that arise following traumatic experiences. Relaxation skills include diaphragmatic (ie, belly) breathing, mindfulness meditation, progressive muscle relaxation (PMR), and other techniques to manage daily stressors and reduce day-to-day impairment when confronted with trauma reminders. After in-session instruction and practice using scripts based on the patient's age, children and adolescents practice the skills between sessions. As children and caregivers practice, they gain mastery of the relaxation skills, which positively contributes to their confidence in managing stressors. The positive benefits of consistently applying the relaxation skills can improve sleep and reduce hyperarousal and muscle tension. Cognitive benefits of children and caregivers practicing relaxation skills include learning to take a nonjudgmental stance towards thoughts, recognizing that they come and go, and learning to allow them to pass, rather than getting stuck thinking about the past or worrying about the future.

AFFECT EXPRESSION AND MODULATION SKILLS

Using this component of TF-CBT, therapists help children and adolescents to identify, label, and express their emotional experiences and range of feelings subsequent to traumatic experiences. Therapists also support caregivers' affective modulation skill development by providing them the space to express their emotions with the therapist rather than to or at their child. In addition to labeling emotions, children learn to manage emotional experiences using thought interruption (ie, stopping unproductive rumination and intrusive thoughts) and positive self-talk (ie, recognizing and labeling the ways they are coping well).

COGNITIVE COPING AND PROCESSING SKILLS

To help children learn how their thoughts, feelings, and behaviors are related, therapists teach them to recognize their internal dialogue (ie, self-talk and automatic thoughts). Therapists provide instruction on the cognitive triangle to teach children/ adolescents and caregivers how changing their perception of a situation changes how they feel and what they do in response. Children and caregivers learn to identify their own unhelpful thinking patterns and challenge or change them to identify more accurate or helpful thoughts. Practice is focused on thoughts related to day-to-day events rather than the traumatic experience. After they create the trauma narrative, children learn to apply cognitive coping skills as they relate to the trauma experience.

TRAUMA NARRATION AND PROCESSING

In the second phase of treatment, therapists guide children and adolescents through developmentally appropriate construction of the trauma narrative and processing of the traumatic experience. Often, the trauma narrative takes the form of a written book with details of the trauma and thoughts, feelings, and sensations experienced or perceived by the child. Depending on a child's developmental level, the therapist may design the trauma narrative using pictures, songs, or other creative art forms. However, a tangible product is not necessary; in TF-CBT, trauma narration is about the child sharing their story and the therapist supporting their processing of traumatic experiences.

The process of developing a trauma narrative leads to children experiencing less hyperarousal and avoidance of trauma reminders (ie, desensitization). With the therapist's support, children describe details of the traumatic experiences and their thoughts and feelings during and after the experience. This, in turn, can lead to correction of the child's inaccurate or unhelpful trauma-related beliefs and thoughts about themself. At this stage, therapists support children in applying cognitive coping and processing skills as they relate to the trauma experience. Therapists use Socratic questioning (ie, gently challenging thoughts through progressively logical inquiry) and introduce different ways for children to think about their trauma-related thoughts and behaviors (eg, children accurately allocating their level of responsibility using the responsibility pie).

In Vivo Exposure

If a child is avoiding inherently safe situations or cues related to trauma reminders, the therapist will introduce in vivo exposure to reduce that avoidance. Therapists collaborate with the child and caregiver to develop an in vivo plan for the child to gradually approach (rather than avoid) feared situations and cues. Children may incorporate previously learned coping skills to manage cognitive and affective distress during exposure exercises. Through consistent practice of approaching feared situations without escaping them, children develop mastery over their fears and fears diminish. In vivo exposure is an optional component of TF-CBT and may not be necessary for all treatment cases.

Conjoint Caregiver-Child Sessions

Conjoint caregiver-child sessions are held periodically throughout treatment when deemed clinically relevant or appropriate. Conjoint sessions are held to create a therapeutic space where children and caregivers can review psychoeducational material and engage in open and positive communication to foster healthy communication around the traumatic event. Conjoint sessions provide an opportunity for caregivers to learn the affect regulation and cognitive coping skills the child is practicing in treatment. Importantly, conjoint sessions are also used for the child to share and process their trauma narrative with their caregiver. This means that conjoint sessions are particularly important near the end of treatment, once the trauma narrative has been completed. As treatment concludes, conjoint sessions can be held to proactively discuss future safety planning with the dyad.

Enhancing Future Safety and Development

The final component of the PRACTICE model addresses enhancing safety. However, therapists address safety concerns from the outset of treatment through effective safety planning when there is a potential for ongoing trauma (eg, in a case of domestic violence where the perpetrator no longer lives in the home, but the child may see them). In the absence of ongoing trauma, therapists conduct regular safety checks to provide support around safety and security. Specific skills training (eg, personal safety skills for a child exposed to abuse or violence, fire safety precautions for a survivor of a house fire) should be postponed until children have started their trauma narrative and processing. If therapists introduce specific safety skills prior to these steps, the children may be reluctant to share their actual responses to traumatic experiences and may experience negative emotions for not having responded to the traumatic experience in the optimal way described. Children may have these reactions even though they did not know these optimal skill responses at the time of the traumatic experience. Therapists teach child safety skills in individual sessions using didactic instruction and role-play, and skills practice is solidified during caregiver-child sessions. Therapists introduce topics related to a child attending to their own feelings, communicating feelings and desires to others, identifying safe people and places to seek support, practicing personal rules and body boundaries, and asking for help until it is received.

CURRENT RESEARCH ON TF-CBT

Since the previous edition of this publication, 5 additional randomized control trials (RCTs) have been published,[18-22] growing the total to more than 20 RCTs. Studies were conducted in the United States and internationally (specifically, in Japan, Kenya, and Tanzania). Sample sizes ranged from 30 to 640 participants and included racially and ethnically diverse children between 3 and 18 years of age. RCTs utilized an individual, dyadic, or combined format for TF-CBT with weekly 50-minute sessions. The studies largely concluded that TF-CBT is superior in decreasing PTSD symptoms, internalizing symptoms, and externalizing behavior problems compared to waitlist or non-directive supportive therapy controls. Available follow-up data suggest that these results were maintained up to 12 months post-treatment.[18]

TF-CBT has been shown to be effective in treating various types of trauma (eg, traumatic grief, sexual and physical abuse, exposure to domestic violence)[2] in a number of diverse populations, cross-culturally, and in a variety of settings. There is growing empirical evidence that it can be applied successfully in residential settings, foster care, schools, and via telehealth.[23-26] TF-CBT materials stress the importance of implementing the intervention with fidelity, while maintaining flexibility to meet the specific needs, and while being culturally sensitive and relevant, of the children and families served.

CONCLUSION

TF-CBT is an intervention with decades of research supporting its efficacy in treating children and adolescents with PTSD symptoms subsequent to trauma exposure. Although this is considered to be a child intervention, if done to fidelity, it will incorporate the child's caregiver throughout treatment with individual and conjoint sessions. This intervention relies on PRACTICE and culminates with the development and processing of a trauma narrative and enhancing future safety for the child. Outcome studies consistently indicate that TF-CBT results in a wide array of improvements in functioning, spanning internalizing and externalizing behavior difficulties, maladaptive cognitions, and distressing memories related to the traumatic experience. Further, by involving the caregiver, TF-CBT improves the use of effective parenting skills and reduces caregiver distress surrounding the traumatic event.

CASE STUDY

Case Study 4-1

Sarah, a 12-year-old Caucasian female, was referred for treatment from the Department of Children's Services (DCS) following reports from her familial foster caregiver (maternal aunt) of nightmares, mood swings, disruptive behavior, and failing grades in school. She was in DCS custody subsequent to substantiated child maltreatment that included physical abuse and neglect by her biological parents. Hers was a pre-adoptive placement, and she had resided in the current placement with her aunt for the past 8 months.

Discussion

Sarah's therapist conducted a thorough intake assessment prior to beginning treatment using a number of standardized assessment tools (eg, Behavioral Assessment Scale for Children; Pediatric ACEs Related Life Events Screener; Trauma Symptom Checklist for Young Children). She included a variety of sources of data in her assessment, including a clinical and collateral interview, behavioral observations, and reliable screeners for measurement of symptoms. After considering a number of diagnoses (eg, OCD and ADHD), Sarah's therapist diagnosed her with PTSD, as her symptoms closely matched diagnostic criteria of the DSM-5-TR. She discussed treatment options and together they decided on TF-CBT, partially due to its strong evidence base in treating PTSD symptoms in populations with similar demographics. Over the course of 15 weeks, Sarah, her foster caregiver, and her clinician worked through the PRACTICE components of PTSD, using developmentally appropriate strategies. During treatment, Sarah's therapist engaged Sarah in imaginal exposure exercises, which culminated in the completion of a trauma narrative in which

Sarah was able to "unpair" fearful associations with previous experiences. This intervention was deemed successful for Sarah, as the therapist noted a reduction in PTSD symptoms and reports generalized to other settings (eg, at home and in the academic setting). Following a discussion on enhancing safety in the future, Sarah graduated from treatment with a clinically significant reduction in her PTSD symptoms.

KEY POINTS

1. TF-CBT has a strong evidence base spanning close to 3 decades for treating diverse, multiple, and complex trauma experiences, children of different developmental levels, and children across various cultures.

2. A short-term treatment model, TF-CBT is shown to be effective in reducing post-traumatic stress symptoms and other trauma impacts. With the incorporation of caregiver-only and conjoint sessions, TF-CBT also has been documented to improve the use of effective parenting skills and reduce caregiver distress surrounding the traumatic event, resulting in a healthier caregiver-child relationship.

3. TF-CBT is a components-based intervention that utilizes the acronym PRACTICE in which each component is administered in order. Components are then practiced at home between sessions to optimize benefits gained in treatment.

RESOURCES

1. Cohen JA, Mannarino AP, Deblinger E. *Treating Trauma and Traumatic Grief in Children and Adolescents*. 2nd edition. The Guilford Press; 2017.

2. National Child and Traumatic Stress Network. Trauma-Focused Cognitive Behavioral Therapy. Updated 2022. https://www.nctsn.org/interventions/trauma-focused-cognitive-behavioral-therapy

3. Oklahoma TF-CBT. Updated 2022. https://oklahomatfcbt.org/

4. The California Evidence-Based Clearinghouse for Child Welfare. Trauma-Focused Cognitive-Behavioral Therapy. https://www.cebc4cw.org/program/trauma-focused-cognitive-behavioral-therapy/detailed

5. Trauma-Focused Cognitive Behavioral Therapy, National Therapist Certification Program. Updated 2022. https://tfcbt.org/

REFERENCES

1. US Department of Health and Human Services, Administration for Children and Families, Administration on Children, Youth and Families, Children's Bureau. *Child maltreatment 2020*. National Data Archive on Child Abuse and Neglect. 2022. https://www.acf.hhs.gov/cb/data-research/child-maltreatment

2. Cohen JA, Mannarino AP, Deblinger E. *Treating Trauma and Traumatic Grief in Children and Adolescents*. 2nd ed. Guilford Press; 2017.

3. Wamser-Nanney R, Vandenburg BR. Empirical support for the definition of a complex trauma event in children and adolescents. *J Trauma Stress*. 2013;26:671-678. doi:10.1002/jts.21857

4. Felitti V, Anda R, Nordenberg D, et al. Relationship of childhood abuse and household dysfunction to many of the leading causes of death in adults: the adverse childhood experiences (ACE) study. *Am J Prev Med*. 1998;14(4):245-258. doi:10.1016/s0749-3797(98)00017-8

5. Silverman AB, Reinherz HZ, Giaconia RM. The long-term sequelae of child and adolescent abuse: a longitudinal community study. *Child Abuse Negl*. 1996; 20(8):709-723. doi:10.1016/0145-2134(96)00059-2

6. Fenton MC, Geier T, Keyes K, Skodol AE, Grant BF, Hasin DS. Combined role of childhood maltreatment, family history, and gender in the risk for

alcohol dependence. *Psychol Med.* 2013;43(5):1045-1057. doi:10.1017/S0033 291712001729

7. Norman RE, Byambaa M, De R, Butchart A, Scott J, Vos T. The long-term health consequences of child physical abuse, emotional abuse, and neglect: a systematic review and meta-analysis. *PLoS Med.* 2012;9(11):1-31. doi:10.1371/journal.pmed.1001349

8. Burns BJ, Phillips SD, Wagner HR, et al. Mental health need and access to mental health services by youths involved with child welfare: a national survey. *J Am Acad Child Adolesc Psychiatry.* 2004;43(8):960-970. doi:10.1097/01.chi. 0000127590.95585.65

9. Vanderzee KL, Sigel BA, Pemberton JE, John SG. Treatments for early childhood trauma: decision considerations for clinicians. *J Child Adolesc Trauma.* 2019;12:515-528. doi:10.1007/s40653-018-0244-6

10. Deblinger E, Mannarino AP, Runyon MK, Pollio E, Cohen JA. Trauma-focused cognitive behavioral therapy for children in foster care: an implementation manual. 2017. https://tfcbt.org/wp-content/uploads/2018/05/FosterCareManual-FINAL.pdf

11. Lieberman AL, Ghosh Ippen S, Van Horn P. *Don't Hit My Mommy! A Manual for Child-Parent Psychotherapy with Young Children Exposed to Violence and Other Trauma.* 2nd ed. National Center for Clinical Infant Programs; 2015.

12. Eyberg SM, Funderburk B. *Parent-Child Interaction Therapy: The Empirically Supported Protocol.* PCIT International, Inc.; 2016.

13. Chaffin M, Silovsky JF, Funderburk B. Parent-child interaction therapy with physically abusive parents: efficacy for reducing future abuse reports. *J Consult Clin Psychol.* 2004;72(3):500-510. doi:10.1037/0022-006X.72.3.500

14. Gurwitch RH, Warner-Metzger CM. Trauma-directed interaction (TDI): an adaptation to parent-child interaction therapy for families with a history of trauma. *Int J Environ Res Public Health.* 2022;19(10):60-89. doi:10.3390/ijerph 19106089

15. Kaminski JW, Claussen AH. Evidence base update for psychosocial treatments for disruptive behaviors in children. *J Clin Child Adolesc Psychol.* 2017;46(4):477-499. doi:10.1080/15374416.2017.1310044

16. National Child and Traumatic Stress Network. Trauma-focused cognitive behavioral therapy. Updated 2022. Accessed 2022. https://www.nctsn.org/interventions/trauma-focused-cognitive-behavioral-therapy

17. The California Evidence-Based Clearinghouse for Child Welfare. Trauma-focused cognitive-behavioral therapy. https://www.cebc4cw.org/program/trauma-focused-cognitive-behavioral-therapy/detailed

18. Dorsey S, Lucid L, Martin P, et al. Effectiveness of task-shifted trauma-focused cognitive behavioral therapy for children who experienced parental death and posttraumatic stress in Kenya and Tanzania: a randomized clinical trial. *JAMA Psychiatry.* 2020;77(5):464-473. doi:10.1001/jamapsychiatry.2019.4475

19. Dawson K, Joscelyne A, Meijer C, Steel C, Silove D, Bryant RA. A controlled trial of trauma-focused therapy versus problem-solving in Islamic children affected by civil conflict and disaster in Aceh, Indonesia. *Aust N Z J Psychiatry.* 2018;52(3):253-261. doi:10.1177/0004867417714333

20. Hitchcock C, Goodall B, Wright IM, et al. The early course and treatment of posttraumatic stress disorder in very young children: diagnostic prevalence and

predictors in hospital-attending children and randomized controlled proof-of-concept trial of trauma-focused cognitive therapy, for 3- to 8-year-olds. *J Child Psychol Psychiatry.* 2022;63(1):58-67. doi:10.1111/jcpp.13460

21. Kameoka S, Tanaka E, Yamamoto S, et al. Effectiveness of trauma-focused cognitive behavioral therapy for Japanese children and adolescents in community settings: a multisite randomized controlled trial. *Eur J Psychotraumatol.* 2020; 11(1). doi:10.1080/20008198.2020.1767987

22. Salloum A, Lu Y, Chen H, et al. Stepped care versus standard care for children after trauma: a randomized non-inferiority clinical trial. *J Am Acad Child Adolesc Psychiatry.* 2022;61(8):1010-1022. doi:10.1016/j.jaac.2021.12.013

23. Cohen JA, Mannarino AP, Jankowski K, Rosenberg S, Kodya S, Wolford II GL. A randomized implementation study of trauma-focused cognitive behavioral therapy for adjudicated teens in residential treatment facilities. *Child Maltreat.* 2016;21(2):156-167. doi:10.1177/1077559515624775

24. Weiner DA, Schneider A, Lyons JS. Evidence-based treatments for trauma among culturally diverse foster care youth: Treatment retention and outcomes. *Child Youth Serv Rev.* 2009;31(11):1199-1205. doi:10.1016/j.childyouth.2009.08.013

25. Stewart RW, Orengo-Aguayo R, Wallace M, Metzger IW, Rheingold AA. Leveraging technology and cultural adaptations to increase access and engagement among trauma-exposed African American youth: exploratory study of school-based telehealth delivery of trauma-focused cognitive behavioral therapy. *J IInterpers Violence.* 2021;36(15/16):7090-7109. doi:10.1177/0886260519831380

26. Stuart RW, Orengo-Aguayo R, Young J, Wallace MM, Cohen JA, Mannarino AP. Feasibility and effectiveness of a telehealth service delivery model for treating childhood posttraumatic stress: a community based open pilot trial of trauma-focused cognitive behavioral therapy. *J Psychother Integr.* 2020;30(2):274-289. doi:10.1037/int0000225

PROMOTING HEALTHY PARENT-CHILD INTERACTIONS

Kaleigh Mancha, MS, LMFT, Certified Full Spectrum Doula

OBJECTIVES

After reading this chapter, the reader will be able to:

1. *Define what (un)healthy interactions between parents and children look like.*

2. *Describe 3 interventions that promote healthy interactions between parents and children.*

3. *Identify 2 trauma-informed therapy models to restore family systems after abuse has occurred.*

BACKGROUND AND SIGNIFICANCE

As understood with the Social Determinants of Health and large-scale events such as COVID-19, there is a deeper understanding that families, communities, institutions, and systems are in a symbiotic and ever-changing relationship that is impacted by cultural norms, social beliefs, socio-economic factors, racism, sexism, and a myriad of other factors. Therefore, there must be a recognition of the interconnectedness of systems and families as it relates to the prevention and treatment of child maltreatment. As stated by Alice Walker,[1] a social activist and writer, "the pain we inflict on children is the pain we endure as a society." It is with this perspective that professionals from all fields can reflect upon the impact of childhood maltreatment on each level of society and be challenged to ponder what it means to respond from a trauma-informed lens and to offer restorative interventions to both children and their parents.

Perinatal mental health conditions (PMHCs) are the number one complication of pregnancy and childbirth, affecting 20% of birthing people or more for specific populations.[2] PMHCs include: postpartum depression, postpartum anxiety, postpartum obsessive-compulsive disorder, postpartum psychosis, and post-traumatic stress disorder. PMHCs can develop any time within the first year after birth or loss, lasting up to 3 years postpartum.

PMHCs can impact anyone who has been pregnant, given birth, or is raising a newborn, including those who have adopted or experienced abortion, miscarriage, and stillbirth. About 10% of male partners will develop a PMHC, though it is believed estimates for men are severely underreported and unknown.[2] Around 40% of military mothers, 50% of Black, Indigenous, and people of color (BIPOC) individuals, and 48% of those living in low-income neighborhoods are affected.[3] The risk of postpartum depression for teen parents is 2 to 3 times higher than the general population, around 60%.[4] Researchers found that lesbian women reported a higher prevalence of PMHCs and increased rates of attempting or considering suicide.[5] This information is clinically significant as studies suggest that less than 50% of women with perinatal mental health challenges are identified by a physician, and 75% of patients experiencing perinatal mental health symptoms go untreated.[6]

If a parent is emotionally unavailable, unable to meet their own basic needs, or lacking the adequate support they need to care for themselves while navigating mental illness, they are less likely to be able to meet the needs of their children. Research shows that parents navigating a PMHC have higher rates in the utilization of corporal punishment on their infants. These parents also tend to have lower rates of breast/chest feeding and schedule fewer visits for well-child care or preventative care appointments. Fewer points of contact with medical professionals means fewer opportunities for screening, education, and support.

SOCIAL NORMS AND THE NORMALIZATION OF AUTHORITARIAN PARENTING

Social norms are established by a society, culture, or group to ascertain and influence what is appropriate behavior under what conditions. This process of normalization can foster an environment that perpetuates or mitigates violence and its deleterious effects.[7] Norms affect how an individual may react to, participate in, or prevent violence.

Under-resourced caregivers may default to compliance-oriented discipline utilizing violence, force, and threats. This style of parenting is minimally responsive to children's needs, emphasizing hyper-independence, deference, and obedience. Some parenting styles can encourage a spectrum of aggressive behaviors, attitudes, and beliefs undermining autonomy and emotional safety for a child, with little awareness or regard for development. Authoritarian parenting, for example, is rooted in beliefs that children are developmentally, cognitively, and emotionally more mature than they are. Assumptions may include that the child is intentional in their unwanted behavior, should know better, and are continuing to not comply out of maliciousness. The caregiver may be misinformed about developmentally appropriate behaviors and are seeking to extinguish the behavior(s) despite its applicability to the child's developmental stage.

Examples of developmentally inappropriate beliefs about infants or children include:

— Expecting an infant to sleep throughout the night and utilizing sleep training methods such as the Ferber Method, that encourage parents to let their infants "cry it out" to teach infants to self-soothe. A parent's consistent lack of response to an infant's cry has been observed to influence infant brain development and cognitive functioning, including issues with self-regulation and challenges with independence and confidence.[8]

— Unwanted behavior being punished by the removal of the child from the parent (eg, time out in a room alone with no time limit or explanation, being sent to their room without support or guidance to process). Co-regulation is a crucial element of increasing positive interactions between caregiver and child, enhancing self-regulation skills, and is supportive of emotional, physiological, and behavioral regulation.[9]

— Children should be punished if they assert their needs, boundaries, or autonomy with adults (eg, forced to hug a relative, required to eat everything on their plate even when they express being full, "children should be seen, not heard"). Autonomy-supportive parenting has been shown to improve both sibling and parent-child relationships, increases positive emotional connections between family members and within the child's social network, and has increased positive reports of parental need fulfillment.[10]

The Child Abuse Prevention and Treatment Act defines child abuse and neglect as, at a minimum: any recent act or failure to act on the part of a parent or caretaker which results in death, serious physical or emotional harm, sexual abuse or exploitation; or an act or failure to act, which presents an imminent risk of serious harm.[11]

THE FIRST FIVE

Children are most vulnerable to maltreatment in the first 5 years of life, with children 5 years of age or younger making up 74.2% of all cases of reported abuse. About 1/4 of total victims are under the age of 2 years old, with the highest rate of victimization being infants (0 to 12 months old). Infants are 2 times as likely as 1 year olds to experience maltreatment, as depicted in **Figure 5-1**.[11]

Reflecting upon the prevalence of PMHCs and social norms regarding violence, as well as parenting philosophies, it is not difficult to understand the correlational and causational impact on children and families. This makes a compelling argument for increased mental health screenings and services as well as investments in quality child care programs and preschool enrichment programs. These investments would offer an opportunity for early intervention after maltreatment has been documented.

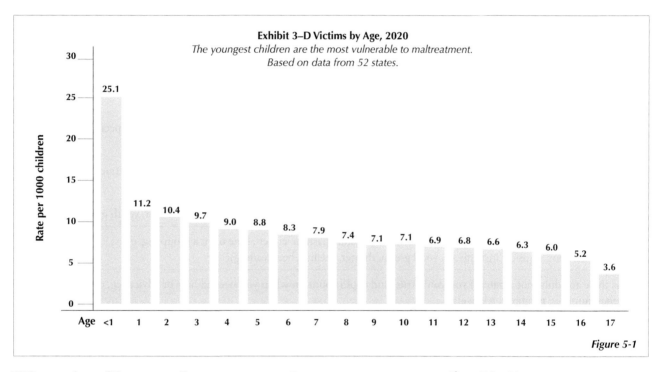

Exhibit 3–D Victims by Age, 2020
The youngest children are the most vulnerable to maltreatment.
Based on data from 52 states.

Figure 5-1

Figure 5-1. *Exhibit 3-D Victims by Age, 2020*

WHAT ARE HEALTHY INTERACTIONS?

While there is no singular definition that can capture the spectrum of healthy interactions between a parent and child, research does indicate that healthy relationships involve ongoing support, affection, and the allowance of the child to experience appropriate autonomy.[12] These elements have been shown to promote good psychological functioning across the lifespan. Sensitive responsiveness is a parent's ability and capacity to observe and respond to the cues of their child. One's responsiveness to an infant's cry, for example, is strongly linked to parental empathy and early attachment behavior. The more parental empathy is present, the more attached the parent and child will be, which in turn facilitates the parent's ability to respond to the child's needs healthfully.[13]

Healthy interactions also include those that facilitate resilience. If a person has navigated adverse childhood experiences (ACEs) (eg, poverty, abuse), the impact of these traumas may be mediated by the restorative or positive interactions that they were also able to experience, both with caregivers and other community members. Much of the work to be done in facilitating and encouraging healthy dynamics between children and their parents rests in the points of contact that community members and providers have with families.

PROTECTIVE AND COMPENSATORY EXPERIENCES

The protective and compensatory experiences (PACEs) questionnaire for adults is designed to assess resilience and calculate the potential to offset ACEs. A PACEs score subtracted from an ACEs score predicts a person's potential for chronic physical ailments, mental and emotional wellbeing, suicidality, the potential for domestic violence, homicide, and substance misuse. The experiences listed in **Table 5-1** involve the consistent engagement of a child with systems outside of their family unit, as well as conditions in the home that require stability, predictability, and basic needs being met.

Positive parenting practices have been studied in an effort to provide robust amounts of psychological protection, regardless of ACEs. This evidence suggests that positive parenting is significant in mediating the impact of abuse, especially for children who are chronically exposed to high levels of adversity.[14]

Table 5-1. Protective and Compensatory Experiences Questionnaire for Adults[15]

Did you have someone who loved you unconditionally (you did not doubt that they cared about you)?
Did you have at least 1 best friend (someone you could trust and had fun with)?
Did you do anything regularly to help others (eg, volunteer at a hospital, nursing home, church) or do special projects in the community to help others (eg, food drives, volunteer)?
Were you regularly involved in organized group sports or other physical activities (eg, soccer, basketball, track, competitive cheer, gymnastics, dance, marching band)?
Were you an active member of at least 1 civic group or a non-sport social group (eg, scouts, church, youth group)?
Did you have an engaging hobby — an artistic or intellectual pastime either alone or in a group (eg, chess club, debate team, musical instrument, vocal group, theater, spelling bee, reading)?
Was there an adult (not a parent) you could trust and could count on when you needed help or advice (eg, coach, teacher, minister, neighbor, relative)?
Was your home typically clean AND safe with enough food to eat?
Overall, did your school provide the resources and academic experiences that you needed to learn?
In your home, were rules clear and fairly administered?
Your PACE score is the total number of checked responses

COMMUNITY-BASED INTERVENTIONS

Before defining research-based therapeutic interventions, it is important to note that all community members, regardless of their training, profession, or experience, can participate in implementing intentional and therapeutic solutions. Preventing child maltreatment is a multifaceted, multi-targeted approach. The Centers for Disease Control and Prevention (CDC) recommends the following strategies for preventing child abuse[16]:

— Strengthen economic supports to families by strengthening household financial security.

— Change social norms to support parents and positive parenting through public engagement, education campaigns, and legislative approaches in order to reduce corporal punishment.

— Provide quality care and education early in life through improved quality of child care programs and preschool enrichment with family engagement.

— Enhance parenting skills to promote healthy child development by offering early childhood home visitation and increasing parenting skills to foster family relationships.

— Intervene to lessen harms and prevent future risk which looks like: enhanced primary care; behavioral parent training programs; treatment to lessen harms of abuse and neglect exposure; and treatment to prevent problem behavior and later involvement in violence.

Prevention in the Prenatal, Perinatal, and Postpartum Period

Strengthening household financial security would include advocacy at the state and federal level regarding income pay gaps for women and policy implementation for paid parental leave. The United States has no national parental leave policy, though 178 other countries around the world do. As of 2021, only 9 states had paid leave programs, with 3 more states (Connecticut, Oregon, and Colorado) expected to add similar policies by 2024. It is estimated there could be in excess of 600 fewer infant deaths per year if the United States mandated national maternal leave, which calculates to a 2% to 3% decline in infant deaths for every guaranteed week of paid maternal leave.[17]

Changing social norms to support parents through educational campaigns and public engagement involves a shift in perceptions around parental mental health and parenting. Addressing parental mental health involves educating both providers and parents in understanding the value of screening for PMHCs as a preventative tool to reduce poor health outcomes of all family members. Screening for PMHCs can be done by any person who provides services to anyone in the perinatal period. Recommended screenings include the Edinburgh Postnatal Depression Screen (EPDS), Patient Health Questionnaire (PHQ-9), or General Anxiety Disorder-7 (GAD-7) screening. Data reveals that screening itself resulted in 22% of women who screened positive for perinatal depression accessing mental health care services.[18] Over the past decade, postpartum parents seeking support for mental health challenges have been met with fear of punishment by the legal system, shame, dismissal, threat of having their children removed from their home, and stigma. Trauma-informed medical offices are key in reaching vulnerable parents and children through routine screening.

Enhancing Parenting Skills Through Education

In understanding the relevance of intentional and healthful parenting strategies, we must acknowledge that evolutionarily, human infants "would not have survived without the care of others, and thus the human infant brain and behavioral systems are programmed to expect input from other people."[19] Regulation of emotions, attention, and behavior is therefore a learned response based on repeated exposure to specific parenting strategies including: supporting exploration and involvement in decision making; paying attention and responding to a child's needs; using effective communication; attending to a child's emotional expression and control; rewarding and encouraging positive behaviors; providing clear rules and expectations; applying consistent consequences for behaviors; and providing adequate supervision and monitoring.[20]

Responsive, authoritative, and attached parenting are all considered interchangeable terms for positive parenting. This style of parenting is heavily rooted in evolutionary practices and encourages behaviors such as baby wearing, breast/chest feeding, and sensitive responsiveness. Regardless of what one calls positive parenting, research indicates that children experience better long-term health outcomes, noting that maternal sensitivity buffers children in high stress environments from developing health issues as adults.[21] Secure attachments protect children from toxic stress and reduce the likelihood for maltreatment.

INTERVENTIONS TO LESSEN HARM AND PREVENT FUTURE RISK: TREATMENT MODALITIES FOR CHILD MALTREATMENT

PARENT-CHILD INTERACTION THERAPY

Parent-child interaction therapy (PCIT) is a family-centered treatment approach that has proven effective for parents and children who were abused or identified as being at-risk for abuse, aged 2 to 7 years. During PCIT, therapists remotely coach parents from another room, while parents interact directly with their children. The therapist teaches and guides parents in learning and practicing strategies that will promote positive behaviors in children who have disruptive or externalizing behavior problems. Unlike other play therapy models, PCIT encourages the parental unit and child(ren) to learn together in a supported environment without the physical presence of the therapist. Research has shown with the implementation of PCIT: parents learn more effective parenting techniques, behavior problems in children decrease, and the quality of the parent-child relationship improves. PCIT is typically provided in 10 to 20 sessions, with an average of 12 to 14 sessions, each lasting about 1 hour. The course of treatment is divided into 2 phases.

Phase I: Relationship Enhancement (Child-Directed Interaction) "PRIDE"

In Phase I (see **Table 5-2**), the focus is on cultivating and strengthening warmth within the parent-child relationship by learning and applying skills that help the child feel secure and supported.

Table 5-2. Child-Directed Interaction Model "PRIDE"	
Praise	Parents praise the child's appropriate behavior to help encourage it and to increase the child's positive feelings about the parent-child relationship
Reflection	Parents repeat and build upon what the child says to show that they are listening, thereby facilitating improved communication
Imitation	Parents mirror the child's gestures and actions, soliciting feelings of approval in the child and reinforcing a desire to play with others
Behavioral Description	Parents narrate the child's activity (eg, "You're building a tower with blocks.") to demonstrate interest and enhance the child's vocabulary
Enjoyment	Parents are enthusiastic and show excitement about what the child is doing

Phase II: Discipline and Compliance (Parent-Directed Interaction)

In this phase, parents learn strategies through coaching and education in order to confidently, calmly, and consistently apply developmentally appropriate discipline.

Multiple studies have shown that PCIT reduces behavioral challenges and decreases maternal distress in parent-child dyads who were exposed to IPV.[22] Decades-long research around PCIT continues to show significant reductions in recurrent child maltreatment, with newer studies indicating in-vivo social regulation during active parenting scenarios as the mechanism for changing behaviors.[23] PCIT may not be appropriate for all parents, including those: with limited or no ongoing contact with their child, with serious mental health problems that may include auditory or visual hallucinations or delusions, with significant expressive or receptive language deficits,

Table 5-3. Time Out Sequence		
Step 1	Parent gives a direct command, child does not follow directions	"Please put your Legos away." (Child ignores parent)
Step 2	Parent counts silently to 5	(Count silently): "One, two, three, four, five." (Child continues to ignore parent)
Step 3	Parent gives warning	"If you don't put the yellow Lego in the box, you are going to have to sit on the chair." (Child continues to ignore parent)
Step 4	Parent counts silently to 5	(Count silently): "One, two, three, four, five." (Child continues to ignore parent)
Step 5	Parent gives explanation	"You didn't do what I asked you to do, so you have to sit on the chair."
Step 6	Parent takes child to time out	(Parent stands up immediately and takes child to the time out chair. Child should be given the option to walk independently to time out chair or to be supported by an adult in getting to the chair.)
Step 7	Parent gives direct ask to sit on chair	"Sit in the chair for x minutes. I'll tell you when you can get up." Number of minutes in time out should be equivalent to age (eg, 3 minutes at 3 years old)
Step 8	Parent waits for 3 minutes plus 5 seconds of quiet	(Child sits quietly for 3 minutes and 5 seconds of quiet)
Step 9	Parent asks child if he/she is ready to return and comply with original ask	"You are sitting quietly in the chair. Are you ready to come back and put away the Legos?" (Child says, "yes.")
Step 10	Parent waits silently for child to show readiness (may point or signal)	(Parent points to the yellow Lego)
Step 11	Parent acknowledges participation	"Thank you."
Step 12	Parent gives follow up command	"Now please put the green Legos in the container." (Child complies)
Step 13	Parent gives enthusiastic praise for desired behavior	"Great job following directions!"

who are sexually abusive, who engage in sadistic physical abuse, or who have substance abuse issues.

An example of an intervention from Phase II includes the Time Out Sequence (see **Table 5-3**).[23] Time outs, when structured and intentionally implemented, can be a developmentally appropriate parenting tool.

ATTACHMENT AND BEHAVIORAL CATCH UP

Attachment and Behavioral Catch Up (ABC) therapy is a strengths-based, solution-focused parenting program that is designed to be taught and practiced in the home, either with a home visitor or via telehealth (**Figure 5-2**). Home visitors are trained to offer 1 hour weekly sessions for 10 weeks. The program focuses on strengthening parent-child relationships, increasing parental skill, and building resilience in families who have been exposed to early adversity, specifically addressing the needs of children aged 0 to 4 years. With this treatment modality, there is a strong emphasis on

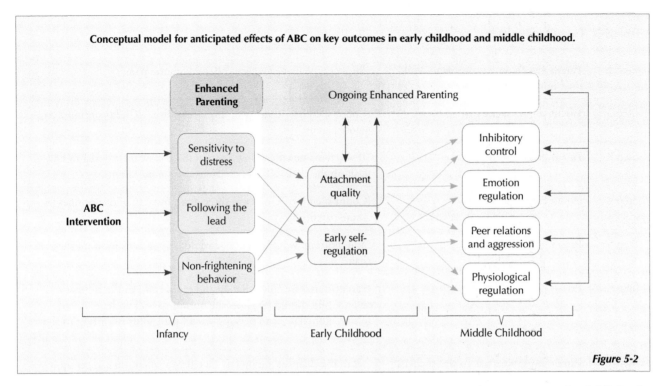

Conceptual model for anticipated effects of ABC on key outcomes in early childhood and middle childhood.

Figure 5-2. Conceptual model for anticipated effects of ABC on key outcomes in early childhood and middle childhood.

cultural humility and cultural responsiveness. Other caregivers in the child's family, including parents' partners, grandparents, and even other children, are encouraged to participate.

The program targets 3 parenting behaviors that facilitate a child's ability to regulate behavior and physiology. The first behavior is nurturing, which invites the parent to behave in nurturing ways when the child is distressed in order to increase healthy attachments. Secondly, the focus shifts to "serve and return interactions" wherein the parent is directed to follow their child's lead with the motivation of teaching co-regulation. Thirdly, in order to aid children in developing adequate capabilities around self-regulation and organized attachment, the parent must reduce "frightening" behaviors. These behaviors are defined as: yelling or screaming, threats, physically preventing the child from moving autonomously (eg, grabbing, pushing, hitting, intruding in the child's space).[24] During each visit, parents will be given feedback by their family's coach, most of which should be positive, about 60 times per session.

ABC therapy has been shown to enhance secure attachment and regulatory capabilities beginning in infancy and toddlerhood, especially for those who have been exposed to problematic or inadequate caregiving. Additionally, this method increases parental sensitivity in order to help reduce cortisol production and improve long-term behavioral outcomes.[24]

CASE STUDY

Case Study 5-1

Cheryl was a 28-year-old single mother of 2 boys, aged 5 years and 1 year. She lost her job 6 months ago and had yet to find steady employment. She had been working part-time as a hostess since, but the pay was low, and she was having trouble making ends meet. She had a number of other stressors in her life and a lack of family support to help financially or with caregiving. Her landlord said she would be evicted if she did not pay her rent within one week. Cheryl's oldest son had some significant behavior problems. He was enrolled in school, but the teachers threatened that he would be expelled for disruptive and defiant behaviors if there was one more incident. Cheryl was increasingly frustrated with her son, and found that she was losing her temper frequently with him. Her discipline strategy for these behaviors was spanking, and two months ago she spanked him and left a bruise on his leg. His teacher reported the bruise to child welfare, and children's services met with Cheryl to discuss the incident shortly after.

Cheryl was mandated to attend parenting classes through the Department of Children's Services. She elected to attend PCIT, where she met weekly with a PCIT therapist and learned skills to improve her relationship with her child as well as some safe and healthy discipline strategies. She and her son were attending weekly sessions with a PCIT therapist for 6 weeks, where the therapist was coaching Cheryl on how to interact with her son in a healthier way.

Discussion

Through PCIT, Cheryl has learned to identify her son's appropriate behaviors. Her use of CDI skills (eg, labeled praises, reflections, behavior descriptions) have improved throughout treatment. She reported that her relationship with her child was getting better, and that she was seeing decreases in his problem behaviors. She has noticed that she enjoys being around him more, and she reports seeing a decrease in his negative behaviors (eg, picking on his brother, talking back, hitting). Additionally, his teacher reports that she has seen improvements in his behavior at school. Cheryl is currently working on practicing safer and healthier discipline strategies in PCIT, including using a structured time out as an alternative to spanking. She practices these strategies at home and in-session. Cheryl reports that she likes getting practice on the procedures in her therapy sessions, with the therapist supporting her in real-time through her headphones. She says that PCIT has helped her to feel calmer, less stressed, and more comfortable parenting her son, and that she is less likely to escalate and use inappropriate discipline in the future because of the skills she has gained.

KEY POINTS

1. About 2/3 of child maltreatment victims are between the ages of 0 and 5 years, meaning most abuse occurs when parents, caregivers, and family members are in the early stages of creating, growing, and forming their family systems.

2. Healthy interactions are responsive, empathic, positive, and nurturing, and they facilitate a child's autonomy.

3. Community interventions for child maltreatment prevention include (but are not limited to): higher quality child care programs that encourage parental engagement, increased screening and treatment of PMHCs, legislation to mandate national parental leave programs, and enhanced targeted parenting education programs for high-risk families.

Table 5-4. Additional Resources

ORGANIZATION	DESCRIPTION	WEBSITE
Child Help	Comprehensive child abuse resource database	https://www.childhelp.org/educator-resources/child-abuse-education-prevention-resources/
Latinx Parenting	Spanish and English resources for decolonizing parenting, specific to Latinx families	https://latinxparenting.org
Love & Logic	Educational online courses and workbooks, for families and agencies	https://www.loveandlogic.com
Our Mama Village	Therapist-curated resources for navigating developmentally appropriate toddler behaviors	https://ourmamavillage.com
Sex Positive Families	Resources for caregivers to discuss sex/puberty with all-aged children	https://sexpositivefamilies.com
Zero to Three	Professional development resources for providers supporting children aged 0 to 3 years	https://www.zerotothree.org/

REFERENCES

1. Williams K. Alice Walker the "PBS American Masters" interview. African American Literature Book Club. February 1, 2014. Accessed April 12, 2022. https://aalbc.com/interviews/interview.php?id=51

2. Perinatal mood and anxiety disorders. Postpartum Support International. 2022. Accessed April 15, 2022. https://www.postpartum.net/learn-more/

3. Hodgkinson S, Godoy L, Beers LS, Lewin A. Improving mental health access for low-income children and families in the primary care setting. *Pediatrics*. 2017;139(1):e2015-1175. doi:10.1542/peds.2015-1175

4. Earls MF; Committee on Psychosocial Aspects of Child and Family Health American Academy of Pediatrics. Incorporating recognition and management of perinatal and postpartum depression into pediatric practice. *Pediatrics*. 2010;126(5):1032-1039. doi:10.1542/peds.2010-2348

5. Darwin Z, Greenfield M. Mothers and others: the invisibility of LGBTQ people in reproductive and infant psychology. *J Reprod Infant Psychol.* 2019;37(4):341-343. doi:10.1080/02646838.2019.1649919

6. Luca D, Margiotta C, Staatz C, Garlow E, Christensen A, Zivin K. Financial toll of untreated perinatal mood and anxiety disorders among 2017 births in the United States. *Am J Public Health*. 2020;110(6):888-896. doi:10.2105/AJPH.2020.305619

7. Addressing the social and cultural norms that underlie the acceptance of violence: proceedings of a workshop—in brief. National Academies of Sciences, Engineering, and Medicine. 2018. Accessed 2022. https://nap.nationalacademies.org/catalog/25075/addressing-the-social-and-cultural-norms-that-underlie-the-acceptance-of-violence

8. Davis A, Kramer R. Commentary: does 'cry it out' really have no adverse effects on attachment? Reflections on Bilgin and Wolke (2020). *J Child Psychol Psychiatry.* 2021;62(12):1488-1490. doi:10.1111/jcpp.13390

9. Lobo FM, Lunkenheimer E. Understanding the parent-child coregulation patterns shaping child self-regulation. *Dev Psychol*. 2020;56(6):1121-1134. doi:10.1037/dev0000926

10. Neubauer AB, Schmidt A, Kramer AC, Schmiedek F. A little autonomy support goes a long way: daily autonomy-supportive parenting, child well-being, parental need fulfillment, and change in child, family, and parent adjustment across the adaptation to the COVID-19 pandemic. *Child Dev*. 2021;92(5):1679-1697. doi:10.1111/cdev.13515

11. US Department of Health and Human Services; Administration for Children and Families; Administration on Children, Youth and Families; Children's Bureau. Child maltreatment 2020. January 19, 2022. Accessed 2022. https://www.acf.hhs.gov/cb/data-research/child-maltreatment

12. Stafford M, Kuh DL, Gale CR, Mishra G, Richards M. Parent-child relationships and offspring's positive mental wellbeing from adolescence to early older age. *J Posit Psychol*. 2016;11(3):326-337. doi:10.1080/17439760.2015.1081971

13. Kaźmierczak M, Pawlicka P, Anikiej-Wiczenbach P, et al. Empathy and hormonal changes as predictors of sensitive responsiveness towards infant crying: a study protocol. *Int J Environ Res Public Health*. 2021;18(9):4815. doi:10.3390/ijerph18094815

14. Yamaoka Y, Bard D. Positive parenting matters in the face of early adversity. *Am J Prev Med*. 2019;56(4):530-539. doi:10.1016/j.amepre.2018.11.018

15. Morris A, Hays-Grudo J, Treat A, Williamson A, Roblyer MZ, Staton J. Protecting parents and children from adverse childhood experiences (ACEs): preliminary evidence for the validity of the PACEs. Paper presented at: Society for Research in Child Development Special Topic Meeting: New Conceptualizations in the Study of Parenting-At-Risk; 2014; San Diego, CA. Accessed September 6, 2022. https://www.srcd.org/sites/default/files/file-attachments/2014_srcd_parenting-at-risk_program.pdf

16. Prevention strategies for child abuse and neglect. Centers for Disease Control and Prevention. 2022. Accessed May 13, 2022. https://www.cdc.gov/violenceprevention/childabuseandneglect/prevention.html

17. Burtle A, Bezruchka S. Population health and paid parental leave: what the United States can learn from two decades of research. *Healthcare (Basel)*. 2016;4(2):30. doi:10.3390/healthcare4020030

18. Byatt N, Levin LL, Ziedonis D, Moore Simas TA, Allison J. Enhancing participation in depression care in outpatient perinatal care settings: a systematic review. *Obstet Gynecol*. 2015;126(5):1048-1058. doi:10.1097/AOG.0000000000001067

19. Dozier M, Bernard K. *Coaching Parents Of Vulnerable Infants*. The Guilford Press; 2019.

20. Farrell AK, Waters TEA, Young ES, et al. Early maternal sensitivity, attachment security in young adulthood, and cardiometabolic risk at midlife. *Attach Hum Dev*. 2019;21(1):70-86. doi:10.1080/14616734.2018.1541517

21. Timmer SG, Ware LM, Urquiza AJ, Zebell NM. The effectiveness of parent-child interaction therapy for victims of interparental violence. *Violence Vict*. 2010;25(4):486-503. doi:10.1891/0886-6708.25.4.486

22. Skowron EA, Funderburk BW. In vivo social regulation of high-risk parenting: a conceptual model of Parent-Child Interaction Therapy for child maltreatment prevention. *Child Youth Serv Rev*. 2022;136:106391. doi:10.1016/j.childyouth.2022.106391

23. McNeil C, Hembree-Kigin T. *Parent-Child Interaction Therapy*. 2nd ed. Springer; 2010.

24. Dozier M, Bernard K. Attachment and biobehavioral catch-up: addressing the needs of infants and toddlers exposed to inadequate or problematic caregiving. *Curr Opin Psychol*. 2017;15:111-117. doi:10.1016/j.copsyc.2017.03.003

ALTERNATIVES FOR FAMILIES: *A COGNITIVE BEHAVIORAL TREATMENT APPROACH FOR FAMILY CONFLICT AND HARSH PHYSICAL PARENTING*

Patrick C. Barton, MA
David T. Solomon, PhD, HSP-P

OBJECTIVES
After reading this chapter, the reader will be able to:

1. *Describe the main elements of Alternatives for Families Cognitive Behavioral Therapy (AF-CBT), including understanding the empirical support behind the treatment and populations for which the treatment is appropriate.*

2. *Identify and describe the role of assessment in AF-CBT, including its use of functional analysis of behavior.*

3. *Identify steps and requirements to become trained in AF-CBT and to attain certification in AF-CBT as a clinician and in-house trainer.*

BACKGROUND AND SIGNIFICANCE
Formerly known as Abuse Focused Cognitive Behavioral Therapy, AF-CBT is a treatment approach designed for families with heightened conflict or anger, caregiver aggression that may range from corporal punishment to child physical abuse, and child behavior problems that may include defiance and aggression.[1] In some of these cases, the severity of the aggression or abuse may warrant court ordered interventions or monitoring by child protective services (CPS). AF-CBT is appropriate for families with a child aged 5 to 17 years and a caregiver, and it can include other members as needed.[2]

While AF-CBT shares many commonalities with traditional CBT (eg, reducing and altering negative thought patterns, teaching skills to replace unhelpful behavior), it also has several unique characteristics.

First, it is focused on the Alternatives for Families Plan, an overarching document that notes useful strategies and helpful actions.[1] The Alternatives for Families Plan is a repository of strategies aimed to reduce overall conflict and provide a framework for continued success and relapse prevention. This document is introduced early in treatment, and as the family learns and practices new skills, the document is updated as they identify which skills appeared most effective for them.

Second, there is a greater emphasis on motivational interviewing (MI) and other techniques (eg, individual goal setting) to increase client engagement, and the manual provides a brief guide to MI in its first phase.[1] There is a clear rationale for incorporating MI with AF-CBT, as many families receiving this treatment may be mandated or have other reasons for feeling pushed into treatment. MI has been shown to improve treatment engagement and adherence in mandated clients for substance misuse[3] and has been found in other research to increase retention in another behavioral caregiver intervention for low-motivation families in the child welfare system.[4] Additionally, it has been found to increase completion of therapy homework and lead to better clinical outcomes in other cognitive behavioral interventions.[5]

Finally, AF-CBT has an emphasis on building caregiver insight through discussion of their own parents' behavior, as well as through the writing of a "clarification letter" to their child. Caregivers are asked to consider how their parents dealt with stress and how their parents disciplined them; then they identify which strategies their parents used that they would like to incorporate or continue using as parents and which ones they would not want to use. Towards the end of treatment, caregivers begin to draft the clarification letter, which should include a description of the conflict or abuse that resulted in them being referred to treatment, praise for the child talking about the conflict or reporting it to someone else (the parent can also praise the child for their other positive attributes), an apology for the conflict and its aftermath, a willingness to discuss the conflict as well as any that may occur in the future, and finally, a statement that they will use nonviolent/nonphysical parenting tactics in the future as well as any other ways that they plan to prevent continued conflict or abuse. It is important for the caregiver to take full responsibility for the abuse or harsh physical punishment that led the family to be referred to treatment, and a statement that the child is not to blame should be included. It is important to convey that a child, regardless of their behavior, is never responsible for any abuse they experience. Once both the caregiver and child have been adequately prepared through treatment, the caregiver will read the letter to their child.[1]

ASSESSMENT

The assessment of individual and family characteristics to determine appropriateness for AF-CBT and to provide a baseline measurement includes 2 sets of procedures identified by Kolko and colleagues.[1] The first procedure involves the use of conventional assessment procedures, such as standardized assessments, record review (eg, records provided by the court or CPS), as well as less structured methodologies such as the clinical interview. Specific items of interest include psychological functioning and illness, specific concerns related to verbal or physical abuse, arguments involving harsh language or swearing, strident disciplinary measures, relevant social skills, anxiety, and general family dynamics.[1]

The treatment model also draws heavily upon assessment procedures that involve the use of functional analysis of behavior common to CBT practice.[1] Functional analysis seeks to understand the behavior in context by conducting ecologically driven observation of the problem behavior and determination of the underlying function of a behavior. To that end, the process follows an ABC format.[6] The A represents the antecedent, or the setting, just prior to the exhibition of the problem behavior. One of the keys in the antecedent is attempting to establish the discriminative stimulus (ie, the signal that portends the onset of the behavior).[6] The B stands for the behavior, which is the action in question that seeks to be modified by the intervention. This can include externalizing behaviors in children, aggressive behavior in adults, or other problematic actions.[1] The behavior must be articulated in descriptive and measurable terms, which can be supplemented by direct observation or standardized assessments.[6]

In the operant conditioning model, a behavior is reinforced either by positive or negative reinforcement.[6] This is C, which is the consequence of the behavior. Positive reinforcement of a behavior implies the acquisition of something desired and includes gaining attention, procurement of material goods, praise, or even reprimands (note that for children, any attention, even negative attention, can be reinforcing and may lead to an increase in difficult child behaviors).[7] Negative reinforcement involves the loss of something unwanted and can include getting out of an assignment, being given fewer chores, or other removal of aversive stimuli.[6] Note also that negative reinforcement is not the same as punishment; negative reinforcement increases a specific behavior while punishment decreases it. The reinforcement of behavior is an essential factor in the maintenance of actions and increases the likelihood of a behavior recurring. In Patterson's Coercion Model,[8] these reinforcement actions and resultant escalations by caregivers and children often lead to a coercive cycle, further entrenching the behaviors.

Specifically, the model posits a reinforcement cycle by which negative child behavior (eg, throwing tantrums, hitting) and negative parental behavior (eg, yelling, using physical punishment) are inadvertently reinforced, sometimes by each other. For example, a child might whine at dinner about having to eat their vegetables, so the parent yells, and the child stops whining and eats. For many parents, a child whining is unpleasant (aversive). Therefore, when the parent yells and the child stops whining, the parent's yelling has been negatively reinforced, and since the whining ended, the parent will be more likely to yell in the future. Suppose the next time, however, the child throws a tantrum, and the parent relents. In this situation, the child's tantrum has negatively been reinforced because the parent relented and now, the child does not have to eat any "dreaded" broccoli. Using functional analysis of these interactions, therapists can help parents change the sequence of events and change the consequences so that negative behaviors are not inadvertently reinforced.[6]

Although Kolko and colleagues[1] recommend the use of a few specific standardized assessment tools, they recognize that it may be useful for clinicians to use assessment tools outside the usual set if they cover specific topics relevant to the family at hand, while still including key points covered in the recommended tools. One of the tools they suggest is the 25-item Strengths and Difficulties Questionnaire (SDQ), which captures broad areas of internalizing and externalizing behavior, as well as peer and social behavior. Likewise, the Trauma Symptom Checklist for Children (TSCC) has been utilized to assess trauma-related symptomology.[9]

Other similar measures can be used at the discretion of the clinician, as many extant measures have excellent reliability and validity and excel in assessing a multitude of psychological and behavioral areas of functioning. Formalized assessment should, at minimum, seek to address areas of problematic functioning exhibited by the client such as anger, anxiety, or depression.

Throughout the treatment process, other methods of assessment of clinical targets should be undertaken as part of the AF-CBT treatment approach. In their manual, Kolko and colleagues[1] provide a wide array of forms and measures that identify target behaviors, beliefs, cognitions, and feelings with subjective units of distress (SUD) associated therein. Use of these forms coincides with specific modules of the program and allows for ongoing assessment of client functioning.[1] Other forms or variations of these assessments, as well as worksheets, are widely available to aid the clinician in ABC and functional behavioral analysis procedures.

Due to the use of AF-CBT in families with aggression, interpersonal violence, and other high-risk behaviors, ongoing assessment of risk and potentially abusive behavior should be conducted at each session. Special care must be exercised in protecting the health and wellbeing of the clients as well as legal liability on the part of the practitioner. Following all state, local, and federal guidelines for mandatory reporting and safety considerations is necessary, and following departmental or agency practices in the same regard is also recommended.[1] Among the recommendations rendered, at each session the clinician is encouraged to engage in a **C**heck-in on **A**ttendance, weekly **S**afety briefing, and at-**H**ome practice adherence (CA$H) procedure. During this check-in, the provider should ask both the child and the caregiver about any conflict that occurred in the home since the last session. Called the Weekly Safety Check In (WSCI), the brief interview is a semi-structured conversation that solicits details about the types of family interactions that occurred since the prior session. Brief questions are asked to learn about any types of conflict, aggression, or distressing situations that occurred between the child and the caregiver. The interview also solicits details about how the caregiver and child responded to the interaction and any follow-up consequences. The clinician is encouraged to differentiate between low-risk occurrences of verbal and lesser physical hostility, which can be targets for discussion, and high-risk incidents that necessitate the development of a safety plan or more urgent action.[1] In addition to safety concerns, the last step of the CA$H procedure involves checking in on any at-home practice (ie, homework) assigned during the last week to help the family determine which skills or behaviors are most effective; this helps families generalize the skills from the sessions into their everyday lives.

OVERVIEW OF THE TREATMENT

The delivery of treatment content is guided by the manual authored by Kolko and colleagues,[1] and it provides a detailed framework of content that should be covered, by which the clinician can guide each session. The manual contains notes, cautions, and suggestions, such as elements of motivational interviewing, as well as recommended topics and language for each section. Broadly, the treatment consists of 3 phases, with the latter sections building upon the successes of the former. Each phase contains several topics that correspond to a specific session of therapy.[1] The treatment, as described in the manual, is designed to be implemented in a stepwise pattern that follows the same basic structure as many manualized CBT protocols, and the topics or interventions are amenable to some degree of individualization to suit the preferences of the practitioner, the client(s), or even the Unified Protocol in CBT.[1] Finally, the manual specifies which sessions and topics are for the child and caregiver together, the child alone, or the caregiver alone.

PHASE 1: ENGAGEMENT AND PSYCHOEDUCATION

The first phase seeks to orient the caregiver and child to the therapeutic modality. This is accomplished first through combined sessions, leading to individual sessions with both parties, and then finishing with a combined session. The first phase seeks to establish rapport with the child and orient the parent and child to upcoming dual sessions.[1] Evidence gathering and understanding the reasoning behind the referral are crucial elements of this phase. The clinician seeks to develop a coherent understanding of the referral that is understood by all parties, as well as introduce the participants to the structure of the sessions and establish ground rules for behavior and goals for treatment.[1] Importantly, Kolko and associates[1] note the need for the introduction of the WSCI and the overview of home practice as necessary elements of the introductory phase. This phase also starts the process of building a therapeutic alliance with the caregiver (some of whom may be there because they are court ordered) through the implementation of MI and other skills, as well as providing psychoeducation about the causes and impact of family conflict.[1]

PHASE 2: INDIVIDUAL SKILL BUILDING

The second phase, following standard CBT procedures, focuses heavily on psychoeducation and cognitive restructuring, along with behavioral interventions to modify problematic child behavior. This phase starts with emotion identification and regulation techniques for the caregiver and child, then moves into cognitive restructuring tactics.[1] From there, the training diverges into focusing more on behavior. The caregiver is instructed in noticing and praising positive child behavior while concurrently managing problematic behaviors. Meanwhile, the child is trained in assertiveness, social skills, and imaginal exposure to address anxious symptoms related to the abuse or conflict.[1] The SUD handouts are used in conjunction with exposure as a metric of success.

Cognitive-behavioral techniques in this phase focus not only on feelings, thoughts, and behaviors, but also seek to understand more traditional behavioral characteristics such as situational cues and the consequences of thoughts, feelings, and actions.[1] This phase constitutes the bulk of the program and contains the majority of sessions. It also contains numerous activities and home practice assignments/experiments in order to detect both working and ineffective strategies for inclusion in the Alternatives for Families Plan. Towards the latter part of this phase, caregivers will also begin drafting the clarification letter to their child, which will be shared with the child during phase 3.

PHASE 3: FAMILY APPLICATIONS

The final module is relatively short and endeavors to build upon the gains made throughout treatment in order to prevent re-occurrence of problematic behaviors and situations. This is accomplished through skill building activities such as healthy communication strategies, clarification of expectations and feelings/actions, and general problem solving techniques.[1] These strategies are also included in the Alternatives for Families Plan, which aims to change family dynamics and communication abilities over the long-term. Likewise, problem solving techniques are designed to reduce familial discord by identifying and implementing proven strategies to mitigate incidents ripe for escalation.[1] The culmination of this module is the graduation ceremony for the child and caregiver. The graduation ceremony is a ritualized event that is spelled out in the manual, and it also follows other termination and relapse prevention plans.[1] Broadly, this is a time of reverence, reflection, and celebration of the substantial gains made by children and caregivers following their hard work and dedication.

EMPIRICAL SUPPORT

A comprehensive list of research publications and a description of key research findings can be found on the AF-CBT website.[10] Further, the California Evidence-Based Clearinghouse for Child Welfare (CEBC) is a registry that reviews and rates the research base on interventions relevant to child welfare on a scale from 1 (well-supported by research evidence) to 5 (concerning practice).[11] As a treatment for caregiver abusive behavior, AF-CBT, according to the CEBC, has a rating of 2 out of 5, indicating that it is "supported by research evidence." This means that the treatment has been subjected to experimental trials under strict methodologies and has yielded consistently reliable and valid results, thereby demonstrating the efficacy and non-maleficence of the intervention.[11] To obtain the coveted rating of 1, the research must be replicated by independent researchers using randomized controlled trials without overlapping samples and, as of the writing of this chapter, that has yet to be accomplished.[11] First author of the treatment, David J. Kolko, consistently spearheads or actively participates in ongoing research regarding AF-CBT and publishes at regular intervals, providing AF-CBT with a robust body of empirical support. While the AF-CBT manual indicates that the treatment is also designed to address child externalizing behavior and trauma reactions,[1] there is currently less research on the effectiveness of AF-CBT for treating child trauma reactions. Specifically, the CEBC rates the evidence for AF-CBT as a trauma treatment at 3 (promising research evidence),[11] and its effectiveness as a treatment for child trauma remains a useful topic for future research. For example, one empirical case study evaluated the application of AF-CBT by an independent practitioner with a child who met criteria for partial PTSD following physical abuse.[12]

The main benefits of AF-CBT have historically been reductions in child abuse potential, parental distress, individualized problems, children's externalizing problems, and family conflict and cohesion.[12] Given the dynamics involved in parent-child relations—and family systems in general—the primary comparison group generally involves some form of family therapy. Early comparisons evidenced varying results that, according to Kolko,[13] necessitated the evolution of both treatment modalities in order to improve outcomes, specifically in the parent-to-child violence aspect and recidivism, a notoriously challenging element. Both treatment modalities, however, demonstrated substantial superiority over a standard community intervention.[13]

A more specific evaluation conducted by Kolko[14] demonstrated that the CBT intervention was superior to the family therapy intervention in the important areas of parental anger, use of harsh discipline, and other forceful parenting methods. The primary evolution was the routine monitoring aspect of clinical progress and at-risk behavior during treatment, which is evidenced by the inclusion of the CA$H system, specifically weekly check-ins on safety and continued monitoring of behavior.[13,14] Additionally, the identification of potential barriers to treatment, including structural barriers but also children's externalizing behaviors and comorbid psychological conditions such as ADHD, necessitated increased attention and inclusion.[14]

More recent studies have continually demonstrated the efficacy of AF-CBT compared to other treatments. Short-term gains for AF-CBT as compared to treatment as usual (TAU) include familial dysfunction and post-traumatic stress in children, with longer-term improvements in individualized treatment goal attainment.[15] Although findings in many outcomes showed reductions in key predictors for both AF-CBT and TAU, results indicated some additional targets for intervention could be useful. A key finding in this study was the potential benefit of tailoring AF-CBT to individual and family presentation, such as anger, aggression, or abusive behavior, which is something that could be a goal for agency or individual practitioner training. In this study, for example, the parental anger element remained largely unchanged, and the reports of physical force used against children after treatment completion mirrored the roughly 5% recidivism rate that still lingers, underscoring a target for treatment.[15] The individuation of the treatment should aid in the reduction of these persistent problems via targeting individual areas of need affecting overall functioning.

TRAINING AND CERTIFICATION

AF-CBT utilizes a manualized treatment protocol,[10] complete with requisite handout materials and assessments.[1] The training model for AF-CBT includes several components. Professionals first complete a brief practitioner's survey and then watch an online video providing a model overview. They then participate in a 1-year learning community that includes a basic training workshop incorporating didactic and experiential components, and then 6 months later, an advanced training that focuses upon augmenting implementation of AF-CBT. Participation requirements include attendance during monthly consultation calls, presentation of 2 cases, and submission of 2 audio files.[10]

Practitioners who complete their training requirements can then apply for a clinician certification in AF-CBT. Outlined on the AF-CBT website, the requirements for certification include passing a knowledge assessment, submitting 2 session samples that reach the minimum fidelity requirement (80%), and submitting a case completion form. Certified clinicians can also apply to become certified as in-house trainers, which similarly involves didactics, fee payment, assessments, provision of letters of recommendation, co-teaching, consultation calls, and module delivery guidelines.[10] Both of these certifications are good for 5 years.

CASE STUDY

Case Study 6-1

A mother and her 8-year-old son were referred to a therapist at a community clinic by CPS for intervention regarding a single incident of excessive discipline whereby the mother spanked the child on his rear with her hand, leaving physical marks. The mother was engaged in treatment but was frustrated both by the necessity for the referral and her seeming inability to effectively manage her son's behavior. Her son showed signs of oppositional defiant behavior which, in the mother's view, continued to escalate, necessitating an ever-increasing disciplinary response on her part. The mother identified a treatment goal of acquiring more effective parenting techniques and mitigating the discord in the household. The child had not been overly engaged in the treatment, and the therapist used rewards to maintain his active participation (eg, allowing him to choose a game to play if he completed all activities each session). Towards the end of the treatment, the therapist noticed his oppositional and defiant behaviors were reducing, showing a pattern of more age-appropriate conduct.

Discussion

In this case, elements of motivational interviewing factored substantially in the acquisition of buy-in on the part of the child's mother. Specifically, the emphasis on personal control and choice via goal setting reframed the treatment away from being just "a mandate from CPS" into a treatment in which the child's mother was engaged and seeking to meet her own goals. The defiant and oppositional behaviors of the child and the escalation in disciplinary measures are cyclical in nature and follow closely the pattern identified by Gerald Patterson in his coercion model that, as referenced in the chapter, are best remediated by de-escalated, clean, and consistent consequences. Although an extinction burst (ie, the child escalating his certain behaviors in response to the new parenting techniques) is likely, adequate psychoeducation and preparation can prepare his mother for this eventuality and, indeed, psychoeducation around the coercive succession is helpful overall. The mother must understand the level of control she exerts over the situation to prevent recurrence, and this will aid her taking full responsibility in her letter to the child in Phase 2 of the protocol. The use of rewards in this situation is appropriate to maintain engagement in the treatment. Allowing the child freedom to choose his own reward at the completion of the session, the therapist should frequently include verbal reinforcements and reflective statements to model and shape/reinforce engaged behavior. Examples of such statements can be found in the AF-CBT manual on pages 14 and 15 or Motivational Interviewing materials proper.

KEY POINTS

1. AF-CBT is an empirically supported treatment for child/caregiver dyads that are experiencing varying levels of conflict, anger, hostility, physical aggression and physical abuse, child behavior problems, and other forms of familial dysfunction.

2. AF-CBT is delivered in 3 interrelated treatment phases that focus on different modules of topical content covered for both children and caregivers. It is adaptable depending on the presentation of symptoms and family dynamics.

3. AF-CBT can be implemented in various settings, including clinics, community agencies, homes, and schools with modifications, and it is amenable to multicultural and individualized needs.

RESOURCES

1. AF-CBT website: https://www.afcbt.org/

2. AF-CBT research and support: https://www.afcbt.org/EvidenceBase/PapersAndResults

3. How to get certified: https://www.afcbt.org/certification/clinician

REFERENCES

1. Kolko DJ, Brown EJ, Shaver ME, Baumann BL, Hershcell AD. *Alternatives for Families: A Cognitive-Behavioral Therapy (AF-CBT), Session Guide.* 3rd ed. Western Psychiatric Institute and Clinic University of Pittsburgh and The PARTNERS Program St. Johns University; 2011.

2. Rahmah S. Abuse-focused cognitive behavioral therapy (AF-CBT) for physical abuse child. In: *International Conference on Early Childhood Education.* 2019; 92-101.

3. Lincourt P, Kuettel TJ, Bombardier CH. Motivational interviewing in a group setting with mandated clients: a pilot study. *Addict Behav.* 2002;27(3):381-391. doi:10.1016/S0306-4603(01)00179-4

4. Chaffin M, Valle LA, Funderburk B, et al. A motivational intervention can improve retention in PCIT for low-motivation child welfare clients. *Child Maltreat.* 2009;14(4):356-368. doi:10.1177/1077559509332263

5. Westra HA, Arkowitz H, Dozois DJA. Adding a motivational interviewing pretreatment to cognitive behavioral therapy for generalized anxiety disorder: a preliminary randomized controlled trial. *J Anxiety Disord.* 2009;23(8):1106-1117. doi:10.1016/j.janxdis.2009.07.014

6. Gresham F, Watson TS, Skinner CH. Functional behavioral assessment: principles, procedures, and future directions. *School Psych Rev.* 2001;30(2):156-172. doi:10.1080/02796015.2001.12086106

7. Fleming AP, McMahon RJ, King KM. Structured parent-child observations predict development of conduct problems: the importance of parental negative attention in child-directed play. *Prev Sci.* 2017;18(3):257-267. doi:10.1007/s11121-016-0672-1

8. Granic I, Patterson GR. Toward a comprehensive model of antisocial development: a dynamic systems approach. *Psychol Rev.* 2006;113(1):101-131. doi:10.1037/0033-295X.113.1.101

9. Kolko DJ, Iselin AM, Gully KJ. Evaluation of the sustainability and clinical outcome of alternatives for families: a cognitive-behavioral therapy (AF-CBT) in a child protection center. *Child Abuse Negl.* 2011;35(2):105-116. doi:10.1016/j.chiabu.2010.09.004

10. Alternatives for families: a cognitive behavioral therapy. Department of Psychiatry; University of Pittsburgh Medicine. Accessed May 28, 2022. https://www.afcbt.org/

11. Alternatives for families: a cognitive behavioral therapy (AF-CBT). California Evidence-Based Clearinghouse for Child Welfare. 2006. Updated September 2021. Accessed July 12, 2022. https://www.cebc4cw.org/program/alternatives-for-families-a-cognitive-behavioral-therapy/detailed

12. Kolko DJ, Fitzgerald M, Laubach J. Evidence-based practices for working with physically abusive families: alternatives for families: a cognitive behavioral therapy. In: Reece RM, Hanson RF, Sargent J, eds. *Treatment of Child Abuse: Common Ground for Mental Health, Medical and Legal Practitioners.* 2nd ed. Johns Hopkins University Press; 2014:59-66.

13. Kolko DJ. Individual cognitive behavioral treatment and family therapy for physically abused children and their offending parents: a comparison of clinical outcomes. *Child Maltreat.* 1996;1(4):322-342. doi:10.1177/1077559596001004004

14. Kolko DJ. Clinical monitoring of treatment course in child physical abuse: psychometric characteristics and treatment comparisons. *Child Abuse Negl.* 1996;20(1):23-43. doi:10.1016/0145-2134(95)00113-1

15. Kolko DJ, Herschell AD, Baumann BL, Hart JA, Wisniewski SR. AF-CBT for families experiencing physical aggression or abuse served by the mental health or child welfare system: an effectiveness trial. *Child Maltreat.* 2018;23(4):319-333. doi:10.1177/1077559518781068

Chapter 7

COMPLEMENTARY INTERVENTIONS: *MINDFULNESS AND YOGA*

Mitzy D. Flores, PhDc, MSN, RN, AHN-BC, CHSE, COI, Caritas Coach©,
    Introspective Hypnosis Practitioner
Kelly Cummings, PhD, RN, 200 RYT, Caritas Coach®

OBJECTIVES

After reading this chapter, the reader will be able to:

1. *Understand the complementary interventions of mindfulness, meditation, and yoga.*

2. *Identify uses and benefits of informal and formal mindfulness practices.*

3. *Understand how mindfulness can improve wellbeing and performance.*

BACKGROUND AND SIGNIFICANCE

Mindfulness is the accepted practice of maintaining a nonjudgmental state of heightened or complete awareness of one's thoughts, emotions, or experiences on a moment-to-moment basis. The goal for the practitioner is to cultivate the practice of being present; allow for a reduction of stress, anxiety, and pain; and create an overall sense of relaxation.[1]

Mindfulness is rooted in Buddhist and Hindu teachings. In a very simplified understanding, Buddhism approaches life as a journey that takes steps toward enlightenment and encompasses attention, awareness, and being present. The practice of mindfulness in Western culture, and its application in psychology, can be traced back to the late 1970s, when Jon Kabat-Zinn developed a program called mindfulness-based stress reduction (MBSR) to treat chronic pain.[2] Through his research, he discovered that patients would often try to avoid pain, but their avoidance would often lead them to experience deeper distress about the situation. He concluded that practicing mindfulness was a more successful approach for pain treatment.[2-4]

As mindfulness shifted into mainstream science and medicine, it became a pivotal therapeutic technique. It has been integrated into practices such as mindfulness-based cognitive therapy, dialectical behavior therapy, and acceptance and commitment therapy, among other modalities.[2] The benefits of its application have also been observed when mindfulness is used in a non-standardized approach, such as walking practices, music therapy, art therapy, and yoga.[5] In a 2018 study released by the Centers for Disease Control and Prevention (CDC), researchers looked at how popular complementary health care (ie, the use of holistic or unconventional health and wellness practices) has become for Americans.[6] The team of researchers from the National Center for Health Statistics, the National Institutes of Health, and the National Center for Complementary and Integrative Health[6,7] examined the rise of the most popular complementary practices (ie, yoga, meditation, and chiropractic care) in the United States over a period of 5 years. The findings revealed that of the

3 main practices, yoga is the most popular, but meditation is identified as the fastest-growing trend, seeing a more than 3-fold leap in those who practice.

MINDFULNESS AND TRAUMA

Studies have shown that mindfulness instruction may benefit individuals with a known trauma, such as an adverse childhood experience (ACE), both by an indirect effect of negating the acute response to trauma and stress and also by inhibiting underlying consequences of chronic exposure to stress and trauma such as psychiatric, metabolic, and cardiovascular disease through the influence on lifestyle choices, underlying biochemistry, and neurobiology (**Figure 7-1-a** and **7-1-b**).[4] Additionally, mindfulness has been modestly associated with alterations in markers of inflammation, cell-mediated immunity, and biological aging. Mindfulness has neurobiological modification potential as demonstrated by enhanced resting state functional connectivity as well as executive control via the dorsolateral prefrontal cortex, both coinciding with decreased peripheral levels of the protein Interleukin 6 (IL-6). Such biomarkers may be modulated by epigenetic changes through histone-modifying enzymes also found to be associated with mindfulness interventions.[7]

Figure 7-1-a. *Lifetime impact of childhood trauma and toxic stress.*

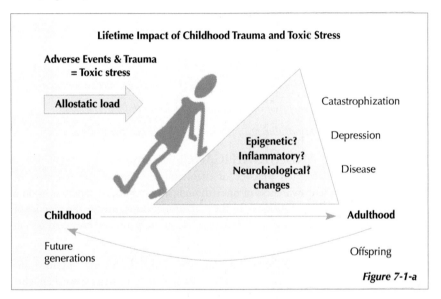

Figure 7-1-b. *Mindfulness is effective in reducing the harmful impacts of trauma and stress.*

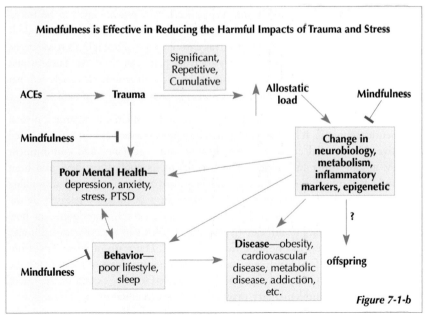

These neurobiological changes may represent modifications that can influence behavior and disease risk factors in adults and possibly the predisposition to disease in children, especially those at higher risk when exposed to stress, trauma, and toxic stress. Though children may be exposed to different types of trauma than adults, these studies collectively suggest that mindfulness may serve to buffer the effects of stress and trauma in children and into adulthood.[5,8,9]

MINDFULNESS AND CHILDREN

Mindfulness-based interventions (MBIs) in cognitive-behavioral therapy have greatly increased over the past years. However, most MBI research with children and adolescents focuses on structured, manualized group programs conducted in school settings, and knowledge about the implementation and effects of MBIs in individual psychotherapy with children and adolescents is scarce.[10] Yet, MBIs in child participant studies were found to be helpful overall and not to carry iatrogenic harm, with the primary omnibus effect size in the small to moderate range indicating the superiority of mindfulness treatments over active control comparison conditions. A significantly larger effect size was found on psychological symptoms compared to other dependent variable types (0.37 versus 0.21, p =.028), and for studies drawn from clinical samples compared to non-clinical samples (0.50 versus 0.20, p =.024).[10]

Mindfulness appears to be a promising intervention modality for children and adolescents (see **Table 7-1**). Although, as of the publication of this book, the majority of studies on mindfulness with children and adolescents engage generally healthy participants recruited from schools, the findings of this meta-analysis suggest that future research might focus on children in clinical settings and target symptoms of psychopathology.[11]

Table 7-1. Observed Beneficial Outcomes Of Mindfulness Programs For Children And Adolescents[5]

OUTCOME

— Decreased anxiety	— Decreased hostility
— Decreased rumination	— Decreased suicidal ideation
— Decreased school-related stress, coping with stress	— Decreased self-harm
— Flatter cortisol curve	— Reduced child abuse potential by parents
— Lower levels of somatization	— Conflict avoidance
— Decreased depressive symptoms	— Improved attention
— Effectiveness in social gains	— Greater wellbeing
— Classroom behavior	— Decreased post-traumatic symptoms severity

THE FUTURE OF MINDFULNESS AND CHILDREN RESEARCH

When it comes to the effects of meditation and related mindfulness practices, the body of research is growing rapidly but is still relatively small. For example, according to the American Mindfulness Research Association[12] the number of papers on mindfulness published in academic journals rose from 10 in the year 2000 to almost 700 in 2016. This indicates that the study of mindfulness is in its infancy.[12,13]

Mindfulness research in the pediatric population is even scarcer. A 2015 meta-analysis suggests that mindfulness as treatment for psychopathology in children and adolescents demands further investigation in the form of controlled clinical trials in clinic settings.[11] In practice, there is a broad range of translational technique, which is to say there is a lack of uniformity in implementation, and it is not extensively reported on in the research literature.

Moreover, findings from 2011 and 2015 suggest resilience can mitigate the negative consequences of trauma.[14,15] Findings such as these have sparked a call to action for pediatricians to both recognize that "many adult diseases should be viewed as developmental disorders that begin early in life and that persistent health disparities associated with poverty, discrimination, or maltreatment could be reduced by the alleviation of toxic stress in childhood" and "to serve as both front-line guardians of healthy child development and strategically positioned, community leaders to inform new science-based strategies that build strong foundations for educational achievement, economic productivity, responsible citizenship, and lifelong health."[5,16] This is an emphatic call to work together to enhance the prevention of ACEs, provide early and accessible interventions, and broadly expand the delivery of trauma-informed care.[5]

MINDFULNESS EXERCISES

Mindfulness exercises are no longer considered unnecessary; rather, 2018 research indicates the integration of mindfulness into traditional health care practices is becoming increasingly more common.[17] Mindfulness benefits the mind, body, and interpersonal relationships by improving mental focus, reducing bias towards others, and decreasing negative thoughts. Some simple mindfulness practices are outlined in **Table 7-2**, while more structured mindfulness practices are outlined in **Table 7-3**.

Table 7-2. Simple Mindfulness Practices[18]

TYPE OF PRACTICE	STEPS TO FOLLOW
Pay attention	It is hard to slow down and notice things in a busy world. Try to take the time to experience the environment with all senses. For example, when eating a favorite food, take the time to smell, taste, and truly enjoy it.
Live in the moment	Try to intentionally bring an open, accepting, and discerning attention to everything being done during the day. Find joy in simple pleasures.
Focus on self-acceptance	Treat yourself like a good friend.
Focus on breathing	When there are negative thoughts, try to sit down, take a deep breath, and close your eyes. Focus on the breath as it moves in and out of the body.

Table 7-3. Structured Mindfulness Practices[18]

TYPE OF PRACTICE	STEPS TO FOLLOW
Body scan meditation	Lie on back with legs extended and arms at sides, palms facing up. Focus attention slowly and deliberately on each part of the body, in order, from toe to head or head to toe. Be aware of any sensations, emotions, or thoughts associated with each part of the body.
Sitting meditation	Sit comfortably with back straight, feet flat on the floor and hands on lap. Breathing through the nose, focus on breath moving in and out of the body. If physical sensations or thoughts interrupt meditation, note the experience and then return focus to breath.
Walking meditation	Find a quiet place 10 to 20 feet in length and begin to walk slowly. Focus on the experience of walking, being aware of the sensations of standing and the subtle movements that keep balance. When reaching the end of the path, turn and continue walking, maintaining awareness of sensations.

MEDITATION

Mindfulness can be cultivated through formal meditation and incorporated into any activity, such as walking, cleaning, or being engaged in conversation.[19] Therefore, one can harness mindfulness by using all the senses to stay in the present and create awareness. Remaining focused on the here and now in turn reduces rumination from past thoughts and reduces anxiety about unknowns of the future. Meditation is a form of mindfulness that utilizes various practices to quiet the mind and attain a higher level of consciousness. Meditation requires a physical act by the practitioner, which in turn creates a singular thought.

THE BENEFITS OF MEDITATION

Meditation has been studied in many clinical trials, and evidence supports the effectiveness of meditation for various conditions, including stress, anxiety, pain, depression, insomnia, and high blood pressure (ie, hypertension).[20] Meditation helps a person navigate stress, both acute and chronic. Mindful breathing can interrupt stress and fight-or-flight reactions. Preliminary research has found that meditation may "quiet" the amygdala, the area of the brain that responds to stress, and it may also help people with asthma and fibromyalgia.[21,22] Meditation can help individuals experience thoughts and emotions with greater balance and acceptance and has been shown to improve attention, decrease job burnout, improve sleep, and improve diabetes control.[23-26]

Studies suggest that meditation boosts compassion, as loving-kindness practices can change responses to suffering, thereby increasing altruistic behavior.[27] Additionally, research on meditators with a long-term practice suggests that the "default mode network" of the brain—where we ruminate and let our thoughts wander when we are not focused on a particular activity—quiets down.[22,28]

YOGA

The word yoga has several meanings including union, yoke, concentration, and relation. The word is commonly associated with the idea of union because the root of the word, "yuj" means to yoke or join. There are 8 "limbs" of yoga which provide lenses through which students can evaluate their levels of engagement with the world, those around them, and their inner self as outlined in **Table 7-4**.[29]

Yoga arrived in the United States in the 1800s with transcendentalists, such as Ralph Waldo Emerson and Henry David Thoreau, who were drawn to yoga and

Table 7-4. The 8 Limbs of Yoga[29]

TYPE OF PRACTICE	STEPS TO FOLLOW
Yama	Non-violence, truth, non-stealing, non-covetousness
Niyama	Cleanliness, contentment, austerity, mantra repetition, surrender to God
Asana	Practice of postures
Pranayama	Practice of breath control
Pratayahara	Withdrawal of the contact of the senses with worldly objects
Dharana	Sustained concentration
Dhyana	Uninterrupted meditation
Samadhi	Experiencing non-difference between seer and seen

Hinduism as forms of resistance to capitalism. Several years later, an Englishman who had been living in India for many years produced what would become the first comprehensive yoga book for Westerners called, *The Serpent Power: The Secrets of Tantric and Shaktic Yoga,* which exposed Europeans and Americans to the foundation of this practice.[30]

Two centuries later, millions of people in the United States practice a very different style of yoga. It is practiced by children in schools, veterans in clinics, patients in rehabilitation facilities, in prisons, in inner cities, and in spas and studios in every state. Old and young, healthy and infirm, all practice yoga because it provides comfort and relief and is truly adaptable to any body type.

Over time, the West has adopted a version of yoga that has been adapted to the culture as a secularized practice of a fitness "workout," despite the ancient heritage and cultural foundation as a mystical practice.[1] Yoga has "proven itself to be beyond religions and beyond religious beliefs, and that is readily seen in the people from a variety of religions and the non-religious who practice yoga because it calms their mind, reduces stress, and makes them more internally clear."[29]

Furthermore, there has been a significant proliferation in the number of yoga schools and yoga teachers. In 2020, Yoga Alliance, the professional credentialing body for yoga, listed over 7000 registered yoga schools and more than 100 000 registered yoga teachers.

More and more Americans are practicing some form of yoga. In 2017, the National Center for Complementary and Integrative Health[31,32] conducted a survey, which found that yoga was the most commonly used complementary health approach for adults (14.3% of adults) and that the percentage of children aged 4 to 17 years who used yoga increased significantly from 3.1% in 2012 to 8.4% in 2017. The study also noted that girls were more likely to practice yoga than boys, and that 4 of the 10 most frequently used complementary and alternative medicine (CAM) interventions by children are yoga practices.[32]

There is a growing trend toward the use of yoga as a mind/body complementary intervention in an effort to improve physical as well as mental health conditions.[33] In 1994, a survey of CAM practices showed that respondents ranked yoga 5th out of 39 therapies in terms of perceived effectiveness.[34] A survey of pediatric chronic pain patients and their parents placed yoga as the 3rd most likely to be helpful complementary approach, and when conventional treatments were included, yoga ranked 4th.[35]

Today, the International Association of Yoga Therapists (IAYT) defines yoga therapy as the "specific application of yogic tools—postures/exercises, breath work, meditation techniques, and more—to address an individual's physical, mental, and emotional needs."[36]

YOGA AND THE NERVOUS SYSTEM

The first dharma (ie, cosmic law of yoga) is the duty to take care of the body. Conscious breathing with asanas (ie, poses) is one of the easiest ways to balance bodies by activating the nervous system, whose function is to "perceive the environment and coordinate the behavior of all the other cells of our vast cellular community."[29] The ability to regulate and activate the nervous system allows individuals to be more resilient, feel energized, and deal with day-to-day challenges. Much attention is currently focusing on the significance of the vagus nerve in relation to overall health and wellbeing. The vagus nerve is the nervous system's "brake," moderating the sympathetic system that keeps us on high alert, while the parasympathetic system regulates growth and repair and is often thought of as the "rest and digest" system.[29]

Studies have shown that improving vagal tone can lead to decreased inflammation, high heart rate variability, better sleep, and positive mood regulation.[29] According to one theory, there are 3 vagal mechanisms: immobilization, mobilization and social engagement, and communication.[37]

The practices of asanas are techniques that are believed to create a safe internal environment to better respond to both inner and outer environments (See **Figure 7-2**, which addresses the the automatic nervous system's (ANS') response to the environment). Practicing asanas allows students to stay still and remain observant, sensitive, and calm. Many postures can be uncomfortable for beginners, but one of the underlying principles of yoga is being with this discomfort calmly while purposefully observing how the body, mind, and nervous system adapt to challenging situations without struggling. Asanas initiate this challenge in a safe place.

Figure 7-2. ANS processes the body's internal and external environments.[37]

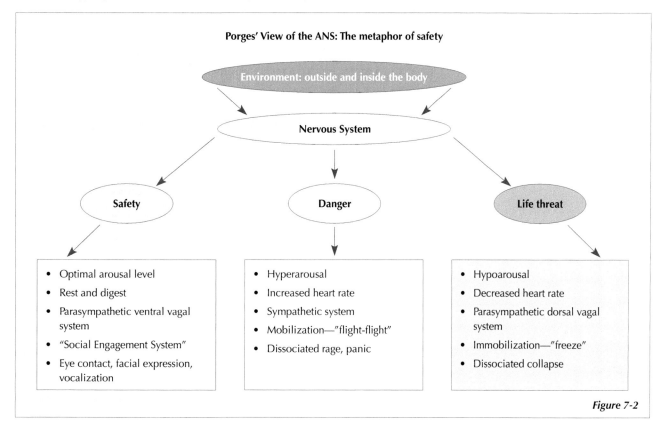

Porges' View of the ANS: The metaphor of safety

Environment: outside and inside the body

Nervous System

Safety

Danger

Life threat

- Optimal arousal level
- Rest and digest
- Parasympathetic ventral vagal system
- "Social Engagement System"
- Eye contact, facial expression, vocalization

- Hyperarousal
- Increased heart rate
- Sympathetic system
- Mobilization—"flight-flight"
- Dissociated rage, panic

- Hypoarousal
- Decreased heart rate
- Parasympathetic dorsal vagal system
- Immobilization—"freeze"
- Dissociated collapse

Figure 7-2

Porges[37] described 4 specific yogic practices that help with regulation/homeostasis and resilience. These practices (**Table 7-5**) work by strengthening vagal tone. Through various practices, yoga can affect the ability to regulate the body, mind, and nervous system, and its effects are compounded through repetitive practice.

Table 7-5. Yogic Practices for Homeostasis[37]	
PRACTICE	EFFECT
Posture	— Changes in posture activate nerves that monitor and control blood pressure and lead to mood changes. — Swaying, rocking, bowing, and prostrating, all stimulate the vagus nerve.
Breathing	— Respiration stimulates the vagus nerve through the larynx. — Audible breathing practices have the ability to regulate the stress response.
Vocalization	— Chanting and singing stimulate the larynx and whole brain function.
Behavior	— Practicing with love, kindness, and compassion has been shown to stimulate vagal tone.

Yoga's Efficacy with Children

A Morbidity and Mortality Weekly Report (MMWR) from the CDC[38] documented the high prevalence of mental health disorders among America's children before COVID-19. Multiple reports led the American Academy of Pediatrics, the American Academy of Child and Adolescent Psychiatry, and the Children's Hospital Association to issue a joint declaration of a national emergency in child and adolescent mental health.[38] MMWR findings also showed that children living in poverty and minority children fare worse than their White, middle class peers in access to care, identifiable risk factors, and prevalence of mental health conditions. Despite the high levels of mental health disorders, MMWR found low rates of treatment (about 11.4% annually for White, 9.8% for Black, and 8.7% for Latinx children).[38] According to the CDC,[39] 1 in 6 children aged 2 to 8 years is diagnosed with a mental disorder, and about 1 in 5 adolescents has a mental disorder with a severe impairment.

According to the CDC, the most common childhood conditions (eg, ADHD, behavior disorders, anxiety, depression), when treated, are treated with approaches using behavior therapy and cognitive-behavior therapy to reduce symptoms. Whether conventional or CAM, there is still limited information about which type of interventions are best for treating each specific childhood mental disorder. Many studies on yoga that have been systematically reviewed are often weak to moderate in terms of research quality; however, most studies show that yoga *generally* leads to some reductions in anxiety and depression and have shown that yoga can have a positive effect on a range of outcomes in cognitive, behavioral, and physiological functioning.[40-46] These studies lack the strength of results to scientifically consider yoga an evidenced-based treatment for childhood mental health disorders.

While there are no certain paths to mental wellbeing or averting mental health disorders, yoga and yoga therapy provide tools for change. Teaching children to slow themselves down through movement and breath helps avoid, derail, or shorten countless crises or meltdowns; teaches awareness of the inner self and outer worlds; and provides a philosophy to approach the world with gentleness and compassion.

Integrating Yoga into the Treatment Plan

Becoming a yoga teacher or therapist requires extensive experience, study, and practice, including a recommended 800 additional hours for those who have already completed the basic 200-hour training. Finding a yoga therapist who works with children can be challenging, as the field is rather young, but the IAYT provides a free search engine to find registered yoga therapists.[36] If yoga is incorporated into treatment plans, the therapist must know their limits and must choose postures and routines that they can teach competently, as it is essential that no harm comes to the child or therapist. Louise Goldberg, author of *Yoga for Children with Autism and Special Needs*,[47] proposed 10 "golden rules" for working with exceptional children, as seen in **Table 7-6**. In yoga, no effort is ever wasted on the part of the teacher and the student. In the end, however, it is the inner work of the student that is the driving force behind transformation.

Table 7-6. 10 Golden Rules of Practicing Yoga with Children[47]	
1. See the whole child	6. Take nothing personally
2. Make yoga fun	7. Be yourself (Satya)
3. Do no harm (Ahisma)	8. Plan to be surprised
4. Maintain enthusiasm	9. Know when to walk away
5. Teach what you are comfortable doing	10. Keep it positive

Key Points

1. Mindfulness is the practice of being present; allowing for a reduction of stress, anxiety, and pain while creating an overall sense of relaxation.

2. Mindful practices such as yoga and meditation have the ability to regulate and activate the nervous system, allowing individuals to be more resilient, feel energized, and deal with day-to-day challenges.

3. Yoga generally leads to some reductions in anxiety and depression and can have a positive effect on a range of outcomes in cognitive, behavioral, and physiological functioning.

References

1. Hofmann SG, Gómez AF. Mindfulness-based interventions for anxiety and depression. *Psychiatric Clin North Am.* 2017;40(4):739-749. doi:10.1016/j.psc. 2017.08.008

2. Mindfulness. Psychology Today. Accessed June 24, 2022. https://www.psychologytoday.com/us/basics/mindfulness

3. Kabat-Zinn J. Mindfulness. *Mindfulness.* 2015;6:1481-1483. doi:10.1007/s12671-015-0456-x

4. Kabat-Zinn J. An outpatient program in behavioral medicine for chronic pain patients based on the practice of mindfulness meditation: theoretical considerations and preliminary results. *Gen Hosp Psychiatry.* 1982;4(1):33-47. doi:10.1016/0163-8343(82)90026-3

5. Ortiz R, Sibinga EM. The role of mindfulness in reducing the adverse effects of childhood stress and trauma. *Children.* 2017;4(3):16. doi:10.3390/children4030016

6. Clarke TC, Barnes PM, Black LI, Stussman BJ, Nahin RL. *Use of Yoga, Meditation, and Chiropractors Among U.S. Adults Aged 18 and Older.* NCHS Data Brief: US Department of Health and Human Services; 2018:1-8. Number 325. https://www.cdc.gov/nchs/data/databriefs/db325-h.pdf

7. Black LI, Barnes PM, Clarke TC, Stussman BJ, Nahin RL. *Use of Yoga, Meditation, and Chiropractors Among U.S. Children Aged 4–17 Years.* NCHS Data Brief: US Department of Health and Human Services; 2018. Number 324. https://www.cdc.gov/nchs/data/databriefs/db324-h.pdf

8. Black DS, Slavich GM. Mindfulness meditation and the immune system: a systematic review of randomized controlled trials. *Ann N Y Acad Sci.* 2016;1373:13-24. doi:10.1111/nyas.12998

9. Stephens MA, Wand G. Stress and the HPA axis: role of glucocorticoids in alcohol dependence. *Alcohol Res.* 2012;34(4):468-483.

10. Kalmar J, Baumann I, Gruber E, et al. The impact of session-introducing mindfulness and relaxation interventions in individual psychotherapy for children and adolescents: a randomized controlled trial (MARS-CA). *Trials.* 2022;23(1):1-14. doi:10.1186/s13063-022-06212-0

11. Zoogman S, Goldberg SB, Hoyt WT, Miller L. Mindfulness interventions with youth: a meta-analysis. *Mindfulness.* 2015;6(2):290-302. doi:10.1007/s12671-013-0260-4

12. American Mindfulness Research Association, LLC. Library. American Mindfullness Research Association. Updated 2024. Accessed February 20, 2024. https://goamra.org/Library

13. van Dam NT, van Vugt MK, Vago DR, et al. Mind the hype: a critical evaluation and prescriptive agenda for research on mindfulness and meditation. *Perspect Psychol Sci.* 2018;13(1):36-61. doi:10.1177/1745691617709589

14. Wrenn GL, Wingo AP, Moore R, et al. The effect of resilience on posttraumatic stress disorder in trauma-exposed inner-city primary care patients. *J Natl Med Assoc.* 2011;103(7):560-566. doi:10.1016/S0027-9684(15)30381-3

15. Chandler GE, Roberts SJ, Chiodo L. Resilience intervention for young adults with adverse childhood experiences. *J Am Psychiatr Nurses Assoc.* 2015;21(6):406-416. doi:10.1177/1078390315620609

16. Shonkoff JP, Garner AS. The lifelong effects of early childhood adversity and toxic stress. *Pediatrics.* 2012;129(1):e232–e246. doi:10.1542/peds.2011-2663

17. Tlalka S. Meditation is the fastest growing health trend in America. Mindful. 2018. Accessed June 24, 2022. https://www.mindful.org/meditation-is-the-fastest-growing-health-trend-in-america/

18. Sparks D. Mayo mindfulness: practicing mindfulness exercises. Mayo Clinic News Network. 2018. Accessed June 24, 2022. https://newsnetwork.mayoclinic.org/discussion/mayo-mindfulness-practicing-mindfulness-exercises/

19. What is mindfulness? Mindful. 2021. Accessed June 24, 2022. https://www.mindful.org/what-is-mindfulness/

20. Meditation and mindfulness: what you need to know. National Center for Complementary and Integrative Health. US Department of Health and Human Services. 2022. Accessed June 24, 2022. https://www.nccih.nih.gov/health/meditation-and-mindfulness-what-you-need-to-know

21. Leung MK, Lau WKW, Chan CCH, Wong SSY, Fung ALC, Lee TMC. Meditation-induced neuroplastic changes in amygdala activity during negative affective processing. *Soc Neurosci.* 2018;13(3):277-288. doi:10.1080/17470919.2017.1311939

22. Desbordes G, Negi LT, Pace TW, Wallace BA, Raison CL, Schwartz EL. Effects of mindful-attention and compassion meditation training on amygdala response to emotional stimuli in an ordinary, non-meditative state. *Front Hum Neurosci.* 2012;6:292. doi:10.3389/fnhum.2012.00292

23. Rusch HL, Rosario M, Levison LM, et al. The effect of mindfulness meditation on sleep quality: a systematic review and meta-analysis of randomized controlled trials. *Annals NY Acad Sci.* 2019;1445(1):5-16. doi:10.1111/nyas.13996

24. Levine GN, Lange RA, Bairey-Merz CN, et al. Meditation and cardiovascular risk reduction: a scientific statement from the American Heart Association. *J Am Heart Assoc.* 2017;6(10):e002218. doi:10.1161/JAHA.117.002218

25. Intarakamhang U, Macaskill A, Prasittichok P. Mindfulness interventions reduce blood pressure in patients with non-communicable diseases: a systematic review and meta-analysis. *Heliyon.* 2020;6(4):e03834. doi:10.1016/j.heliyon.2020.e03834

26. Anheyer D, Leach MJ, Klose P, et al. Mindfulness-based stress reduction for treating chronic headache: a systematic review and meta-analysis. *Cephalalgia.* 2019;39(4):544-555. doi:10.1177/0333102418781795

27. Zeng X, Chiu CP, Wang R, Oei TP, Leung FY. The effect of loving-kindness meditation on positive emotions: a meta-analytic review. *Front Psychol.* 2015;6:1693. doi:10.3389/fpsyg.2015.01693

28. Mascaro JS, Darcher A, Negi LT, Raison CL. The neural mediators of kindness-based meditation: a theoretical model. *Front Psychol.* 2015;6:109. doi:10.3389/fpsyg.2015.00109

29. Stern E. *One Simple Thing: A New Look at the Science of Yoga and How it Can Transform Your Life.* North Point Press; 2020.

30. Avalon A. *The Serpent Power: The Secrets of Tantric and Shaktic Yoga.* Dover Publications; 1974.

31. National Health Interview Survey 2017. National Center for Complementary and Integrative Health. 2018. Accessed June 24, 2022. https://www.nccih.nih.gov/research/statistics/nhis/2017

32. Birdee GS, Legedza AT, Saper RB, Bertisch SM, Eisenberg DM, Phillips RS. Characteristics of yoga users: results of a national survey. *J General Intern Med.* 2008;23(10):1653-1658. doi:10.1007/s11606-008-0735-5

33. Kaley-Isley LC, Peterson J, Peterson E. Yoga as a complementary therapy for children and adolescents: a guide for clinicians. *Psychiatry.* 2010;7(8):20-32.

34. Furnham A, Forey J. The attitudes, behaviors, and beliefs of patients of conventional vs. complementary (alternative) medicine. *J Clin Psychol.* 1994;50(3):458-469. doi:10.1002/1097-4679(199405)50:3<458::aid-jclp2270500318>3.0.co;2-v

35. Tsao JC, Meldrum M, Bursch B, Jacob MC, Kim SC, Zeltzer LK. Treatment expectations for CAM interventions in pediatric chronic pain patients and their parents. *Evid Based Complement Alternat Med.* 2005;2(4) 521-527. doi:10.1093/ecam/neh132

36. What is yoga therapy? International Association of Yoga Therapists. 2022. Accessed June 24, 2022. https://yogatherapy.health/what-is-yoga-therapy/

37. Porges SW. *The Polyvagal Theory: Neurophysiological Foundations of Emotions, Attachment, Communication, and Self-regulation.* W.W. Norton; 2011.

38. Shim R, Szilagyi M, Perrin JM. Epidemic rates of child and adolescent mental health disorders require an urgent response. *Pediatrics.* 2022;149(5):e2022056611. doi:10.1542/peds.2022-056611

39. Data and statistics on children's mental health. Centers for Disease Control and Prevention. 2022. Accessed June 24, 2022. https://www.cdc.gov/childrensmentalhealth/data.html

40. Therapy to improve children's mental health. Centers for Disease Control and Prevention. 2022. Accessed June 24, 2022. https://www.cdc.gov/childrensmentalhealth/parent-behavior-therapy.html

41. Hagen I, Naya US. Yoga for children and young people's mental health and wellbeing: research review and reflections on the mental health potentials of yoga. *Front Psychiatry.* 2014;5:35. doi:10.3389/fpsyt.2014.00035

42. Galantino ML, Galbavy R, Quinn L. Therapeutic effects of yoga for children: a systematic review of the literature. *Ped Phys Ther.* 2008;20(1):66-80. doi:10.1097/PEP.0b013e31815f1208

43. Coeytaux RR, McDuffie J, Goode A, et al. *Evidence Map of Yoga for High-Impact Conditions Affecting Veterans.* Department of Veterans Affairs; 2014. https://www.hsrd.research.va.gov/publications/esp/yoga.pdf

44. Miller S, Mendelson T, Lee-Winn A, Dyer NL, Khalsa SBS. Systematic review of randomized controlled trials testing the effects of yoga with youth. *Mindfulness.* 2020;11(6):1336-1353. doi:10.1007/s12671-019-01230-7

45. Ferreira-Vorkapic C, Feitoza JM, Marchioro M, Simoes J, Kozasa E, Telles S. Are there benefits from teaching yoga at schools? A systematic review of randomized control trials of yoga-based interventions. *Evid Based Complement Alternat Med.* 2015;2015:345835. doi:10.1155/2015/345835

46. James-Palmer A, Anderson EZ, Zucker L, Kofman Y, Daneault J. Yoga as an intervention for the reduction of symptoms of anxiety and depression in children and adolescents: a systematic review. *Front Pediatr.* 2020;8:78. doi:10.3389/fped.2020.00078

47. Goldberg L. *Yoga Therapy for Children with Autism and Special Needs.* W.W. Norton & Company; 2013.

Relational Resilience

Sarah H. Buffie, MSW, LSW
Adrienne N. Kennedy, DSW
C. Danae Riggs

Objectives
After reading this chapter, the reader will be able to:

1. *Define relational resilience as the result of feeling predictably physically, emotionally, and psychologically safe in relationships with others.*

2. *Explain how relational templates are set in childhood.*

3. *Recognize how adults can develop skills to impact positive relational templates.*

Background and Significance

Over the past 30 years, the notion of "relationship building" has been a much talked about and necessary element for any learning or healing context. When Drs. Felitti and Anda completed the first adverse childhood experiences (ACEs) study,[1] they found that an important protective factor for those experiencing ACEs was having at least one positive, safe adult that they could rely on. Naturally, this positive, safe relationship did not take away anyone's past, nor did it heal all the trauma that one might have experienced; however, the capacity to feel safe in a relationship with another was the bedrock for building self-esteem, sense of self, and experiences of belonging. It is in this context of relationship that regardless of degree, clinical licensure, intervention, or strategy competency that people have an opportunity to heal. Dr. Bruce Perry[2] states, "there is no more effective neurobiological intervention than a safe relationship." From this framing we have come to understand "relational resilience" as the capacity to achieve a good outcome following adversity through the experience of predictable physical, emotional, and psychological safety in relationships with others (**Figure 8-1**).

Over decades of working and consulting in the foster care, education, developmental disability, and mental health systems, it has been found that relational resilience is what should be emphasized or regarded as a priority in human service systems. Oftentimes, service and support workers are encouraged to be procedural, clinical, and transactional in their engagements with the people they support, which leads to the relational context being skewed, cold, and detached. When this relational aspect is omitted from the interaction under the guise of "professional boundaries," more harm than good is done, and the element of healing is not present. When providers can understand themselves and their own regulated nervous system as an instrument of resilience, they are invited to learn deeply about a person's history, culture, interests, and passions. Learning this allows for the design of support, routines, and healing interventions that come from a place of compassion, empathy, and creativity rather than focusing on the pathologizing labels, which fall short in describing the true root of challenges people face. This missing element is simple, though not always easy to achieve: nervous system to nervous system, right brain to right brain[3]; this is how individuals heal, and now that more is known about the field of neuroscience,

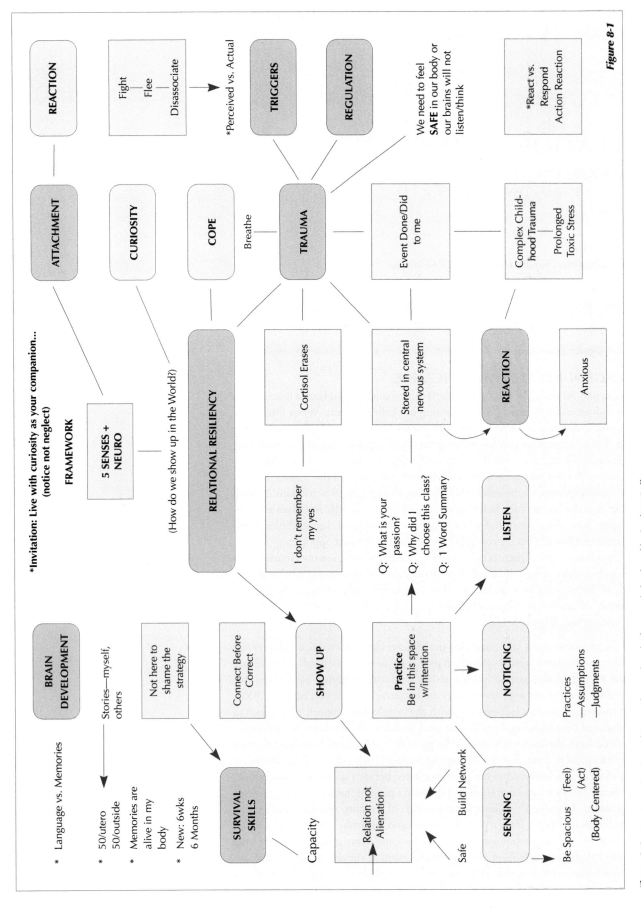

Figure 8-1. *The relational resiliency framework. Based on the framework developed by Sarah H. Buffie.*

there is a deeper understanding that when people enter a space, their nervous systems are reading one another before words are formed and before interactions are carried out. When individuals cultivate the first aspect of relational resilience, which is the capacity to feel safe in one's own body and the ability to truly know themselves and how they regulate and co-regulate with others, there is a greater capacity to signal safety to the other nervous systems that any given individual may encounter.

THE IMPACT OF TRAUMA ON THE BRAIN

Relational resilience is the capacity to achieve a good outcome following adversity due to experiencing predictable physical, emotional, and psychological safety in relationships with others. To appreciate the benefits of relational resilience, it is important to first recognize and respect the impact of trauma on the brain. The brain constructs a framework for how relationships work based on interactions with others. When the brain experiences toxic stress, particularly in childhood, it becomes flooded with cortisol, the stress hormone. Learning to deal with stress is a normal part of healthy development; however, when stress becomes toxic, the stress response stays activated and releases cortisol even when there is no apparent risk of harm.[4] Overloading the stress response system can severely affect a child's developing brain. Negative relational experiences and the accompanying stress cause the brain to change.[5] In addition to having a stress response system that is constantly on high alert, neural connections that support learning and reasoning can lessen and become weaker. During this time, children learn what connections with others look and feel like through the developing framework. Frameworks that perceive relationships as potentially hazardous can be constructed by negative experiences and interactions such as abuse, neglect, family turmoil, neighborhood violence, extreme poverty, racial discrimination, historical trauma, and other hardships. Even infants and young children are affected adversely when significant stresses threaten their family and caregiving environments.[3]

The negative impact of toxic stress can be avoided when adults provide children with positive interactions. Interactions and experiences with adults that are safe, predictable, and non-threatening support the brain in developing a relational framework that regards relationships as nurturing, and they lay the foundation for relational resilience to flourish. Caring and supportive relationships alter the brain in the same way stress does. It is impossible to erase a person's adverse prior experiences, but it is feasible to provide new secure and connected experiences. Over time, the repetition of new experiences alters the relational framework, and one's ability to form positive relationships with others improves.

Human brains are wired for connection, and human beings are dependent on others for survival. Throughout their lifespan, human beings constantly interact with stimuli that can have safe or unsafe impact on the ability to attach to and rely on others. In infancy, the attachment relationship between child and caregiver directly impacts that infant's ability to cope with stress.[6] Warm, responsive, and predictable relationships increase one's ability to cope with hardship and develop the skills to stay within their window of tolerance when stressful experiences arise. In 1992, Judith Jordan first used the language of relational resilience to encourage helping professionals evolve beyond the "separate self" model of development[7] and into an understanding that developed into relational templates through the relational context. Jordan's[8] work is grounded in relational-cultural theory (RCT), which asserts that "all psychological growth occurs in relationships and that movement out of a relationship (chronic disconnection) into isolation constitutes the source of much psychological suffering."

As neuroscience has evolved and deepened societies' collective understanding of the developmental implications of this psychological suffering, the focus has shifted from managing a child's behavior to creating more predictable environments to nurturing relational resilience. Polyvagal theory posits that learning and growth require nervous system state regulation.[9] When one's vagus nerve senses a real or perceived threat in the environment or in the relational field (ie, neuroception), it is designed to increase sympathetic arousal leading to the fight or flight response or activate the dorsal vagal shutdown leading to the freeze response. The third branch of the vagus nerve, called the ventral vagal system, is activated when there are more cues of safety present than cues of danger. For a child who has had repeated and prolonged stress response activation in the context of unsafe relationships, their vagus nerve is primed to neurocept danger and continually activate the stress response, even if there is no clear and present danger in the environment. This neuroception of danger can lead to challenging behavioral expression that is often dismissed or pathologized as "oppositional," "manipulative," or "aggressive" behavior. Having a strong "no" or not feeling safe enough to engage with a person in a position of power can look like "opposition" or "defiance" when in actuality it is a sign of a dysregulated nervous system. Attempting to meet needs in any way other than in a direct manner can be interpreted as "manipulative" when the child is quite simply in survival mode. The sympathetic response that mobilizes the young person into fight or flight mode can be perceived as aggression, when it is simply the amygdala overfiring due to past stressors. When adults perpetuate these misunderstandings and blame or shame children for their innate survival strategies, they become unsafe for the child, thereby eroding or affirming a negative relational template. There are great consequences for the mental, emotional, psychological, and physical health of children when their caregivers disregard the impact of trauma on the developing brain, body, and behavioral patterns that emerge towards the biological need for protection and connection.

How Relational Resilience is Cultivated

The ability to adapt and thrive despite adversity develops within the context of supportive relationships. Family members and other adults who play an essential role in children's lives, including helping professionals such as early childcare providers, social workers, nurses, and coaches, can develop relationships that promote resilience. This is because children require relationships to develop resilience, not individualism. The essential building blocks for boosting the ability to do well in the face of considerable adversity are the dependable presence of at least one supportive relationship and multiple opportunities for the child to develop practical coping skills. The quality and stability of a relationship are more important than the number of relationships, and they affect virtually all aspects of development—intellectual, social, emotional, physical, and behavioral—and lay the foundation for various outcomes later in life.[4] Therefore, developing relational resilience in childhood and adolescence, adults can begin with a focus on their interactions with children as an opportunity to set a new relational template.

Safe Adults Creating Relational Resilience in Children

Taking the time to build safe and nurturing relationships prepares children to succeed academically and behaviorally in their interactions with others. Connections are created in the moment-to-moment interactions that adults have with children, such as allowing children to try new actions or activities. Interactions with adults who keep them safe lay the groundwork for resilience development. Teachers, coaches, and other adults in the community, including helping professionals with whom children have the opportunity to form relationships, can all play a part in assisting a child in developing resilience. Reflecting on past experiences and how they may have affected the relational framework when attempting to establish a connection that supports resilience is critical.

Professionals in helping roles should consider the public perception of individuals in their field as trustworthy, safe, and non-threatening. Understanding cultural ways of being/interacting and the child's historical events that may have eroded their trust will aid in determining experiences that shape a child's relational framework.

Barriers to Relational Resilience

Knowing how to cultivate relational resilience supports healthy child development. However, systemic barriers can prevent children from accessing these relational benefits. Administrative burdens[10] such as too little pre-service and ongoing professional development, overwhelming paperwork requirements, and the stress, frustration, anxiety, and secondary traumatic stress that can occur when working with individuals who have experienced trauma can often hinder the development of relationships that foster resilience. These burdens can harm how professionals in helping roles perceive and experience their work and even perpetuate inequities. Understanding the impact of administrative burdens and how to reduce them will help promote resilience through more effective relationships. While clinicians and human service professionals can be a key element in a child or adolescent's healing journey, caregivers and family members are oftentimes the ones spending the most time with the child. In addition to the challenges noted above, there are significant barriers in the areas of accessible trauma-informed health care, racism, mental health challenges, limited paid leave, and lack of trauma-informed respite supports that also greatly impact children's ability to connect with adults who can foster relational safety.

Lack of Training, Professional Knowledge, and Skill Development

A lack of training, professional knowledge, and skill frequently create difficulty when professionals endeavor to develop the type of relationship needed to foster resilience. To create the conditions for developing relational resilience, professionals in helping roles need to possess foundational knowledge, mindsets, and capacities that support the development of healthy relationships. Consequently, professionals in helping roles need pre-service and ongoing high-quality professional learning opportunities structured around social and emotional skills targeted to their role. Scaffolded learning opportunities that include modeling, observation, and real-time feedback are particularly helpful in developing these core capabilities and mindsets within child-serving professions. Effective professional learning ensures that helping professionals have the foundational knowledge, mindsets, and capacity needed to create strategies that can be implemented to promote relational resilience.

Overwhelming Administrative Burden

Administrative tasks, such as paperwork, take time and impact all professionals' workload. Therefore, systemic rules that impose a paperwork burden are a significant source of dissatisfaction that impacts professionals' ability to develop quality relationships with the people they serve. Professionals overwhelmed by documentation requirements tend to work longer hours and can experience a disconnect between one's preferred relationship-building work and their daily work. This disconnect is a key contributor to adverse physical and mental health consequences, leading to alienation, isolation, depersonalization, cynicism, emotional exhaustion, and burnout.[11] The psychological and physical costs to the professional and the relational cost to the person served that arise from responding to the bureaucratic demands of many human service systems is critical when formulating documentation policy. When eliminating administrative tasks is not an option, regular reviews, revision, alignment, and streamlining must be done to minimize the burden.[12]

Negative Emotional Consequences

Negative consequences, such as stress, frustration, anxiety, and secondary traumatic stress, are inherent to working within systems that serve individuals who have experienced trauma. Organizational support is essential in buffering the effect of stress and burnout. Interventions that continually monitor the wellbeing of professionals in helping roles and intervene when stress, burnout, or secondary traumatic stress emerge are promising practices.[12] Brief interventions, such as monthly screenings for burnout, help organizations understand how helping professionals are experiencing their role and establish when other mitigations for adverse impacts are needed. In addition, interventions used during work hours incorporating preventive and assistive measures, such as supervision, training, mentoring, or coaching, can help professionals manage work-related stress.

Another helpful intervention is training professionals to detect and monitor the signs and symptoms of stress, burnout, or secondary traumatic stress within themselves. Pre-service training, positive psychology interventions, and stress management programs have had favorable effects on the self-efficacy, resilience, optimism, and hope that individuals in helping professions experience.[12] A significant offering from Dr. Beth Barol[13] is the incorporation of the Biographical Timeline framework in order for clinicians and caregivers alike to put the child(ren)'s current challenges in the context of their early life experiences. This framework offers teams the space and clarity to address the root causes of stressors instead of getting distracted by symptomology, therefore alleviating the impacts of stress, frustration and anxiety.

THE CIRCLE OF SECURITY: IMPORTANT LESSONS FOR CAREGIVERS AND CLINICIANS

Parenting and providing therapeutic care to children can be a complex and challenging journey. Parents and providers all strive to meet the needs of children, help them grow, and create a secure environment. In this pursuit, The Circle of Security offers valuable lessons for caregivers and clinicians.[14] Based on decades of attachment research, it provides relationship tools and a new perspective on understanding and meeting children's attachment needs. By applying these lessons, caregivers and clinicians can foster lasting security and satisfaction for both children and themselves.

— *Recognizing Attachment Needs.* The first important lesson from The Circle of Security is recognizing the attachment needs of children. Attachment needs can be divided into 3 categories: Going Out on the Circle, Coming In on the Circle, and Hands on the Circle. By understanding these needs, caregivers and clinicians gain insights into providing appropriate support and meeting children's emotional requirements.

— *Providing a Secure Base.* The concept of a secure base is central to The Circle of Security. Caregivers and clinicians learn to create an environment where children feel safe, seen, and supported as they explore the world. Encouragement, attentive presence, and offering assistance when needed are essential aspects of providing a secure base. By striking a balance between allowing independence and ensuring support, caregivers and clinicians help children develop a sense of confidence while still knowing they have a reliable source of comfort and protection to return to.

— *Creating a Safe Haven.* Caregivers and clinicians are encouraged to provide emotional support, comfort, and understanding when children seek solace. This involves being available, listening attentively, and offering a sense of security and connection. By creating a safe haven, caregivers and clinicians foster trust and help children regulate their emotions, which is crucial for their overall wellbeing.

— *Balancing Independence and Support.* Caregivers and clinicians must be in charge in a kind and loving manner. Setting appropriate boundaries, offering guidance, and promoting autonomy while still providing necessary guidance and structure are essential. Striking this balance allows children to develop self-confidence, while receiving the necessary support for their growth and development.

— *Reflecting on Parenting Style.* The Circle of Security prompts caregivers and clinicians to reflect on their own parenting styles and attachment patterns. Understanding how their own experiences and beliefs impact their interactions with children is crucial. By gaining insights into their own attachment experiences, caregivers and clinicians can enhance their understanding of children's needs and develop more responsive and nurturing caregiving or therapeutic practices.

— ***Embracing Imperfection.*** One of the most comforting aspects of The Circle of Security is the acknowledgment that no one is a perfect parent or caregiver. The approach emphasizes "good enough" parenting and recognizes that everyone will inevitably miss meeting a child's needs at times. The focus is on constantly striving to meet those needs and building a secure and supportive relationship over time.

The Circle of Security provides invaluable lessons for caregivers and clinicians working with children. By understanding and applying the principles of attachment theory, caregivers and clinicians can enhance their ability to meet children's needs, create secure relationships, and promote healthy development. These lessons emphasize the importance of being attuned to children's attachment needs, providing a secure base and safe haven, maintaining a balance between independence and support, reflecting on one's own parenting style, and embracing imperfection. By incorporating these lessons into their caregiving or therapeutic practices, caregivers and clinicians can positively impact the lives of children and foster their emotional wellbeing.

CONCLUSION

Relational resilience results from feeling predictably physically, emotionally, and psychologically safe in relationships with others. Relational resilience is impacted by the relational templates set in childhood and may be altered or influenced throughout the lifespan through safe relational experiences with warm, responsive adults. There are environmental, historical, psychological, and systemic barriers to building relational resilience among children who have experienced maltreatment; however, despite these barriers, helping professionals and social service organizations have the capacity to address policy and alter practices in order to create the context for relationships to be prioritized. For relational resilience to flourish among individuals, families, communities, and within educational and human service systems, social/emotional learning needs to be prioritized for both children and adults. Adults must become aware of relational templates and deeply understand how their own self-regulation impacts others; using this awareness to make choices that center on the relational field will significantly impact children who survive threatening environments and systems.

CASE STUDIES

Case Study 8-1

Emily, aged 9 years, exhibited an extremely difficult interpersonal style during therapy sessions. Emily engaged in frequent name-calling, refused to participate or speak, and displayed an inconsistent engagement with the clinician. Additionally, she exhibited intense mistrust toward the provider, making it challenging to establish a therapeutic rapport.

Emily's difficult interpersonal style posed significant challenges for the clinician. The constant name-calling and refusal to participate created a hostile and resistant atmosphere during sessions, which hindered the therapeutic process. The inconsistent engagement further added to the difficulty, as it became challenging to predict and maintain Emily's involvement in treatment activities. Moreover, Emily's intense mistrust of the clinician presented a significant barrier to building a therapeutic relationship based on trust and collaboration. This mistrust may have stemmed from past negative experiences or a general mistrust of adults. As a result, the clinician needed to approach therapy with patience, empathy, and understanding to gradually earn Emily's trust and create a safe therapeutic space.

Discussion

Clinicians working with children like Emily need specialized training and support to effectively manage the challenges posed by the child's difficult interpersonal style.

They may employ a variety of therapeutic techniques, such as play therapy, art therapy, or trauma-informed approaches to help the child gradually open up and engage in the therapeutic process. Collaborating with the child's caregivers or involving family therapy may also be beneficial in addressing underlying issues contributing to difficult behavior. Recognizing the stressors associated with working with children who have challenging interpersonal styles is crucial. Clinicians should receive ongoing supervision and access to resources supporting their wellbeing and resilience. By acknowledging and addressing these challenges, clinicians can enhance their ability to provide effective and compassionate care, ultimately helping children like Emily overcome their difficulties and experience relational resilience through positive therapeutic outcomes.

Furthermore, providers must prioritize their own self-care and emotional regulation to effectively navigate the complexities of working with challenging populations. Clinicians and caregivers should practice self-reflection and self-regulation techniques before attempting to regulate the child's behavior to create a calm and grounded presence during therapy sessions. Taking intentional pauses to assess their own emotional state, engaging in perspective-taking, and employing self-regulation strategies such as deep breathing exercises or mindfulness practices can help clinicians regulate their own stress or frustration. By cultivating a state of calm within themselves, clinicians are better equipped to respond to the child's challenging behaviors with patience and understanding.

Case Study 8-2

Bryan, a 13-year-old boy with a long history of abuse and neglect from his biological aunt and uncle, was placed for the second time in an unstable and abusive foster placement. After surviving there for several months, the circumstances became so unbearable that Bryan resorted to one of his highly adaptive survival strategies and ran away, causing him to be labeled as a missing person. At team meetings, his human service workers displayed their frustration by focusing on the demands of the paperwork that Bryan "made them do because of his behavior" and other burdensome administrative duties that took priority over Bryan and his needs as a child who was attempting to alleviate the pain from his abuse.

Discussion

Fostering relational resilience in Bryan would have a higher probability of happening if his team modeled predictable and safe emotional, physical, and psychological interactions with him to the best of their abilities. Everyone on Bryan's team is human, so they are bound to have bad days, become dysregulated themselves, or miss the relational mark—rupture will not always be avoided, but developing the capacity for repair, especially in the relational context, is a skill worth nurturing. When the team was finally able to reunite with Bryan, he was met with a team that had been nurtured and coached to center safety, reduce judgment, maintain consistency and predictability, and behave in a trauma-responsive manner.

Over time, the team was coached to understand their role was to become the safe adults that Bryan always needed. It was not a simple task, but it started with their behavior change—not Bryan's. Bryan wanted to get a job, he wanted to consistently see his siblings, and, like most boys his age, he also wanted a girlfriend. Bryan expressed wanting new clothes so that he did not get bullied, and he wanted to play a sport and have a membership at the Boys and Girls Club so he could hang out and shoot hoops. His big dream was to record his music in a studio and have a phone to use to record his beats and write down his lyrics. Before their coaching and internal transformation, the robust social services team wanted him to take his medications, stop being so angry, and behave. When they identified what Bryan valued and wanted for his life through motivational interviewing techniques, it was shared that very few members of his team had ever heard these things before. That was not surprising, as all of their evaluations, behavior plans, and team meetings were focused on what was wrong with Bryan, not what happened and certainly not learning about his survival strategies.

As a group of professionals charged with Bryan's care, it was imperative that his team consistently and predictably worked on their own behavioral patterns in order to understand themselves as instruments of resilience. This understanding, and the self- and co-regulation practices that followed, supported his team in helping Bryan develop new relational templates based on trauma-informed and responsive interactions that began to develop relational resilience.

KEY POINTS

1. Feeling predictably physically, emotionally, and mentally safe in interactions with others builds relational resilience.

2. The relational templates that are established in childhood have an impact on relationship resilience, which can be changed or influenced throughout life by having safe relational experiences with kind, attentive adults.

3. Helping professionals and social service organizations must recognize and address the environmental, historical, psychological, and structural policies and practices that obstruct the development of relational resilience.

REFERENCES

1. Cronholm PF, Forke CM, Wade R, et al. Adverse childhood experiences: expanding the concept of adversity. *Am J Prev Med.* 2015;49(3):354-361. doi:10.1016/j.amepre.2015.02.001

2. Szalavitz M, Perry BD. *Born for Love: Why Empathy Is Essential-and Endangered.* William Morrow, an imprint of Harper Collins Publishers; 2011.

3. Cozolino LJ. *The Neuroscience of Human Relationships: Attachment and the Developing Social Brain.* W.W. Norton & Company; 2014.

4. From best practices to breakthrough impacts: a science-based approach to building a more promising future for young children and families. Center on the Developing Child at Harvard University. 2016. http://www.developingchild.harvard.edu

5. Kochanska G, Boldt LJ, Goffin KC. Early relational experience: a foundation for the unfolding dynamics of parent–child socialization. *Child Dev Perspect.* 2018;13(1):41-47. doi:10.1111/cdep.12308

6. Frewen P, Brown M, DePierro J, D'Andrea W, Schore A. Assessing the family dynamics of childhood maltreatment history with the Childhood Attachment and Relational Trauma Screen (CARTS). *Eur J Psychotraumatol.* 2015;3(6):27792. doi:10.3402/ejpt.v6.27792

7. Jordan J. Relational resilience. Academia. February 17, 2022. Accessed May 25, 2022. https://www.academia.edu/71780352/Relational_Resilience

8. Jordan JV. Relational resilience in girls. In: Goldstein S, Brooks R, eds. *Handbook of Resilience in Children.* Springer; 2013.

9. Slonim T. The polyvagal theory: neuropsychological foundations of emotions, attachment, communication, and self-regulation. *Int J Group Psychother.* 2014; 64(4):593-600. doi:10.1521/ijgp.2014.64.4.593

10. Herd P, Moynihan DP. *Administrative Burden: Policymaking by Other Means.* Russell Sage Foundation; 2019.

11. Ommaya AK, Cipriano PF, Hoyt DB, et al. Care-centered clinical documentation in the digital environment: solutions to alleviate burnout. *NAM Perspectives.* 2018;8(1). doi:10.31478/201801c

12. Vîrgă D, Baciu E-L, Lazăr T-A, Lupşa D. Psychological capital protects social workers from burnout and secondary traumatic stress. *Sustainability.* 2020; 12(6):2246. doi:10.3390/su12062246

13. Barol B. Learning from a person's biography: an introduction to the biographical timeline process. *Positive Approaches.* 2001;3(4):20-29.

14. Circle of Security International. Accessed June 27, 2023. https://www.circleofsecurityinternational.com/

Primary, Secondary, and Tertiary Prevention of Childhood Maltreatment

Caelan Soma, PsyD, LP, LMSW

Objectives

After reading this chapter, the reader will be able to:

1. Describe how child maltreatment affects brain function, cognitive issues, emotions, and behavior.

2. Identify risk and protective factors for child maltreatment.

3. Describe the 3 levels of child maltreatment prevention.

Background and Significance

Child maltreatment is a significant problem associated with long-term adverse effects. Despite the increased awareness of child maltreatment and its economic burden, over 600 000 children are maltreated each year. The United States Department of Health and Human Services' 2020 report[1] indicated the estimated number of childhood maltreatment victims in 2020 was 618 000. It is important to highlight that child maltreatment is tremendously underreported, and therefore, these statistics are likely much higher than the provided estimates.[2,3] The national rounded number of children who received a child protective services (CPS) investigation response or alternative response in 2020 was 3 145 000.[1] Data show that 76.1% of victims experienced neglect, 16.5% were physically abused, 9.4% were sexually abused, and .2% were sex trafficked. The national estimate of victims who died from abuse and neglect decreased from 1830 for the Federal Fiscal Year (FFY) 2019 to 1750 for FFY 2020, decreasing the mortality rate from 2.48 per 100 000 children to 2.38 per 100 000 children in the population.[1]

Impact of Child Maltreatment

The profound, negative impact of child maltreatment on brain development and functioning is well documented. Child maltreatment impacts all aspects of a child's health, and the effects are observable in behavior, emotional wellbeing, interpersonal relationships, cognitive functioning, and physical and mental health outcomes.

Effects on Brain Function

Research that links child maltreatment and changes in the brain structure and development has been growing consistently. Evidence shows that early relational trauma (eg, abuse and neglect) results in a broad range of consequences on brain function, including deficits in the deep and outer portions of the brain (ie, the regions responsible for processing social-emotional information, language, motor skills, and cognitive functions).[4]

Both positive and negative experiences affect brain development. Strong brain connections and functions are established when infants are cared for in ways that meet their physical and emotional needs. However, when caregivers respond with abuse or do not respond to infants' needs at all, brain pathways are impaired. This impairment is a result of prolonged and exaggerated stress responses, which cause intense dysregulation of the brain and central nervous system. The earlier in a child's life abuse occurs, the more severe the effects are on brain development and functioning, as much of the brain's development occurs between infancy and age 3. By 3 years of age, a child's brain has reached almost 90% of its adult size.[5]

Statistics indicate that the younger a child is, the more they are at risk of experiencing maltreatment, with 1 in 40 infants victimized by abuse every year.[5] With early prevention and interventions, however, the brain can heal over time. This is due to the unique plasticity of a child's brain and its ability to create new neuronal pathways by replacing older, negative experiences with newer, positive ones. Exposing a maltreated child to consistent, repeated, positive experiences with others can change their brain chemistry in positive ways and build resilience.[5]

COGNITIVE ISSUES

Most childhood trauma has been shown to significantly compromise cognitive development and can occur at any age. Cognitive deficits such as difficulties with focus and concentration and poor problem solving have been linked to traumatic life events.[4,6,7] This is because trauma causes a reduction in the volume of the hippocampus, the region of the brain central to learning and memory. Furthermore, stress induces the release of glucocorticoids, such as cortisol, that can damage the hippocampal area of the brain, further decreasing cognitive functions.[8]

EMOTIONAL AND BEHAVIORAL IMPACT

Childhood trauma has significant adverse emotional consequences. For example, maltreatment can lead to low self-esteem, depression, loss of future orientation, and hopelessness, and it can greatly deteriorate one's ability to regulate overall stress. The dysregulation of emotions often leads to aggression, agitation, withdrawal, loss of small motor activities, and an inability to sleep.[9] Behavioral changes in children with a history of trauma are often misread as willful resistance, stubbornness, impulsiveness, or confrontational, and the children are commonly diagnosed with anxiety, mood disorders, or disruptive behavior disorders. The overlapping symptoms and reactions between trauma and other mental health disorders are significant.

LONG-TERM PERSONAL AND SOCIETAL CONSEQUENCES

The landmark Adverse Childhood Experiences (ACEs) study conducted in 1998 was the first of its kind to find a graded relationship between the number of categories of childhood exposure to adversity and each of the adult health risk behaviors and diseases that were studied. Since this time, hundreds of researchers have investigated and found similar connections between childhood adversity and later adverse mental and physical health outcomes. In the initial study, persons who had experienced 4 or more of 7 possible categories of adverse childhood exposure had a 4 to 12 times increase in health risks for alcoholism, drug abuse, depression, and suicide attempts when compared to those who had not experienced any. They also had a 2 to 4 times increase in smoking and poor self-rated health, as well as a 1.4 to 1.6 times increase in physical inactivity and severe obesity. The number of categories of adverse childhood exposures also showed a graded relationship to the presence of adult diseases, including ischemic heart disease, cancer, chronic lung disease, skeletal fractures, and liver disease. The 7 categories of ACEs were strongly interrelated, and persons with multiple categories of childhood exposure were likely to have multiple health risk factors later in life. Maltreatment, both direct and indirect, has tremendous negative effects on public health due to its resulting increase in medical and mental health issues such as eating disorders, altered immune function, anxiety, and aggressive behavior.[10]

These outcomes in turn correlate with social problems such as homelessness, parenting difficulties, unemployment, and the increased utilization of public and private resources.[2] According to the National Child Abuse and Neglect Data System (NCANDS),[2] child maltreatment statistics for 2015 estimated the United States population's economic burden of child maltreatment based on *substantiated* incident cases (482 000 nonfatal and 1670 fatal) was $428 billion, which represented the lifetime costs incurred by the victims of the aforementioned incident cases. Using the estimated incidences of *investigated* annual incident cases (2 368 000 nonfatal and 1670 fatal), the estimated economic burden was $2 trillion. Evidence-based prevention efforts that reduce maltreatment incidence might offset these costs.[3]

CHILDHOOD MALTREATMENT RISK AND PROTECTIVE FACTORS

It is widely recognized that several risk factors are associated with the occurrence of child maltreatment. Risk factors for overall maltreatment, including abuse and neglect, include stress and negative life events, death of either parent, mental health issues, substance abuse, low socioeconomic status, unstable housing, poor parental skills, young maternal age, large family, single-parent family, parental childhood experience of maltreatment, spousal violence between parents, lack of social support, and unplanned pregnancy. Risk indicators specific to sexual abuse include living in a family without a biological parent, growing up in a family with poor marital relations between parents, living with a non-biological caregiver (eg, a step-parent), poor child-parent relationships, unhappy family life, and maternal employment out of the home.[1,11] Child risk factors include being younger than the age of 5, having behavior problems, and having developmental delays.

Factors that protect or buffer children from being maltreated are known as protective factors. Supportive family environments and social networks consistently emerge as protective factors; other factors such as parental employment, adequate housing, and access to health care and social services may also serve to protect against child abuse and neglect. These factors are protective because they help support children's self-regulation skills, social competence, adaptive functioning, and self-esteem.[11]

PREVENTION LEVELS

Prevention science is grounded in the concept that adverse health, developmental, mental health, and life course outcomes are attributable to a variety of empirically-based risk and protective factors. Thus, to be effective, prevention strategies need to reduce risk factors and enhance protective factors among individuals, families, and their social ecologies.[12]

Many described efforts to prevent child maltreatment fall on a continuum from broad to specific, labeling the points on this continuum as primary, secondary, and tertiary prevention.[2,13-15] Primary services are for all families, regardless of risk level, and are designed to prevent child maltreatment in the same way that taking multivitamins prevents colds or other illnesses. In contrast, secondary prevention services target a certain population of children because of their perceived elevated risk level and documented exposure to maltreatment. Secondary prevention is initiated much like crisis intervention or first aid. While the targets for this type of prevention have been exposed to violence—either as witness or victim—they are not perceived as suffering from apparent reactions to or symptoms of the exposure of maltreatment. Prevention services for child maltreatment at the tertiary level are the most comprehensive. These services are directed at groups that are suffering from the consequences of child maltreatment and are exhibiting signs of traumatic exposure. Therefore, tertiary prevention functions much like when an individual receives medical treatment or undergoes surgery in attempt to minimize the symptoms and reactions of their illness or injury.[16]

Although shutdowns due to COVID-19 affected the delivery of child maltreatment prevention programs, the technology-mediated approaches that emerged reduced the time and training associated with implementing new practices and are promising.[17] For example, web-based programs that provide video-based psychoeducation and modeling directly to parents have been established. Data strongly support its feasibility and indicate that providers spend significantly less time on several activities in preparation for and during sessions, as well as during follow-up sessions compared to in-person sessions.[17]

Primary Prevention

Primary prevention activities are directed at the general population and aim to prevent maltreatment before it occurs or strive to reduce, control, or eliminate maltreatment. Primary prevention activities with a universal focus seek to raise awareness among the public, service providers, and decision makers about the scope of child maltreatment and the problems associated with it. This approach aims to prevent maltreatment by promoting protective factors for optimal family functioning.

Universal approaches to primary prevention include[18]:

— Public service announcements that encourage positive parenting

— Parent education programs and support groups that focus on child development, age-appropriate expectations, and the roles and responsibilities of parenting

— Family support and family strengthening programs that enhance the ability of families to access existing services and resources that support positive interactions among family members

— Public awareness campaigns that provide information on how and where to report suspected child abuse and neglect

— Early childhood education programs (ECEPs)

— Routine primary prevention programs in pediatric care clinics

— School-based programs

— Community education

ECEPs are excellent resources for preventing child maltreatment, as they aim to promote healthy development and prevent negative outcomes for children. These programs are listed as primary prevention because they benefit all families, helping to prevent child maltreatment by addressing multiple problems at multiple levels across multiple settings. While the content and structure of programs vary, they all share the common goal of providing early intervention in the form of education to parents and caregivers about human development and the kinds of environments in which children flourish.[12]

There has been an increase in the delivery of clinic-based, routine primary prevention programs in pediatric care clinics. During pediatric visits, a child development specialist or social worker provides parenting guidance and case management services. Clinic-based models show promise with respect to preventing maltreatment and promoting positive parenting practices within pediatric care.[19]

Schools are also an excellent place to share information about prevention, as they are safe spaces to communicate with children, often before they are affected by maltreatment. Many programs are aimed at preventing sexual abuse and involve discussions, modeling, and interactive learning with role-play or behavioral skills rehearsal. Findings conclude that school-based programs can have a positive effect on self-protection, personal safety knowledge, awareness of others' behavioral intentions, and knowledge about abusive behaviors. The programs that are longer in length and include an experiential component for children are the most effective.[20]

Community education and mobilization is the final primary prevention tactic, with strategies including media campaigns and global parenting education about topics such as abusive head trauma and shaken baby syndrome. Results from community education programs documented enhanced parental self-efficacy and knowledge of concepts and actions relevant to preventing child abuse. However, findings from evaluations of media campaigns to prevent child sexual abuse are somewhat mixed.[21] Community mobilization efforts to prevent child maltreatment often utilize volunteers and community members to support families. Benefits often include decreases in parental stress, substantiated child maltreatment, and childhood injuries related to maltreatment, as well as enhanced social support, collective efficacy, child safety, and parenting practices.

SECONDARY PREVENTION

Secondary prevention seeks to identify and stop child maltreatment at its earliest stage, before noticeable symptoms arise, to reduce the recurrence of maltreatment and any related impairment. Secondary prevention activities with a high-risk focus are offered to families with one or more risk factors, and the programs target services for the communities and neighborhoods that have high incidence of any and all risk factors. Approaches to prevention programs that focus on at-risk populations include[18]:

— Parent education programs located in high schools which focus on teen parents or those in substance abuse treatment programs for mothers and families with young children

— Support groups that help parents deal with their everyday stresses and meet the challenges and responsibilities of parenting

— Home visitation programs that provide support and assistance to expecting and new mothers in their homes

— Respite care for families that have children with special needs

— Family resource centers that offer information and referral services to families living in low-income neighborhoods

Home visitation programs involve home visits between a family and a professional home visitor (eg, a nurse or social worker). Typically, issues like parenting skills, health care, and child development education are addressed, and some programs also provide employment education support. One of the strongest advantages of home visitation programs is the elimination of common barriers to receiving services for children at risk for maltreatment. Research documents the positive impact of several high-quality home visitation programs on global parenting and maltreatment-specific outcomes.[11,12,22]

Home visitation programs are incredibly beneficial for families. In the secondary tier of prevention, these visits address at-risk family functioning and may focus on improving parenting and child outcomes. Typically, they are also longer in duration than those in the first tier of prevention. Many have a foundation in attachment theory and focus on promoting positive parent-child interaction. Research demonstrates the benefits of several high-quality home visitation models with respect to maltreatment risk, specifically in increased sensitive and responsive parenting, strengthened relationships, less physical punishment, improved child safety, and reduced child abuse recidivism.[12]

Intervention programs are also part of secondary prevention and fall into 2 categories. The first addresses parental risks, focusing on specific risk factors for maltreatment. Typically, they focus on parents with substance abuse problems and parents affected by intimate partner violence.[23]

The second type of intervention focuses on parent interventions. Parent management intervention programs are typically grounded in social cognitive theory with the aim to reduce maltreatment by increasing parent behavior management skills. Research has found these interventions to be effective at reducing harsh parenting behaviors, thereby lessening reports of physical abuse and child welfare recidivism.[24] Some argue that any maltreatment results in symptomology; however, if maltreatment is identified at this level and intervention is initiated, positive outcomes are likely.

TERTIARY PREVENTION

Tertiary prevention is initiated when maltreatment has taken place and symptomology is present. Treatment and intervention are intended to facilitate healing, reduce negative consequences of the maltreatment, and prevent its recurrence. These prevention programs include services such as[18]:

— Parent mentor programs with stable, non-abusive families acting as role models and providing support to families in crisis

— Trauma-focused cognitive behavioral therapy (TF-CBT)

— Mental health services for children and families affected by maltreatment to improve family communication and functioning, including Alternatives for Families – Cognitive Behavioral Therapy (AF-CBT), Attachment, Self-regulation and Competence (ARC), and Child-Parent Psychotherapy (CPP)

TF-CBT is used with children and adolescents who have experienced one or more traumas in their life in a variety of settings, including parental homes, foster care, kinship care, group homes, outpatient behavior health care, and residential programs. TF-CBT has proven successful with children and adolescents who have significant emotional problems, trauma symptomology, anxiety, and depression.[24] Evaluations of relationship-based programs have also shown benefits for families in regard to maltreatment risk. CPP has resulted in increases in secure attachment and decreases in disorganized attachment, behavior problems, and trauma-related symptoms. Additionally, there have been decreases in parenting stress, maternal psychopathology, and fewer families involved with CPS.[25]

AF-CBT is a trauma-informed, evidence-based treatment designed to improve the relationships between children and caregivers in families involved in arguments, frequent conflict, physical force/discipline, child physical abuse, or child behavior problems. It is appropriate for use with physically coercive/abusive parents and their school-age children. It is used primarily in outpatient and in-home settings.

ARC is a framework for intervention with children and families who have experienced multiple or prolonged traumatic stress. ARC identifies 3 core domains that are both frequently impacted among traumatized children and relevant to future resiliency. Designed to be applied flexibly across child-serving and family-serving systems, ARC provides a theoretical framework, core principles of intervention, and a guiding structure for providers. ARC is designed for children and adolescents and their caregivers or caregiving systems.

CPP is an intervention model for children aged 0 to 6 years who have experienced at least one traumatic event and are experiencing mental health, attachment, or behavioral problems, including post-traumatic stress disorder. The treatment is based in attachment theory but also integrates psychodynamic, developmental, trauma, social learning, and cognitive behavioral theories. Therapeutic sessions include the child and parent or primary caregiver. The primary goal of CPP is to support and strengthen the relationship between a child and their caregiver as a vehicle for restoring the child's cognitive, behavioral, and social functioning. Treatment also focuses on contextual factors that may affect the caregiver-child relationship.

Case Study

Case Study 9-1

Patricia and Mark Allen were a couple raising 3 children between the ages of 2 and 6. The family was struggling financially, with Mark working full-time at night and Patricia working 2 part-time jobs in addition to caring for their children. They noticed that their oldest child, Charlie, had developed behavioral issues at home, and recently begun refusing to get up for school, causing his mother to take him to school late several times after he missed the bus. His parents tried raising their voices, threatening to take away his video games, and spanking Charlie several times, but his behavior did not improve. One morning, when bringing him late to school, Patricia noticed a flyer in the office for free parenting classes offered at a local community center, and she decided to attend.

Discussion

The Allen family has several stressors and other factors that may put them at risk for experiencing maltreatment. For example, financial struggles, having a greater number of children, and already utilizing physical discipline are all risk factors for child maltreatment. Assuming the parenting classes are offered to all members of the community, they could represent primary prevention by helping parents manage stress, find more effective, non-physical discipline techniques, and foster positive parent-child relationships. For example, Patricia may find it is more effective to consistently follow through with more effective punishment than to simply threaten a punishment, and the program could likewise help Patricia be more mindful of noticing and praising Charlie's positive behavior. The program may be more effective if it is time-limited, as families such as the Allens may have barriers to attending many sessions and may be looking for quick tips that can be implemented right away. The program may also be more effective if it provides referrals to other resources (eg, to help reduce the family's financial needs) or services (eg, more intensive secondary prevention efforts if the parenting classes are not sufficient to meet the needs of the family). Finally, the program may be more effective if both parents are able to attend. However, this may not be possible due to barriers such as work schedules. In such cases, the parent who attends the program should be encouraged to share handouts and other information with their partner.

Key Points

1. The long-term benefits of child maltreatment prevention include improved overall wellbeing and saving millions of dollars in the United States alone.

2. Primary prevention activities with a universal focus seek to raise awareness of the public, service providers, and decision makers about the scope and problems associated with child maltreatment.

3. Secondary prevention activities with a high-risk focus are offered to populations that have one or more risk factors associated with child maltreatment, such as poverty, parental substance abuse, young parental age, parental mental health concerns, and parental or child disabilities.

4. Tertiary prevention is initiated when maltreatment has taken place and symptomology is present.

References

1. Children's Bureau. *Child Maltreatment 2020*. US Department of Health and Human Services; January 2022. Updated June 2023. https://www.acf.hhs.gov/sites/default/files/documents/cb/cm2020.pdf

2. Peterson C, Florence C, Klevens J. The economic burden of childhood maltreatment in the United States, 2015. *Child Abuse Negl*. 2018;86:178-183. doi:10.1016/j.chiabus.2018.09.018

3. Klika JB, Rosenzweig J, Merrick M. Economic burden of known cases of child maltreatment from 2018 in each state. *Child Adolesc Social Work J*. 2020; 37(3):227-234. doi:10.1007/s10560-020-00665-5

4. Austin AE, Lesak AM, Shanahan ME. Risk and protective factors for child maltreatment: a review. *Curr Epidemiol Rep*. 2020;7(4):334-342. doi:10.1007/s40471-020-00252-3

5. Child maltreatment and brain development: a primer for child welfare professionals. Children's Bureau. US Department of Health and Human Services. March 2023. https://www.childwelfare.gov/pubs/issue-briefs/brain-development/

6. Kennedy JM, Lazoritz S, Palusci VJ. Risk factors for child maltreatment fatalities in a national pediatric inpatient database. *Hosp Pediatr.* 2020;10(3):230-237. doi:10.1542/hpeds.2019-0229

7. Bremner JD, Wittbrodt MT. Stress, the brain, and trauma spectrum disorders. *Int Rev Neurobiol.* 2020;152:1-22. doi:10.1016/bs.irn.2020.01.004

8. Bakermans-Kranenburg MJ. The limits of the attachment network. *New Dir Child Adolesc Dev.* 2021;180:117-124. doi:10.1002/cad.20432

9. Sherin JE, Nemeroff CB. Post-traumatic stress disorder: the neurobiological impact of psychological trauma. *Dialogues Clin Neurosci.* 2011;13(3):263-278. doi:10.31887/DCNS.2011.13.2/jsherin

10. Kisely S, Abajobir AA, Mills R, Strathearn L, Clavarino A, Najman JM. Child maltreatment and mental health problems in adulthood: birth cohort study. *Br J Psych.* 2018;213(6):698-703. doi:10.1192/bjp.2018.207

11. Child maltreatment: Risk and protective factors. Centers for Disease Control and Prevention. 2015. https://www.cdc.gov/violenceprevention/childabuseandneglect/riskprotectivefactors.html

12. Harden B, Simons C, Johnson-Motoyama M, Barth R. The child maltreatment prevention landscape: where are we now and where should we go? *Ann Am Acad Pol Soc Sci.* 2020;692(1):97-118. doi:10.1177/0002716220978361

13. Self-Brown S, Reuben K, Perry E, et al. The impact of COVID-19 on the delivery of an evidence-based child maltreatment prevention program: understanding the perspectives of SafeCare providers. *J Fam Violence.* 2020;37(5):825-835. doi:10.1007/s10896-020-00217-6

14. Fortson B, Klevens J, Merrick M, Gilbert LK, Alexander SP. *Preventing Child Abuse and Neglect: A Technical Package for Policy, Norm, and Programmatic Activities.* National Center for Injury Prevention and Control, Centers for Disease Control and Prevention; 2016. https://www.cdc.gov/violenceprevention/pdf/can-prevention-technical-package.pdf

15. Children's Bureau. *Child Maltreatment 2019.* US Department of Health and Human Services; January 2021. Updated June 2023. https://www.acf.hhs.gov/sites/default/files/documents/cb/cm2019.pdf

16. Preventing multiple forms of violence: a strategic vision for connecting the dots. National Center for Injury Prevention and Control, Centers for Disease Control and Prevention; 2016. https://www.cdc.gov/violenceprevention/pdf/strategic_vision.pdf

17. Chen M, Chan KL. Effects of parenting programs on child maltreatment prevention: a meta-analysis. *Trauma Violence Abuse.* 2016;17(1):88-104. doi:10.1177/1524838014566718

18. Child Maltreatment. Children's Bureau, Administration for Children and Families. US Department of Health and Human Services. Updated June 2023. https://www.acf.hhs.gov/cb/data-research/child-maltreatment

19. Walsh K, Zwi K, Woolfenden S, Shlonsky A. School-based education programs for the prevention of child sexual abuse. *Res Soc Work Pract.* 2018;28(1):33-55. doi:10.1177/1049731515619705

20. Mikton C, Butchart A. Child maltreatment prevention: a systematic review of reviews. *Bull World Health Org.* 2009;87:353-361. doi:10.2471/blt.08.057075

21. Stronach EP, Toth SL, Rogosch F, Cicchetti D. Prevention intervention and sustained attachment security in maltreated children. *Dev Psychopathol.* 2013;25 (4.1):919-930. doi:10.1017/S0954579413000278

22. Curry SJ, Krist AH, Owens DK, et al. Interventions to prevent child maltreatment: US Preventive Services Task Force recommendation statement. *JAMA.* 2018;320(20):2122-2128. doi:10.1001/jama.2018.17772

23. Weber L, Kamp-Becker I, Christiansen H, Mingebach T. Treatment of child externalizing behavior problems: a comprehensive review and meta-meta-analysis on effects of parent-based interventions on parental characteristics. *Eur Child Adolesc Psychiat.* 2019;28(8):1025-1036. doi:10.1007/s00787-018-1175-3

24. Farina V, Salemi S, Tatari F, et al. Trauma-focused cognitive behavioral therapy a clinical trial to increase self-efficacy in abused the primary school children. *J Educ Health Promot.* 2018;7:33. doi:10.4103/jehp.jehp_80_17

25. Celano M, NeMoyer A, Stagg A, Scott N. Predictors of treatment completion for families referred to trauma-focused cognitive behavioral therapy after child abuse. *J Trauma Stress.* 2018;31(3):454-459. doi:10.1002/jts.22287

II

INTERSECTIONAL CONSIDERATIONS AND APPLICATIONS

CHILDREN WITH DISABILITIES: A SYSTEMIC RESPONSE FOR SERVICING CHILDREN AND ADOLESCENTS WITH COMPLEX BEHAVIORAL SUPPORT NEEDS

Nancy Thaler, MHOS
Beth I. Barol, PhD, LSW, BCB, NADD-CC

OBJECTIVES

After reading this chapter, the reader will be able to:

1. *Identify the root causes for children and adolescents with developmental disabilities being classified as "complex cases."*

2. *Become acquainted with clinical and support services that prioritize a healthy environment and stable relationships.*

3. *Recognize the value of cross-systems collaboration and identify how resources can be braided and blended to help a child or adolescent get the care and support they need.*

BACKGROUND AND SIGNIFICANCE

The words "No provider will serve them" often indicates that the service system is failing a young person in great need. "People with complex behaviors" is the language commonly used to describe individuals who are "difficult" to serve. They may present challenging behaviors and, typically, they are dually diagnosed with intellectual and developmental disability (ID) and co-occurring mental illness. Regardless of the label, the challenge is the same, as these individuals present behavior that is often dangerous to themselves or others around them. They have behaviors they cannot control, and these behaviors may be perceived as strange or frightening. This chapter will explore the dynamics of complex cases and the systemic responses that are in place to address this shortfall.

Professionals in the field are learning from the many children and adults who have challenged and pushed them to find ways to help each individual. Many providers have expanded their knowledge base, individualized services, and learned to serve people with creativity and commitment. However, there are still many children and adults who are underserved and at risk of becoming what is termed a "complex case."

New knowledge and additional resources have been acquired over time; professionals know more about diagnoses such as autism spectrum disorder (ASD), anxiety, and bipolar disorder, and there are new medications that are diagnostically driven, often replacing the traditional use of neuroleptic medications targeted towards sedation and behavior control. Additionally, more is known about trauma—which those with disabilities suffer at a higher rate than those without—and the profound impact it has on a person's ability to function. There are new therapeutic interventions designed for trauma that show positive results.

Less than a year after the Pennsylvania Department of Human Services (DHS)[1] published its *Bulletin on Complex Case Planning for Children and Youth Under Age 21,* more than 50 children and teenagers across the commonwealth were referred to DHS with an urgent request for assistance. An analysis of the information about these first 50 individuals tells us something about who they are and what their needs are. This group was not a random sample; they were simply the first referrals sent to DHS after the bulletin's implementation. However, because there are similarities in their histories and needs, information can be gleaned regarding the efforts to improve services for children and adolescents with similar needs. The most significant information gleaned from a review of available records follows.[2] Behavior is the issue that was always identified as the reason a provider was not willing to serve a child. The most common descriptions of problematic behavior include:

— Hyperactivity

— Failure to bond

— Aggression/hurting others

— Screaming

— Sleep disturbance

— Property destruction

— Fire setting

— Refusal to cooperate

— Elopement

— Theft

— Cannabis use

— Enuresis/feces smearing

— Pica (an eating disorder where a person eats non-food items)

— Suicidal ideation

— Self-harm (eg, self-hitting, head banging, self-mutilation, running into traffic, attempted suicide)

— Sexual acting out (eg, public masturbation, promiscuity, predatory behavior)

A majority (77%) of these behaviors were exhibited by teenagers and young adults aged 14 to 19 years, with more than half (65%) being boys. A majority (76%) of those teens had at least 5 out-of-home placements at the time of referral, some having as many as 20. Many of these children (38%) were from adoptive or foster families. Furthermore, most of them were served by multiple systems of care, as all were eligible for services from the Office of Children, Youth and Families (OCYF), the Office of Mental Health and Substance Abuse Services (OMHSAS), the Office of Developmental Programs (ODP), and in a few cases, the justice system. Many also received services from local programs such as shelters designed to serve children and adolescents.

A significant majority (84%) of these individuals had at least 1 mental health diagnosis combined with 1 or more developmental disabilities. 68% had a history of ***complex trauma***, which is defined as trauma that occurs early in life and is persistent. The trauma experienced was most often identified as neglect and physical or sexual abuse. Over 36% of the cases had diagnoses but no histories in the records. Diagnoses were based on the presenting behaviors alone. When one considers the lived experience of these children, they can surmise that there were in fact significant traumatic instances in each of their lives that would warrant a trauma-informed approach to their treatment. Complex presenting behaviors, and the fact that the services systems had exhausted their resources and run out of options, indicated that the traumas in these children's lives had been compounding for years. Therefore, the actual percentage of children and adolescents presenting as complex cases is considered to be closer to 100%, all with a history of complex trauma.

Most older adolescents that are considered complex cases do not have a home or family to go to. They generally do not meet the criteria for admission to a hospital or residential treatment facility (RTF) either, so they are placed in temporary placements, such as homeless shelters, in hotel rooms staffed by OCYF personnel, extended stays in hospitals and RTFs, and are pending a suitable plan. Additionally, 16% have chronic physical health problems such as type 1 and type 2 diabetes, hypothyroidism, or epilepsy.[2]

Some children and adolescents that receive services have been identified as having issues that require special attention. These include sexual identity exploration and problematic sexual behavior (ie, self-exposure, "sexualized behavior," aggression, and suicidal ideation).

PRINCIPLES FOR HELPING AN INDIVIDUAL
A SUCCESSFUL ORIENTATION
In the case of the Pennsylvania's DHS study, interviews with DHS regional staff, county staff, and case managers provided insights on what worked for the children as a result of their collaboration. Counties, managed care organizations, and providers in many areas of the state reported working together and innovating new treatments. Success, as defined by the problematic behavior subsiding and the child engaging in school and in the broader community, is more likely when cross-system teams work together to understand the needs of these children and adolescents as well as develop solutions. When local systems collaborate and work as a team (eg, using a system of care approach with the principles of the children and adolescent service system program [CASSP]), it is far more likely that a solution, such as the child being provided a place to live enriched by well trained and supportive staff, will be found. Collaboration would include professionals from agencies according to the needs of the child needing support (eg, supports coordinator, medical social worker, nurse, psychotherapist, psychiatrist, speech therapist, teachers, representatives from the Home and Community Based Service System).[3]

CREATING A POSITIVE SCHOOL AND HOME ENVIRONMENT
A positive environment typically involves[3]:

— A setting for just a few or for a single individual.

— A setting that is trauma-informed to assure there is no inadvertent re-traumatizing. This, of course, requires knowing an individual's trauma history.

— Enhanced staffing at a 1:1, sometimes 2:1 ratio, until the person is stable and resilient with no more threat of danger to themself or others.

— Routines and activities to match the individual's emotional state.

— Activities that build on the individual's strengths and preferences so that they experience success and develop self-confidence and self-esteem.

— Treatment, including for trauma, that is aligned with the individual's diagnoses.

It is vital here to focus on some of the key elements for success. Children and adolescents thrive when their providers focus on building trust and relationships. This includes, when possible, strengthening supportive ties with friends and relatives and developing and maintaining consistent, trained staff and caregivers who are committed to those in their care.

In many cases, the system itself must make modifications in order to provide a restorative environment and effective treatment. Negotiated or enhanced rates are often necessary to support more individualized living arrangements, higher staffing ratios, and specialized services that are evidence-based but not typically available.

Trauma and its Effects

Trauma is a major factor in the lives of most of the children and adolescents who have been referred to DHS. Their trauma generally begins in early childhood and often goes unrecognized as the root cause of their behavior. Despite descriptions of extensive trauma in their records, rarely will that trauma be identified as a diagnosis or be factored into their treatment plan.

Trauma that occurs in childhood is commonly known as developmental trauma, complex trauma, or neurodevelopmental trauma. Developmental trauma differs considerably from post-traumatic stress disorder (PTSD), as an adult who experiences trauma and develops PTSD has—presumably—a "normal" childhood to fall back on. However, when the trauma happens during a child's development, it severely undermines the child's ability to form secure relationships with adults and peers, and it interrupts their development in terms of emotion expression and management.[4] The diagnosis "dysregulation," which refers to an inability to manage thoughts and emotions, thereby giving a person difficulty in controlling their impulses and behaviors, often appears somewhere in the affected child's chart.

How a patient behaves, learns, and relates to people is rooted in their early childhood experiences. A child raised in the security of a loving environment will develop healthy relationships, trust adults, and learn from their environment. A child who experiences serious neglect and abuse will often develop survival behaviors that may be functional in the environment where the trauma has occurred but are dysfunctional in other environments. Fight, flight, or freeze are the words used to describe the response to trauma. Behaviors such as running away, hitting, or lying can be functional survival strategies, but they do not work in healthier, non-traumatic environments.[5]

Trauma and Developmental Disabilities

All forms of trauma affect brain development. Trauma to the head itself, such as a diagnosed concussion or traumatic brain injury, can damage the brain and compromise the full range of cognitive functions and adaptive skills.[4,5] Childhood emotional trauma that causes a dominant flight or fight response within the developing brain is often linked to a developmental delay across several domains, including cognitive functioning and language and motor development, as it makes survival the dominant mode in the brain rather than allocating brain development resources to social and cognitive development and functioning.[6]

Children born with a developmental disability are 1.5 to 10 times more likely to be victims of trauma than children without disabilities, and they are more profoundly affected by it, as their difficulties in understanding, problem solving, and communicating can intensify the trauma.

The behavior in traumatized children and adolescents with developmental disabilities is often not recognized as trauma-related but is instead interpreted as "negative behavior" that stems from their disability, thereby needing to be controlled and modified. It is vital to understand that in addition to the typical behaviors seen from traumatized children and adolescents without developmental disabilities (eg, elopement, drug use, stealing, self-harm), face slapping, head banging, feces smearing, self-stimulating, and self-soothing behaviors are also observed from traumatized children and adolescents with developmental disabilities. Once this is understood, the presence of trauma can be better identified, and the development of appropriate supports and interventions can begin.[6-8]

It is important to acknowledge, however, that self-abusive behaviors are not always the result of trauma. Particularly in neurodiverse children with ASD, the behavior may be a response to stress or anxiety, or it may be an effort to communicate when the child does not have verbal communication capabilities. It is important to conduct a full functional assessment as well as a social history (such as a biographical timeline, as discussed in Volume 1, Chapter 6: Biographical Timelines) to determine the reason for the behavior.

Conventional treatment modalities utilized for neurotypical adults with PTSD are often not effective with children with developmental disabilities. One of these, cognitive behavioral therapy (CBT), is an intervention frequently used for adults and can require a level of interaction that children and adolescents with developmental disabilities can find difficult or impossible. However, eye movement desensitization and reprocessing (EMDR),[8] is an evidence-based therapy that does not require cognition-based interaction, and therefore can be effective. Other models of therapy that are widely used to treat developmental trauma include play therapy, art therapy, therapies using animals, occupational therapy, neurofeedback, various approaches of developmental psychotherapy, and group activities ranging from peer discussion groups to sports or singing.

FETAL ALCOHOL SYNDROME AND LEAD POISONING
Both fetal alcohol syndrome (FAS) and lead poisoning are often underidentified external/chemical/substance insults that affect brain development and can result in poor reasoning and judgement, difficulty with attention, impaired memory, irritability, deficits in adaptive behavior, or problems with socialization or self-regulation. A child may have these conditions without having a developmental disability diagnosis, and yet the challenges are the same. Recognizing the presence of either of these conditions is important to securing the right physical health services and behavioral health supports.

DOING WHAT WORKS: PRACTICES THAT SUPPORT THE RECOVERY OF CHILDREN FROM THE SEQUELAE OF THE EXPERIENCE OF TRAUMA
SITUATING THE CONTEXT OF COMPLEX CASES
Not all children with problematic behavior have experienced trauma, nor do they all have both mental health and developmental disability diagnoses. However, a plethora of children and adolescents with problematic behavior *do* have multiple diagnoses and trauma, so it is vital to make sure that social histories are exhaustive in an effort to rule out conditions before assumptions are made.

Dr. Daniel Hughes states it plainly in his often used quotation, "Don't ask what the child is doing, ask what has happened to the child."[9] Asking what happened, when it happened, and how long it happened for will lead to an understanding of the behavior and the best method of support. Furthermore, providers should ask:

What was the trauma experience? Who were the perpetrators? What was the location? The answers to these and other questions are critical in developing a treatment plan and a trauma-informed environment. Knowing and consistently sharing the trauma history with direct support staff builds empathy and helps them understand behavior, encouraging them to "hang in there."[10]

FACILITATING RECEPTIVITY

To be open to treatment, an individual must be receptive, and receptivity is dependent on a sense of comfort and trust. The environment should not present them with difficult sounds, experiences, stressors, or interactions, but rather, it should calm the flight/fight/freeze response. Ensuring that nothing triggers the trauma response of the person receiving treatment is of the utmost importance. Providers should keep in mind that the number of people with whom the patient lives and their behaviors will affect the patient's recovery. Providing a living arrangement with a small number of other residents has been effective for many patients, and in instances of extreme behavior, temporarily providing patients with an individual home has also been effective.

EFFECTIVE TEACHING, TREATMENT, AND SUPPORTIVE INTERVENTIONS

The specific diagnoses should be the basis for the type of teaching strategies, treatment, and support approaches that are used. There is an array of options, many of which can be woven into daily life and may be used simultaneously, such as: trauma-focused cognitive behavioral therapy (TF-CBT); applied behavior analysis (ABA); individual therapy; social stories; group therapy; peer counseling; internal family systems therapy (IFST); intensive systems therapy (IST); sex education and counseling; education about the mind and body; mindfulness training; neuroaffective relational model therapy; dyadic developmental psychotherapy[11]; sensory interventions that calm (eg, breathing exercises, weighted blankets, warm baths), swinging; EMDR; bio/neurofeedback; neural entrainment; play therapy; art therapy; music therapy; psychodrama; animal therapy; movement therapy (eg, yoga, tai chi, exercise); and group activities that involve movement with others (eg, drumming, dancing, singing).

THERAPEUTIC CAREGIVING

Whether a child is supported in or out of their family home, the quality of their caregiving is crucial. Staffing ratios must allow for spontaneous, frequent, and responsive interaction. Staff and family members must also be well trained, mentored, and emotionally supported in order to understand the individual's experiences, the reasons for the behavior, and how best to interact with them. Direct supporters must be full members of the interdisciplinary team because they are the ones who spend the most time with the individual; therefore, they can help with trauma recovery and learning new behaviors. Emotionally responsive caregiving will lead to positive change.

CHILDREN IN FOSTER CARE OR ADOPTIVE FAMILIES

38% of children and adolescents who present as having complex behavior to DHS have been in foster care or adoptive families.[2] This raises the question: Are adequate training and supports being provided for alternate families to ensure success for the family and the child? Training, in-home supports, and adequate respite care can be determinant factors of success. If the individual has thoughts like "no one wants me" or "I am not good enough to have a family," it will add to their trauma history and undermine healing interventions. Interventions for children with disabilities in foster care or adoptive families can be found in **Table 10-1**. Additionally, providers must recognize that the cost for care may be greater than the standard reimbursement rate allows, so offering tiered payment plans can directly impact the access children have to care.

Table 10-1. Interventions for Children in Foster Care and Adoptive Families	
INTERVENTION	RELATIONSHIP TO CHILD OUTCOMES
Establish routines and meaningful activities	— Routines create stability and reduce uncertainty. — Stability leads to feelings of competence and success.
Establish healthy eating habits	— Good nutrients encourage mental and physical growth. — Too much caffeine, sugar, and highly processed foods can trigger enzyme and hormonal reactions that interfere with thought processes, sleep, self-control, and the brain's capacity to heal from trauma.[12]
Establish healthy interpersonal relationships	— Having a caring adult increases resilience. — The adult or adults who have this permanent relationship should be considered primary members of the interdisciplinary team.[13]
Establish long-term supports and living arrangements	— Temporary placements and forced relocations can be a trigger for past traumas and reinforce a feeling of homelessness and hopelessness. — Older children and young adults who have been in numerous out-of-home living arrangements and treatment programs often have no family to go back to and are not eligible for a medical facility.

CASE STUDY

Case Study 10-1

Joe, aged 13, lived in a single-parent household with 4 older siblings. His father was no longer around, but when he lived with the family, he used to beat Joe's mother, siblings, and Joe. As the youngest sibling, Joe was the most vulnerable to the abuse and a constant witness of violence in his early years. Joe was not very articulate, was seen as having attention-deficit/hyperactivity disorder (ADHD) and reacted violently under many circumstances. Joe was assessed as having a lower IQ and was placed in "special-ed" classes.

Joe's mom had 2 jobs to keep food on the table. As a result, the siblings had to raise each other. Their mom frequently resorted to punishment to have any control in the household.

At one point, Joe and his siblings had all been placed in foster care due to their mother's inability to care for and provide for them. A case manager connected the family with other systems of support that helped the family get their basic necessities met, including housing, food, and transportation. Eventually, Joe's siblings were allowed to move back home. Joe remained in foster care and was not allowed to move back home. Abandoned by everyone he knew and loved, he was highly reactive, defensive, and hostile. He was moved to several foster homes, often only lasting a couple of weeks before having to move again. After 4 "failed placements," he was moved to an RTF. Joe was seen by caregivers as a "bad kid" who used challenging behaviors to manipulate people. The only approach that was employed by caregivers was a punishment-based behavior modification program, and his challenging behaviors increased in response.

In desperation, a team was convened by Joe's specialized (System of Care) case manager, including his teacher, the school psychologist, and social worker, as well as key staff at the RTF, Joe's mother, a representative from the public behavioral health services, and from the developmental disabilities services system. The group reflected on the child's biographical timeline and recognized the devastating effects of his early traumas, abuse, neglect, and feeling abandoned by the family. Working from the trauma paradigm, they were able to design and advocate for an entirely different treatment model, including somatic regulation, family therapy, reintegration into his family, in-home supports such as an in-home direct supporter (ie, a social therapist) trained in trauma healing to provide guidance, coaching, and reinforcement through creative interactions and meaningful activities. Supports were made available in school as well as at home. Growth and improvement were seen in a short amount of time.

Discussion

The system of care recognized that ongoing support was needed to imbed and continue Joe's progress. They used a person-centered evaluation process to determine when he and his family would be ready to fade the additional supports once everyone was confident that the new lifestyle and resulting positive behaviors were deeply embedded.

KEY POINTS

1. Children and adolescents with co-occurring IDs and mental illness who are considered "complex cases" are often discarded by care systems due to the overshadowing ID diagnosis. However, when it is established that developmental trauma is the root cause of their challenging behaviors, a collaborative, interdisciplinary team, if trained in trauma treatment, can rally to provide effective treatment.

2. While there are many helpful clinical interventions for traumatized children, they are all adjunctive to a healthy relationship with caregivers and supporters. Resilience and healing are built through a healthy lived experience.

3. Cross-systems collaboration, including team building and contributing resources on the micro through the macro intervention level, is vital to ensure that the treatment teams can carry out the agreed upon interventions and keep them in effect over time.

REFERENCES

1. Complex case planning for children and youth under age 21. Pennsylvania Department of Health and Human Services. 2021. https://www.dhs.pa.gov/Services/Children/Pages/Complex-Case-Planning.aspx

2. Thaler N. Serving children and youth with complex behavioral support needs: "No provider will serve him." *Positive Approaches J.* 2021;10(3):58-74.

3. Schober M, Harburger D, Sulzbach D, Zabel M. A Safe Place to Be: Crisis Stabilization Services and Other Supports for Children and Youth. Technical Assistance Collaborative Paper No. 4. Alexandria, VA: National Association of State Mental Health Program Directors. 2022. https://store.samhsa.gov/sites/default/files/nasmhpd-a-safe-place-to-be.pdf

4. The basics of infant and early childhood mental health: a briefing paper. Zero to Three. 2017. https://www.zerotothree.org/resources/1951-the-basics-of-infant-and-early-childhood-mental-health-a-briefing- paper

5. Hambrick E, Brawner T, Perry BD, et al. Restraint and critical incident reduction following introduction of the Neurosequential Model of Therapeutics (NMT). *Resid Treat Child Youth.* 2018;35(2):2-23. doi:10.1080/0886571X.2018.1425651

6. D'Andrea W, Ford J, Stolbach B, Spinazzola J, van der Kolk BA. Understanding interpersonal trauma in children: why we need a developmentally appropriate trauma diagnosis. *Am J Orthopsychiatry.* 2012;82(2):187-200. doi:10.1111/j.1939-0025.2012.01154.x

7. Charlton M, Kliethermes M, Tallant B, Taverne A, Tishelman A. Facts on traumatic stress and children with developmental disabilities. National Child Traumatic Stress Network. 2004. https://www.nctsn.org/resources/facts-traumatic-stress-and-children-developmental-disabilities

8. Barol B, Seubert A. Stepping stones: EMDR treatment of individuals with intellectual and developmental disabilities and challenging behavior. *J EMDR Pract Res.* 2010;4(4):156-169. doi:10.1891/1933-3196.4.4.156

9. Hughes D. Building trust with children who have been hurt in relationships. Pennsylvania Care Partnership. 2021. https://www.pacarepartnership.org/community-partners/webinar-series/dan-hughes-hold-page

10. Barol B. Revisiting the fourfold positive approaches paradigm: environment, communication, assessment, and hanging in there. *Positive Approaches J.* 2019; 1(1):13-26.

11. Hughes DA, Golding KS, Hudson J. *Healing Relational Trauma with Attachment-Focused Interventions*. Norton & Company; 2019.

12. Kharrazian D. *Why Isn't My Brain Working?* Elephant Press; 2013.

13. Sroufe LA, Egeland B, Elizabeth A, Carlson A, Collins WA. *The Development of the Person: The Minnesota Study of Risk and Adaptation from Birth to Adulthood.* Guilford Press; 2005.

Childhood Maltreatment and Trauma-Informed Care in the LGBTQIA+ Community

Ash Moomaw, MA
David T. Solomon, PhD, HSP-P

Objectives

After reading this chapter, the reader will be able to:

1. *Describe the impact of child maltreatment on the LGBTQIA+ community.*

2. *Apply culturally competent skills to working with LGBTQIA+ individuals.*

3. *Apply trauma-informed care principles to their work with LGBTQIA+ survivors of childhood maltreatment.*

Background and Significance

Children and adolescents who are lesbian, gay, bisexual, transgender, queer, intersex, asexual, another sexuality (LGBTQIA+) or are a gender minority (eg, pansexual, gender nonbinary) are at an elevated risk for interpersonal trauma and traumatic systemic discrimination. This vulnerable population makes up around 9.5% of the population between the ages of 13 and 17, according to a survey conducted in 2020. This percentage represents only those individuals who are comfortable reporting their identity, meaning there are likely more children who identify as belonging to the LGBTQIA+ community.[1] Part of understanding these children is understanding the typical experiences of LGBTQIA+ children and adolescents. Negative interpersonal experiences are common for these individuals. LGBTQIA+ children and adolescents may experience more personal discrimination like bullying, harassment, intimate partner violence (IPV), physical and sexual abuse, and traumatic forms of societal stigma, bias, and rejection.[2] In a 2022 national survey,[3] 73% of LGBTQIA+ individuals reported experiencing discrimination based on their identity. This especially affected lesbian, gay, and bisexual individuals as they have been shown consistently over the past several decades to have a higher risk of childhood maltreatment, including physical and sexual abuse.[4-7] Outside of explicit maltreatment, LGBTQIA+ children may also face parental rejection of their identity. Only approximately 30% of LGBTQIA+ children and adolescents identify their home as an affirming space for their sexuality or gender identity. Children and adolescents who reported feeling supported by parents and friends also reported lower rates of suicide attempts, indicating the importance of parental support for LGBTQIA+ children's mental health.[3]

In a national sample of 1177 LGBTQIA+ middle and high school students,[8] nearly 80% reported having experienced some form of child maltreatment. In another large North American survey of 3598 adolescents aged 14 to 18 years, 58% of participants reported a history of emotional neglect, 56% reported emotional abuse, and 43% reported having experienced 4 or more adverse childhood experiences.[9] A 2022 survey reported that 1 out of every 3 LGBTQIA+ children have been physically threatened or harmed due to their identity, and 17% of LGBTQIA+ individuals have experienced or were threatened with conversion therapy, a treatment modality that has been deemed abusive, often occurring to those younger than 18 years of age, by many professionals.[3,10] Additionally, LGBTQIA+ individuals have higher overall rates of sexual assault, particularly transgender individuals and bisexual women.[11]

For individuals with these abusive experiences, their identity as an LGBTQIA+ child decreases the likelihood that others will believe them. This is demonstrated in a study by Miller & London,[12] wherein they asked participants to assume the role of jurors in a hypothetical child sexual abuse legal case. Participants read a vignette where the victim was described as either a cisgender or a transgender child. When the victim was described as transgender, mock jurors were less likely to "convict" the perpetrator and rated the victim as less credible. This was especially true when the victim was described as a transgender girl compared to a transgender boy.

Another important area for professionals to be aware of is the systemic barriers LGBTQIA+ children face. While systemic barriers have always existed for children in this vulnerable community, recently there has been more attention on the impact of discriminatory laws and legislation, such as bills that do such things as: prohibit or criminalize health care for transgender youth; bar transgender youth from being able to participate in sporting events; ban LGBTQIA+ education in schools; and allow health care providers to deny treatment to LGBTQIA+ individuals due to religious beliefs.[13] For these reasons, it is vital that any professional who works with LGBTQIA+ individuals understands the unique needs and experiences of this community, as these laws have increased in number and severity within the year that this book was published, impacting many children and their families' ability to seek out care that best fits their needs. These laws are changing regularly and by state, so each provider should make themselves aware of their state's legislation and keep up to date on how it impacts the LGBTQIA+ children and adolescents they serve.

For LGBTQIA+ children and adolescents, systemic discrimination[3] and traumatic experiences, such as childhood maltreatment or other types of interpersonal trauma, compound each other and can leave lasting impacts on the mental health of children within the LGBTQIA+ community. Additionally, disparities in mental health and substance use are emerging earlier in life, as LGBTQIA+ children are starting to disclose their identities earlier.[14] One study[15] reported mental health disparities between LGBTQIA+ children and cisgender, heterosexual children begin at the age of 10 years, and substance use differences begin at the age of 12 years. These disparities are indicative of the differences in levels of victimization, discrimination, and other traumas reported between LGBTQIA+ children and their peers. The additional stress faced by LGBTQIA+ children and adolescents may be referred to as minority stress, a term that is used to describe the additional stress marginalized individuals face due to systemic factors, such as heterosexual/cisgender normativity, or the assumption that "normal" is any individual who is not LGBTQIA+.[16] In addition, minority stress theory identifies additional proximal and distal stressors such as discrimination, perceived stigma, and internalized biases against one's own identity. For those with multiple marginalized identities, there may be more than one marginalized identity contributing to this stress level.[17] The culmination of these minority stress factors has been shown to act similarly to trauma; a recent review suggested that minority stress experienced by sexual minority individuals leads to neural changes similar to those seen in individuals with post-traumatic stress disorder.[18] A 2022 national survey[3] also reported that 45% of LGBTQIA+ children and adolescents had attempted suicide, a 3% increase from recent years. In a large study of Chinese emerging adults,[19] for LGBTQIA+ participants in particular, a history of suicide attempts was higher for those with a high prevalence of emotional and sexual abuse in childhood. Furthermore, in another study of emerging adults,[20] those with a history of emotional abuse and neglect had heightened levels of depression and anxiety. This is higher in children with multiple adverse experiences, such as being in the welfare system. For example, LGBTQIA+ children in the child welfare system report a higher level of suicidal ideation, suicide attempts, and depression, compared to heterosexual, cisgender children in the child welfare system.[21] LGBTQIA+ children also have an elevated risk of post-traumatic stress disorder due to the abuse and discrimination they experience because of their identity.[22]

The data surrounding the experiences of LGBTQIA+ children and adolescents exemplifies the vital importance of sensitive and competent care from providers for this community. With continued education, understanding, and compassion, professionals within health care fields can hopefully limit the harm done to LGBTQIA+ children and help them to lead healthier lives.

TRAUMA-INFORMED CARE AND LGBTQIA+ CHILDREN

When providing care to LGBTQIA+ children and adolescents who have experienced maltreatment, providers should integrate identity-affirming practices and trauma-informed care. The latter refers to an approach developed by mental health and public health care professionals to create guidance for a constructive way to approach trauma. Trauma-informed care attempts to understand the traumatic experiences an individual has had and respond in a way that accommodates the unique vulnerabilities and needs of those who have experienced trauma.[23] This includes not only recognizing signs and symptoms of trauma an individual may have but also how clients perceive services and how to limit possible re-traumatization.[24] Implementing this care includes the individual actions of clinicians but also larger organizational efforts to create an accommodating and considerate space for patients with trauma.[24] In this section, each area of trauma-informed care will be discussed as well as examples of what this may look like in relation to LGBTQIA+ individuals.

Affirmative care refers to when professionals understand and take into consideration the systemic and social stress factors, like minority stress factors, that negatively impact a client due to their identity. This includes limiting perpetuating these stressors and approaching a client with knowledge of all their identities that may lead them to be marginalized and at increased risk (eg, race, ethnicity, sexual orientation, gender, ability status, etc.)[25] While a full discussion of affirmative practices is beyond the scope of this chapter, more comprehensive reviews are provided by Heck and colleagues[25] and Solomon and colleagues.[26]

Some general recommendations for affirmative care specifically for LGBTQIA+ individuals include:

— Being up to date on terminology for various identities (see Additional Resources section)

—Avoiding the words "preferences" or "preferred" (eg, ask "What are your pronouns?" as opposed to "What are your preferred pronouns?")

— Avoiding deadnaming (ie, calling a transgender or gender nonbinary patient by the name they were assigned at birth that is no longer used)

— Not over-pathologizing their identities by assuming all their struggles are identity-related

Additionally, affirmative practices should be used with *all* clients, as opposed to "turning them on" when a client has identified themselves as LGBTQIA+. For example, if a practitioner assumes that all clients are heterosexual and cisgender, they may ask questions that reflect these assumptions, which could then impact the therapeutic relationship and create a less safe environment for LGBTQIA+ individuals to disclose their identity.

THE PRINCIPLES OF TRAUMA-INFORMED CARE

In trauma-informed care, there are 5 principles outlined by Fallot & Harris[27] that should be understood and implemented: safety, trustworthiness, choice, collaboration, and empowerment. There is some variability in what others may consider to be the core principles of trauma-informed care, but research reviews have identified that key components of all trauma-informed care principles include awareness of trauma, safety, opportunities to rebuild control, and use of the individual's strengths[28] (which are included within the 5 aforementioned principles). With the understanding and use of trauma-informed care principles, LGBTQIA+ children and adolescents who have experienced childhood maltreatment and other trauma may feel more comfortable in health care spaces, thereby allowing for more opportunities for treatment and increased quality of life. Furthermore, trauma-informed care is compatible with other affirmative practices suggested for LGBTQIA+ individuals, given that both approaches focus on collaboration and are egalitarian in the therapeutic relationship.[29] It should be noted that there is some overlap between the principles described below. For example, increasing collaboration with the client may involve offering them choices in treatment and both may increase a client's sense of safety.

The first principle of trauma-informed care is safety. When discussing safety, those who practice trauma-informed care should consider both the physical and emotional safety of the individuals they care for.[30] LGBTQIA+ children may not feel safe in health care spaces for a variety of reasons, including past traumatic experiences with providers. For LGBTQIA+ children and adolescents, negative interactions with health care professionals are not uncommon and may result in increased fear, avoidance, or discomfort in health care settings. In order to communicate physical safety, having an inviting and safely located physical space, as well as taking the necessary precautions for the safety of patients and clients (eg, outside doors that lock to increase safety if there are threats to a client's physical safety, easily accessible restrooms, and adequate space), is the first step in creating an environment that is more welcoming for individuals who have experienced trauma.[23] Additionally, to increase emotional safety, staff should be trained in cultural sensitivity, and paperwork, such as background and demographic questionnaires, should use appropriate language (eg, asking for a client to identify their pronouns without using the word "preferred"). Many therapeutic modalities for individuals who have experienced child maltreatment involve incorporating caregivers into therapy; it is useful to explain to children and adolescents, at the onset, when and how caregivers will be involved as well as the rationale for including caregivers in the process. For LGBTQIA+ children, there are a few ways to incorporate a safer environment, which include things like having gender neutral bathroom options and having LGBTQIA+ support indicated throughout the office (eg, fliers, flags, pronouns pins).[30] Additionally, feedback from LGBTQIA+ patients may be useful in creating a safer environment as well.

Trustworthiness is the second principle of trauma-informed care, and it involves creating transparency as to the procedures, expectations, and boundaries of a care facility or therapeutic relationship. To do this, clear instructions and documentation should be provided to all clients regarding what they should expect from their care providers, and this may include who their care provider will be, goals, methods of treatment, how long they should expect to be there, and any other information that provides clarity into the individual's expected experience.[23] For LGTBQIA+ children, this is a particularly difficult topic to navigate as each state may require differing levels of parental knowledge in different settings. Professionals should stay up to date on their local, state, and federal legislation requirements and update their policies to limit any harm these rules may cause to these vulnerable children.

Professionals should consider having conversations with colleagues and supervisors related to procedures for LGBTQIA+ clients. Additionally, these procedures should be discussed openly and should allow LGBTQIA+ children and adolescents to understand and ask questions related to confidentiality such as what name or pronouns are included in notes, what parents may or may not have to know regarding session content, how much support they have in their identity at home and at school, parental access to notes, and when safety concerns may lead to disclosure of information regarding the client's identity.[31] Additional resources on this topic are provided by Lothwell and colleagues[31] and the publication by the Substance Abuse and Mental Health Services Administration related to serving LGBTQIA+ children (see Additional Resources section).

Furthermore, experts agree that LGBTQIA+ clients should be granted full autonomy in making decisions related to disclosing their identities to others,[32] but this consideration is complicated when the client is a minor. Specifically, for LGBTQIA+ children, it is necessary that the patient be given a clear indication about the possibility of disclosing identity-related matters to their parents. For example, some LGBTQIA+ children may have traumatic experiences with disclosure of their identity that may resurface in a health care space. It is important for clinicians working with children and adolescents to understand the laws related to disclosure and confidentiality for minors, as they can often vary from location to location and include nuanced rules. In many places, if a caregiver has provided consent for the minor to enter treatment, they have a right to inquire about what is said in treatment. However, many states have regulations in place that allow minors, in certain situations, to provide legal consent for treatment and often this allows the minor a greater amount of confidentiality. At the same time, even when a parent has a right to the information about their child's treatment, many states allow provisions to not disclose any information that could reasonably lead to harm to the minor. Thus, if disclosing a child's identity to their parent could lead to maltreatment of the child, then the therapist would be legally and ethically clear to not make such a disclosure. In addition, there is often little reason to spontaneously disclose information about a patient's identity to a caregiver, especially if the patient is not engaging in any potentially harmful behavior related to their identity. Such disclosures should only be made after consideration of the regulations related to the confidentiality of minors as well as the potential benefit or harm to making that disclosure.

The rules related to disclosure and confidentiality should be explained to the patient and the caregiver, and they should have the opportunity to ask questions. In some situations, it may be helpful to have the conversation about confidentiality with both parties at the same time so that everyone knows exactly what was said and can be "on the same page."

When children and adolescents have some involvement with child welfare agencies, therapists may have to update the family's case worker on their progress. In such cases, it is important to establish with all parties what will be included in the progress updates. When confidentiality must be broken, this should be discussed with the patient ahead of time, and the provider should allow them as much autonomy in the process as possible. For example, if any suicidal ideation was expressed that would need to be conveyed to a caregiver to keep the patient safe. The provider should remind the patient of the rules related to confidentially, explain why confidentiality needs to be broken, and provide them with some options as to how the disclosure will occur (eg, if the patient would like to tell their caregiver or rather the provider make the disclosure). Finally, when caregivers do have a right to information discussed with their child in therapy, it may be helpful to mitigate potential issues by *requesting* that the caregiver agree to grant the minor some privacy in treatment. The therapist may say something like: "As a parent, you have a right to ask any questions about what is going on in your child's treatment. However, therapy is likely not going to be as effective if your child is concerned that I am going to tell you the things they say in session. They may even avoid bringing up important topics because of this worry. What I can guarantee you is that if there is anything you need to know to keep your child safe, such as if they are thinking about hurting themself or somebody is hurting them, I will share it with you. What I am asking is that you allow them some privacy with the other topics they bring up in sessions with me. How would you feel about that?"

This conversation is not legally binding, however. The caregiver can always agree and change their mind, but at the very least, this outlines the rationale for privacy, reassures the caregiver that safety will still be maintained, and encourages the caregiver to allow privacy.

Choice is the third principle of trauma-informed care and one that may seem difficult given the legal standing of LGBTQIA+ children as dependents of their caregivers. Individuals who have experienced trauma often feel a lack of control or choice regarding that experience. To create a trauma-informed care environment, the team of providers should examine and communicate to the patient what opportunities for choice and control they can provide within the limits of their care.[33] An example for an LGBTQIA+ child is the choice to discuss their gender identity at length. A provider may ask the child how they identify, then allow them to choose to explain this identity, have the provider do their own research, or limit further conversation on the topic. This gives the child a choice in their communication around their identity and will provide increased control about how they choose to interact with their care provider. It may be that any given topic is revisited later, but allowing choice empowers the child by knowing that they have control over themselves and what they communicate. Furthermore, both small and large choices can be incorporated into the care process. For LGBTQIA+ children, this may look like choosing their own name, pronouns, identity exploration, and topics of conversation; these then may lead to conversations around larger choices, such as gender-affirming care, wherein caregivers may have to be included in the discussion.[33] Even in this instance, the provider can allow the child a choice as to how to approach this topic with their caregivers, even if the discussion itself is not avoidable.

The fourth principle of trauma-informed care is collaboration. Collaboration is the extent to which the facility or provider works with their clients towards limiting the power differential and creating a collaborative care experience. Collaboration may include feedback and incorporation from the person being served into the delivery or a say on the services, rules, practices, and regulations of the facility.[30] Not only does this allow improved care for the current patient, but it also allows for the improvement of care for any future patients.

To reduce the power differential that exists in health care settings, providers should let patients know that they are the experts on their own experience, are respected for these experiences, and therefore are key in constructing and deciding upon goals and priorities in treatment for themselves as individuals and for the facility at large.[23] An example of this approach would be involving a patient in the setting of their goals and priorities for treatment. An LGBTQIA+ child may prioritize creating peer relationships before coming out to family or vice versa. They may also choose to prioritize the immediate effects of mental health concerns such as flashbacks, panic attacks, or suicidality, before exploring their gender identity. Through collaboration, a trauma-informed practitioner would allow the child this choice and would tailor treatment to fit their priorities. Additionally, this provider may continue to ask about priorities in future sessions with LGBTQIA+ children in order to continue the process of collaboration with all clients.

For individuals who are receiving treatment, it is necessary that they are provided with the skills and the fifth principle, empowerment, as they continue their journey. LGBTQIA+ children are part of a stigmatized group, and therefore, they may encounter a variety of difficult life experiences due to their identities. Health care professionals should aim to have a positive impact on these children and provide them with resiliency skills and self-efficacy in an effort to take care of themselves. To do this, professionals should strive to allow for the individual to provide input regarding treatment and goals, create realistic expectations of positive growth, recognize the strength of the individual, and validate and affirm the individual in their experiences and thoughts, especially those that are related to the impact of holding a stigmatized identity.[30] This will provide a positive basis for care that allows continued growth, both during and after health care interactions. For treating an LGBTQIA+ child, this may look like focusing on their strengths and interests and heavily incorporating those into treatment. These strengths can include their strong sense of self and identity gained from being a part of the LGBTQIA+ community or the joy they find in authentically representing their gender identity. By focusing on the positive qualities of an individual while accepting and validating their experiences, health care professionals can create positive experiences that will be the foundation of a healthier person and one that may be more comfortable seeking care when needed.

Providers should use these core principles in order to best fit the needs of the populations they serve, including factors of intersectionality such as race, ethnicity, socioeconomic status, ability status, and various other identity pieces that may factor into the traumatic experiences that an LGBTQIA+ child has had.[33] It is important to have continued collaboration with individuals within these communities so that the provider may better understand the needs of their community, thereby incorporating those needs into a trauma-informed care and practice facility.

CASE STUDY

Case Study 11–1

Dr. Smith had his first appointment with a 14-year-old bisexual child due to concerns related to the child's symptoms of depression and anxiety. The child's mother reported emotional abuse and a lack of acceptance from the child's father related to the child's bisexuality. Upon the child's arrival with their mother, they were provided paperwork and sat in a comfortable and inviting office to complete these documents, which asked several appropriately-worded questions about identity and pronoun use. After finishing the paperwork, both the child and mother were invited back by Dr. Smith where they then shared a brief conversation about the adolescent's needs. Dr. Smith noticed that the child was quiet and looked at their feet often when their mother discussed their identity or past experiences. Dr. Smith, noticing these cues, asked if the client would prefer to talk to Dr. Smith alone for a time about their concerns. The client agreed, and Dr. Smith invited the client's mother back to the waiting room for a moment. Dr. Smith reminded the client about the rules of confidentiality for minors and informed them about things that may or may not need to be shared with their caregiver. After this conversation, the child disclosed that he is a bisexual, transgender boy, and his parents were not aware of his gender identity due to their negative reaction regarding his sexuality. Dr. Smith affirmed the child in his difficult experiences related to the disclosure and thanked him for sharing something that was uncomfortable to discuss. After allowing the client time to share his experiences, Dr. Smith asked the client what his goals for therapy were. Dr. Smith allowed for transparency by giving the child time to ask questions about this process and what his parents would know about his time in therapy.

Discussion

The first trauma-informed care principle of safety is exhibited through the paperwork's questions regarding pronoun use, identity aspects, and various LGBTQIA+ support materials throughout the office. Dr. Smith exemplifies the principle of choice when asking the client if he would like to talk to Dr. Smith without his mother present for a time. Transparency and trustworthiness are used when further discussing confidentiality and allowing the client to ask questions. Empowerment was used when praising the client for his difficult disclosure and through the collaboration of patient and provider to solidify goals that the adolescent is comfortable with.

KEY POINTS
1. LGBTQIA+ children are at a higher risk of trauma and child maltreatment compared to the general population.

2. For LGBTQIA+ survivors of child maltreatment, an integration of identity-affirming practices and trauma-informed care is recommended.

3. The principles of trauma-informed care include safety, trustworthiness, choice, collaboration, and empowerment.

ADDITIONAL RESOURCES

— https://pflag.org/glossary is a helpful resource for up-to-date information on proper terminology related to LGBTQIA+ identities.

— https://www.wpath.org/publications/soc provides the current standards of mental and physical health care for gender minority individuals developed by the World Professional Organization for Transgender Health.

— https://store.samhsa.gov/sites/default/files/pep22-03-12-001.pdf

REFERENCES

1. Conron KJ. LGBT Youth Population in the United States. The Williams Institute, UCLA. 2020. https://williamsinstitute.law.ucla.edu/wp-content/uploads/LGBT-Youth-US-Pop-Sep-2020.pdf

2. McCormick A, Scheyd K, Terrazas S. Trauma-informed care and LGBTQ+ youth: considerations for advancing practice with youth with trauma experiences. *Fam Soc.* 2018;99(2):160-169. doi:10.1177/1044389418768550

3. 2022 National Survey on LGBTQ+ Youth Mental Health. The Trevor Project. 2022. Accessed May 18, 2022. https://www.thetrevorproject.org/survey-2022/

4. Austin SB, Jun H, Jackson B, et al. Disparities in child abuse victimization in lesbian, bisexual, and heterosexual women in the nurses' health study II. *J Womens Health.* 2008;4:597-606. doi:10.1089/jwh.2007.0450

5. Balsam KF, Rothblum ED, Beauchaine TP. Victimization over the life span: a comparison of lesbian, gay, bisexual, and heterosexual siblings. *J Consult Clin Psychol.* 2005;73:477-487. doi:10.1037/0022-006X.73.3.477

6. Corliss HL, Cochran SD, Mays VM. Reports of parental maltreatment during childhood in a United States population-based survey of homosexual, bisexual, and heterosexual adults. *Child Abuse Negl.* 2002;26:1165-1178. doi:10.1016/s0145-2134(02)00385-x

7. Hughes T, McCabe SE, Wilsnack SC, West BT, Boyd CJ. Victimization and substance use disorders in a national sample of heterosexual and sexual minority women and men. *Addiction.* 2010;105(12):2130-2140. doi:10.1111/j.1360-0443.2010.03088.x

8. Sterzing PR, Gartner RE, Goldbach JT, McGeough BL, Ratliff GA, Johnson KC. Polyvictimization prevalence rates for sexual and gender minority adolescents: breaking down the silos of victimization research. *Psychol Violence.* 2019;9(4):419-430. doi:10.1037/vio0000123

9. Craig SL, Austin A, Levenson J, Leung VWY, Eaton AD, D'Souza SA. Frequencies and patterns of adverse childhood events in LGBTQ+ youth. *Child Abuse Negl.* 2020;107. doi:10.1016/j.chiabu.2020.104623

10. Mercer J. Evidence of potentially harmful psychological treatments for children and adolescents. *Child Adolesc Social Work J.* 2017;34(2):107-125. doi:10.1007/s10560-016-0480-2

11. Sexual Assault and the LGBTQ+ Community. Human Rights Campaign. 2022. https://www.hrc.org/resources/sexual-assault-and-the-lgbt-community

12. Miller QC, London K. Mock jurors' perceptions of child sexual abuse cases involving sexual and gender minority victims. *Psychol Sex Orientat Gend Divers.* 2021. doi:10.1037/sgd0000541

13. Legislation Affecting LGBTQ+ Rights Across the Country 2021. American Civil Liberties Union. 2021. https://www.aclu.org/legislation-affecting-LGBTQ+-rights-across-country-2021

14. Fish J. Future directions in understanding and addressing mental health among LGBTQ+ youth. *J Clin Child Adolesc Psychol.* 2020;49(6):943-956. doi:10.1080/15374416.2020.1815207

15. Fish J, Bishop M, Russell S. Developmental differences in sexual orientation and gender identity–related substance use disparities: findings from population-based data. *J Adolesc Health.* 2021;68(6):1162-1169. doi:10.1016/j.jadohealth.2020.10.023

16. Tan KKH, Treharne GJ, Ellis SJ, Schmidt JM, Veale JF. Gender minority stress: a critical review. *J Homosex.* 2020;67(10):1471-1489. doi:10.1080/00918369.2019.1591789

17. Meyer, IH. Prejudice, social stress, and mental health in lesbian, gay, and bisexual populations: conceptual issues and research evidence. *Psychol Bull.* 2003;129(5):674-697. doi:10.1037/0033-2909.129.5.674

18. Nicholson AA, Siegel M, Wolf J, et al. A systematic review of the neural correlates of sexual minority stress: towards an intersectional minority mosaic framework with implications for a future research agenda. *Eur J Psychotraumatol.* 2022;13(1). doi:10.1080/20008198.2021.2002572

19. Wang Y, Feng Y, Han M, et al. Methods of attempted suicide and risk factors in LGBTQ+ youth. *Child Abuse Negl.* 2021;122. doi:10.1016/j.chiabu.2021.105352

20. Charak R, Villarreal L, Schmitz RM, Hirai M, Ford JD. Patterns of childhood maltreatment and intimate partner violence, emotion dysregulation, and mental health symptoms among lesbian, gay, and bisexual emerging adults: a three-step latent class approach. *Child Abuse Negl.* 2019;89:99-110. doi:10.1016/j.chiabu.2019.01.007

21. Scannapieco M, Painter KR, Blau G. A comparison of LGBTQ+ youth and heterosexual youth in the child welfare system: mental health and substance abuse occurrence and outcomes. *Child Youth Serv Rev.* 2018;91:39-46. doi:10.1016/j.childyouth.2018.05.016

22. Mustanski B, Andrews R, Puckett J. The effects of cumulative victimization on mental health among lesbian, gay, bisexual, and transgender adolescents and young adults. *Am J Public Health.* 2016;106(3):527-533. doi:10.2105/ajph.2015.302976

23. Butler LD, Critelli FM, Rinfrette ES. Trauma–informed care and mental health. *Directions in Psychiatry.* 2011;31:197-210.

24. U.S. Department of Health and Human Services. Developing a Trauma-Informed Child Welfare System - Child Welfare Information Gateway. Childwelfare.gov. 2018. www.childwelfare.gov/pubs/issue-briefs/trauma-informed/

25. Heck NC, Flentje A, Cochran BN. Intake interviewing with lesbian, gay, bisexual, and transgender clients: starting from a place of affirmation. *J Contemp Psychother.* 2013;43(1):23-32. doi:10.1007/s10879-012-9220-x

26. Solomon DT, Heck N, Reed OM, Smith DW. Conducting culturally competent intake interviews with LGBTQ youth. *Psychol Sex Orientat Gend Divers.* 2017;4(4):403-411. doi:10.1037/sgd0000255

27. Fallot RD, Harris M. Creating cultures of trauma-informed care (CCTIC): a self-assessment and planning protocol. 2009. http://www.annafoundation.org/CCTICSELFASSPP.pdf

28. Hopper E, Bassuk E, Olivet J. Shelter from the storm: trauma-informed care in homelessness services settings. *Open Health Serv Policy J.* 2010;3(1):80-100. doi:10.2174/1874924001003010080

29. Ellis AE. Providing trauma-informed affirmative care: introduction to special issue on evidence-based relationship variables in working with affectional and gender minorities. *Practice Innovations.* 2020;5(3):179-188. doi:10.1037/pri0000133

30. Levenson JS, Craig SL, Austin A. Trauma-informed and affirmative mental health practices with LGBTQ+ clients. *Psychol Serv.* 2021. doi:10.1037/ser0000540

31. Lothwell LE, Libby N, Adelson SL. Mental health care for LGBT youths. *Focus (Am Psychiatr Publ).* 2020;18(3):268-276. doi:10.1176/appi.focus.20200018

32. Solomon DT, Reed OM, Sevecke JR, O'Shaughnessy T, Acevedo-Polakovich ID. Expert consensus on facilitating the coming-out process in sexual minority clients: a Delphi study. *J Gay Lesbian Ment Health.* 2018;22(4):348-371. doi:10.1080/19359705.2018.1476279

33. Boudreau D, Mukerjee R, Wesp L, Letcher LN. Trauma-informed care. In: Mukerjee R, Wesp L, Singer R, eds. *Clinician's Guide to LGBTQIA+ Care: Cultural Safety and Social Justice in Primary, Sexual, and Reproductive Healthcare.* Springer Publishing Company; 2022:69-81.

Family Maltreatment and Military Families: *Prevention and Response Efforts*

Ann C. Eckardt, PsyD, ABPP
Anna Segura, PhD
Amy M. Smith Slep, PhD

Objectives

After reading this chapter, the reader will be able to:

1. *Describe the prevention efforts and maltreatment systems that are in place for military families.*

2. *Summarize the research supporting family maltreatment determinations in the military.*

3. *Recognize common military acronyms, abbreviations, and terms.*

Background and Significance

Military families are best served when their unique features are identified and understood, especially when maltreatment is involved. One way to increase understanding is through fluency in military acronyms, abbreviations, and terms. Another way to develop military family knowledge is to know the structure of the military, including the branches and related components. As of 2020,[1] 6 branches of the military exist: the Army, Navy, Marine Corps, Air Force, Coast Guard, and Space Force. "Soldier" is often heard as a catch-all for a person serving in the military; however, there are specific terms for each branch. Soldiers are in the Army, sailors are in the Navy, marines are in the Marine Corps, airmen are in the Air Force, coast guardians are in the Coast Guard, and guardians are in the Space Force.[2]

Aside from the basic structures, it is essential to recognize that the military is a high stress occupation that affects both service members (SMs) and their families. Children in military families face routine separations from their parents, frequent moves, and parental safety risks. Although separation from family members and deployment appear to impact the mental health of children, the outcomes related to moving are unclear.[3] These stressors are amplified when there are increased demands on the military, such as mobilization or deployment and high operations tempo (OPSTEMPO). When a parent is deployed, young children often exhibit behavioral problems and are more at risk of suffering neglect; parents experience an increase in their stress,[4] and children and adolescents typically have higher rates of mood symptoms, aggression, and overall problems.[5] As violence within military families remains a challenging problem, it is key to identify military families' risk and protective factors so child maltreatment prevention efforts can be tailored to their needs.

In 2018, there were approximately 3 500 000 military personnel, including Department of Defense (DoD) SMs, Coast Guard SMs, reservists for DoD and Coast

Guard, retired and standby reserve, and civilian personnel; roughly 40% of these SMs are parents.[6] Military families share many similarities with civilian families, though there is still a "civilian-military divide," as many civilians do not understand military life. However, one has to remember that it is challenging to formally assess the number of people who would identify as a military family, given the multi-faceted definition of "family."[7]

Developing targeted programs and systems and actively managing alleged maltreatment incidents are cornerstones for the DoD. The DoD's programs achieve this through a variety of face-to-face or remote delivery services and through engaging in coordinated responses to handle alleged maltreatment with law enforcement, educational partners, and community members.[8] The bulk of addressing maltreatment is through the Family Advocacy Program (FAP). In accordance with DoD Instruction (DoDI) 6400.01, FAP is tasked with family maltreatment response and prevention efforts for both children and adults, and it is the largest federal maltreatment agency, making it a tremendous vector for change.[9] The preventative and comprehensive (ie, dealing in both child and partner cases) mission of FAP differs from civilian maltreatment protection agencies, as the Child Abuse Prevention and Treatment Act (CAPTA)[10] outlines that child abuse and neglect incidents be investigated following a report. Additionally, in 2021, there were an estimated 19 000 000 military veterans,[11] to whom these services also apply. Overall, FAP offers a robust and multi-layered family prevention and maltreatment response system by working with SMs and their families to address child abuse and neglect, as well as intimate partner abuse.[12]

The research covered in the next section of this chapter was used as the foundation for work in civilian sectors. The advances made in the military have been translated into efforts with the state of Alaska,[13] criteria in the *Diagnostic and Statistical Manual of Mental Disorders, 5th edition* (DSM-5), and the *International Classification of Diseases, 11th edition* (ICD-11).[14]

EVIDENCE BASE AND RESEARCH

Historically, the military and FAP have conducted research on preventive approaches and policies related to family maltreatment, which has resulted in the implementation of changes based on research findings in the military family maltreatment system.[15] In this section, the authors will outline the evidence base and research behind FAP's efforts to prevent and respond to family maltreatment.

NEW PARENT SUPPORT PROGRAM

The New Parent Support Program (NPSP) is one example of FAP's evidence-supported practices. NPSP is a universal, free, and voluntary child maltreatment prevention program that offers home visitation services, including referral, education, and support to SMs and their families who have children younger than 3 years or are expecting a baby.[15,16] This program is modeled on empirically-supported early home visitation and strengths-based model programs.[17] NPSP aims to create a safe and nurturing environment for children by promoting resilient families and healthy parenting attitudes and skills (eg, nurturing and attachment, knowledge of parenting and child and adolescent development, concrete supports for parents).[16] Home visitors provide services tailored to each family's and parent's needs, such as breastfeeding support, lessons on effective and safe parenting of infants and toddlers (eg, sleeping habits, nutrition), and tips for new fathers.[16] The implementation of NPSP varies across all military branches and installations but offers similar education tools and personalized services to all SMs and their families.[15,18]

DECISION TREE ALGORITHM AND INCIDENT DETERMINATION COMMITTEE

FAP's development and implementation of empirically-supported practices is also shown through their approach to substantiating maltreatment incidents.[15] The authors of this chapter are members of a research team that has been involved in the operationalizing of maltreatment definitional criteria and processes for more than 20 years at the time of this publication.[19-22] At the start of this work, and presently, the field struggles to find reliable and agreed-upon ways to define and measure maltreatment.[23] The team sought to develop and test criteria for defining family maltreatment and procedures for applying those definitional criteria that could be consistently implemented in the field.[15,24] This has been a multistage process that included the review of family maltreatment definitions, the development of an operationalized diagnostic criteria and decision making processes that promote reliable decision making, and the study of factors that influence these substantiation decisions.[19-24] All of this development has resulted in well-tested, evidence-based practices to guide content and processes for substantiating maltreatment incidents.

In terms of evidence-based practices to guide the content of the substantiation decisions, Heyman & Slep[24] created the Decision Tree Algorithm (DTA), which includes operationalized definitions of partner and child physical, emotional, and sexual abuse as well as child neglect that were field tested with hundreds of cases to fine-tune the criteria.[19,24] Studies showed that

> "sensitivity, specificity, and predictive values are consistently good across all forms of maltreatment, suggesting that the definitions and determination procedures performed well on both sides of the determination coin, substantiating maltreatment when it was there and not substantiating when it was not."[21]

Implementing standardized definitions of family maltreatment and procedures allowed decreased variability among military bases, promoted reliable decision making,[19,24] and resulted in a high level of agreement between master reviewers' expert case determinations and field sites' determinations.[21] The definitions implementation also resulted in a secondary preventive effect on family maltreatment by reducing the 1-year recidivism (ie, substantiated re-offense).[22] Furthermore, stakeholders rated high levels of acceptability and fairness regarding the definitions and processes.[21] For the most part, the substantiation of a maltreatment incident requires 2 separate decisions: whether the act/omission of maltreatment occurred and whether the impact of the act/omission resulted in an actual impact or the reasonable potential of an impact.[24] The definitions have been adopted and are being used by all branches of the military in order to determine whether allegations of maltreatment cross the threshold and should be labeled as abuse.[25]

Evidence-based practices extend to how the DTA is applied when considering family maltreatment incidents. Studies with the US Air Force (USAF) and the Army showed that the Field-tested Assessment, Intervention-planning, and Response (FAIR) system, when implemented with fidelity, led to more correct decisions and had a preventive effect in maltreatment recidivism compared to the former system.[26,27] One element of this approach (in addition to the DTA) is the Incident Determination Committee (IDC). The IDC is an administrative process that results in a decision about whether an allegation of abuse/neglect meets or does not meet the DTA criteria. The substantiation decision is made by a committee that includes the FAP clinical representative, a lawyer from the Judge Advocate General office, a representative from the Military Police, the manager of the FAP prevention branch (ie, a nonvoting member in FAIR [only in the Army where FAP is divided in this way]), a high-ranking enlisted representative, and a representative from the involved SM's leadership. The committee is led by a high-ranking officer. Research has found that unit representatives perceived the new approach as fairer to both offenders and victims and were more likely to attend IDCs.[27]

Another empirically-based element of this system is the use of the standardized decision processes that guide committees through the definitional criteria, voting on each element in succession. This process is supported by an automated algorithm or computerized decision tree that: 1) directs the decision making for each criterion by guiding a step-by-step process for discussion and voting on the incident rather than asking the committee for an overall summary decision, and 2) reports the overall summary decision to the committee on the basis of the votes to the specific criteria presented.[15,19,20,27]

Studies focusing on the implementation of the FAIR system showed the need to focus the FAP's collected information in the individual and confidential psychosocial assessment interviews[23]; thus, standardized assessment protocols were built to support assessments.[15] In this system, supervisors present the clinical assessment findings at the IDC after carefully reviewing them, and the assessing social worker ensures that the assessment fully addresses potentially relevant criteria.[27]

CLINICAL CASE STAFFING MEETING AND INCIDENT SEVERITY SCALES

The current system also includes a separate Clinical Case Staffing Meeting (CCSM) for social workers (who have clinical expertise in maltreatment) to collaborate on and get supervisory approval for treatment plans.[27] In addition to monitoring maltreatment and responding to allegations when they arise, FAP also includes prevention and treatment services in its mission that are available to all SMs and their families, regardless of the substantiation decision.[12] Services that SMs and families are referred to are driven by the risk assessment and clinical presentations of the family.

The authors' research team has extended the work on developing criteria and processes for making reliable and valid substantiation decisions by applying the same blueprint to developing and piloting severity rating criteria for cases that have already met criteria for maltreatment.[28] The team developed a classification system for maltreatment severity (ie, mild, moderate, or severe) that could be applied across types of maltreatment, raters, and clinics.[28] This classification system was later refined and field-tested, and a computerized clinical decision support tool for the criteria was also created. This was implemented across the DoD and is known as the Incident Severity Scales (ISS).

CONCLUSIONS AND FUTURE DIRECTIONS

In many ways, families in the military have access to more and better prevention and intervention services than non-military families. However, needs remain. Future efforts to engage and serve high-needs families before maltreatment occurs and ensure high quality and responsive services when it does occur are critical. Continuing to improve the quality and consistency of the services and systems addressing maltreatment in military families will support families and may also inform civilian service enhancements.

DIAGNOSTIC ASSESSMENT – STRUCTURED INTERVIEW FOR RELATIONAL PROBLEMS – CHILD PHYSICAL ABUSE

Below is the Child Physical Abuse Section of the Structured Interview for Relational Problems.[29] This is one of many tools clinicians can use to assess for maltreatment.

CHILD PHYSICAL ABUSE

As you conduct the interview, please rate the answers using the following criteria based on the obtained information

— ? = inadequate information

— 1 = the assessed statement is absent or false

— 2 = the assessed statement meets the subthreshold

— 3 = the assessed statement is true or meets the threshold

Table 12-1. Structured Interview for Relational Problems – Child Physical Abuse[29]					
CHILD PHYSICAL ABUSE	CHILD PHYSICAL ABUSE CRITERIA				
"Now I'm going to ask you some questions about things that sometimes go on between a parent and a child at some time or another."					
					(continued)

Table 12-1. Structured Interview for Relational Problems – Child Physical Abuse *(continued)*

CHILD PHYSICAL ABUSE	CHILD PHYSICAL ABUSE CRITERIA				
In the last year... ..."Have you done any of these things to your child?" (Show category 1 CHILD physical force list to interviewee)	A. Non-accidental use of physical force by a child's parent/caregiver: spanking with hand; dropping; pushing; shoving; slapping; grabbing or yanking limbs or body; throwing; poking; hair-pulling; scratching; pinching; restraining or squeezing; shaking; biting	?	1	2	3
"OK, how about any of these?" (show category 2 CHILD physical force list to interviewee)	Throwing objects at; kicking; hitting with fist; hitting with a stick, strap, belt, or other object; scalding; burning; poisoning; stabbing; applying force to throat; strangling or cutting off air supply; holding under water; using a weapon	?	1	2	3
"What about anything similar but not listed here?"	Any other non-accidental use of physical force	?	1	2	3
"Think about what you would consider to be the most serious incident. I'm going to ask you some questions about your child. You may not know some of these details, but just answer to the best of your ability."	B. Significant impact on the child as evidenced by any of the following:	?	1	2	3
"Sometimes, when things get physical, people notice marks, bruises, or cuts. Did your child have any?" If NO: "What about pain? (How long did that last?)" If NO: "What about any other injury?"	(1) More than inconsequential physical injury	?	1	2	3
"Again, I'd like you to think about the most serious physical incident in the last year. I'd like you to tell me exactly what happened in the incident. Please be as detailed as if you were watching it on a video screen and describe for me everything that you see, from the beginning to the end." ("Where were you when this happened?") ("How hard was [act] on a scale of 1-10, with 1 being feather-light and 10 being as hard as possible?")	(2) Reasonable potential for more than inconsequential physical injury given the inherent dangerousness of the act, the degree of force used, and the physical environment in which the acts occurred An injury involving any of the following: (a) Any injury to the face or head (b) More than superficial bruise(s) (c) More than superficial cut(s) /scratch(es) (ie, requires pressure to stop bleeding) (d) Bleeding (e) Welts (f) Loss of consciousness (g) Loss of functioning (including, but not limited to: sprains, broken bones, detached retina, loose or chipped teeth) (h) Heat exhaustion or heat stroke (i) Damage to internal organs (j) Disfigurement (including scarring) (k) Swelling lasting at least 24 hours (l) Pain felt (a) in the course of normal activities and (b) at least 24 hours after the physical injury was suffered.	?	1	2	3

(continued)

Table 12-1. Structured Interview for Relational Problems – Child Physical Abuse *(continued)*					
CHILD PHYSICAL ABUSE	CHILD PHYSICAL ABUSE CRITERIA				
"Was your child afraid, either during or after the incident? (What was s/he afraid of?) (How long did it last?)"	(3) More Than Inconsequential Fear Reaction (a) Child's fear (verbalized or displayed) of bodily injury to self or others AND	?	1	2	3
If YES to fear: "I'm going to ask you some questions about specific ways that the(se) incident(s) may have affected your child."	(b) At least one of the following signs of fear or anxiety lasting at least 48 hours				
"Did your child think about the incident(s) when s/he didn't want to or did thoughts about it come to him/her suddenly when s/he didn't want them to? (Tell me about that...)"	(i) Persistent intrusive recollections of the incident	?	1	2	3
"Did s/he go out of his/her way to avoid people, places, or things related to the incident? (Tell me about that...)"	(ii) Marked negative reactions to cues related to incident, as evidenced by any of the following: (a) Avoidance of cues	?	1	2	3
"What about getting very upset when something reminded him/her of the incident(s)?"	(b) Subjective or overt distress to cues	?	1	2	3
"What about physical symptoms — like breaking out in a sweat, breathing heavily or irregularly, or his/her heart pounding or racing?"	(c) Physiological hyperarousal to cues	?	1	2	3
"What about finding him/herself acting or feeling as if s/he were back in the incident?"	(iii) Acting or feeling as if incident is reoccurring	?	1	2	3
Since the incident(s)...	(iv) Persistent symptoms of increased arousal, as evidenced by any of the following:				
..."Has your child had trouble sleeping?"	(a) Difficulty falling or staying asleep	?	1	2	3
..."Has your child been unusually irritable? What about outbursts of anger?"	(b) Irritability or outbursts of anger	?	1	2	3
..."Has your child had trouble concentrating?"	(c) Difficulty concentrating	?	1	2	3
..."Has your child been watchful or on guard even when there was no reason to be?"	(d) Hypervigilance	?	1	2	3
..."Has your child been jumpy or easily startled, like by sudden noises?"	(e) Exaggerated startle response	?	1	2	3
	B1 IS CODED 3 OR B2 IS CODED 3 OR (B3a IS CODED "3" AND AT LEAST ONE OF B3b (1-4) IS CODED "3")		1		3

(continued)

Table 12-1. Structured Interview for Relational Problems – Child Physical Abuse *(continued)*

CHILD PHYSICAL ABUSE	CHILD PHYSICAL ABUSE CRITERIA			
"You said that you have [ACTS] and that, as a result, your child had [IMPACTS]. In any of these incidents, did your [ACTS] come after s/he had already used physical force?" (IF YES, "In what percentage of the incidents had s/he used force first?") (IF 100% - "In what percentage of the incidents was s/he still in the act of using force when you [ACT]?") (IF 100%, "Was there ever a time that your [ACTS] occurred for some other reason than to stop your child's use of force?") (IF NO, "Did you ever do more than was necessary to stop your child from using force?")	C1. Act(s) DID NOT OCCUR ONLY to protect self from imminent physical harm because child was in the act of physical force.		1	3
	a. There exists an incident when the child DID NOT use force first or WAS NOT still in the act of using force when self's act(s) occurred.		1	3
	b. Self's act(s) was/were NOT SOLELY to stop child's use of physical force.		1	3
	c. Self's act(s) used MORE THAN minimally sufficient force to stop child's use of physical force.			
	C1. Act(s) by self DID NOT OCCUR ONLY to protect self from imminent physical harm because child was in the act of physical force.		1	3
(If not clear from prior questions) "In any of the times you have [ACTS] and that, as a result, your child had [IMPACTS], were your [ACTS] happening in play?" (If YES, "In what percentage of the incidents did your [ACTS] happen in play?")	C2. Act(s) by self DID NOT ALWAYS occur in developmentally appropriate play.		1	3
(If not clear from prior questions) "In any of the times you have [ACTS] and that, as a result, your child had [IMPACTS], did you [ACTS] to protect your child or someone else from physical harm?" (If YES, "Tell me about such a time.") ("In what percentage of the incidents did your [ACTS] happen to protect your child or someone else?")	C3. Act(s) by self WERE NOT ALWAYS to directly protect child or another person from imminent physical harm (including, but not limited to: pushing child out of the way of a car, taking weapon away from suicidal child, stopping child from inflicting injury on another person). Note: Subsequent actions that were not directly protective (eg, whipping child for running into the street) would not meet this criterion.		1	3

KEY POINTS

1. The NPSP is a prevention effort, and the IDC is a maltreatment system in place for military families.

2. The DTA was developed, piloted, and disseminated with high agreement rates, and there is evidence the system reduced recidivism.

3. Some common military acronyms, abbreviations, and terms are: active duty, SM, OPSTEMPO, and FAP.

ADDITIONAL RESOURCES

— Chandra A, Lara-Cinisomo S, Jaycox LH, et al. Children on the homefront: the experience of children from military families. *Pediatrics.* 2010;125(1):16-25. doi:10.1542/peds.2009-1180

— Clearinghouse for military family readiness. The Pennsylvania State University. 2002. https://militaryfamilies.psu.edu/

— Domestic abuse victim advocate locator. Military One Source; Department of Defense. 2022. https://www.militaryonesource.mil/leaders-service-providers/child-abuse-and-domestic-abuse/victim-advocate-locator/

— The family advocacy program. Military One Source; Department of Defense. 2020. https://www.militaryonesource.mil/family-relationships/family-life/preventing-abuse-neglect/the-family-advocacy-program/

— The new parent support program. Military One Source; Department of Defense. 2020. https://www.militaryonesource.mil/family-relationships/parenting-and-children/parenting-infants-and-toddlers/the-new-parent-support-program/

— Child maltreatment in military families: a fact sheet for providers. National Child Traumatic Stress Network. https://www.nctsn.org/sites/default/files/resources/child_maltreatment_military_families_providers.pdf

— Understanding child trauma and resilience: For military parents and caregivers. https://www.nctsn.org/resources/understanding-child-trauma-and-resilience-for-military-parents-and-caregivers

— Working effectively with military families: 10 Key concepts all providers should know. National Child Traumatic Stress Network. https://www.nctsn.org/sites/default/files/resources/working_effectively_with_military_families_10_key_concepts_providers.pdfhttps://www.nctsn.org/sites/default/files/resources/working_effectively_with_military_families_10_key_concepts_providers.pdf

REFERENCES

1. Johnson S. How many military branches are there and what does each branch do? United Service Organizations. September 23, 2020. Accessed May 23, 2022. https://www.uso.org/stories/2855-how-many-military-branches-are-there-and-what-does-each-do

2. Garamone J. Space Force personnel to be called guardians. US Department of Defense. December 19, 2020. Accessed May 23, 2022. https://www.defense.gov/News/News-Stories/Article/Article/2452910/space-force-personnel-to-be-called-guardians/

3. Cramm H, McColl MA, Aiken AB, Williams A. The mental health of military-connected children: a scoping review. *J Child Fam Stud.* 2019;28:1725-1735. doi:10.1007/s10826-019-01402-y

4. Trautmann J, Alhusen J, Gross D. Impact of deployment on military families with young children: a systematic review. *Nurs Outlook.* 2015;63(6):656-679. doi:10.1016/j.outlook.2015.06.002

5. Cunitz K, Dölitzsch C, Kösters M, et al. Parental military deployment as risk factor for children's mental health: a meta-analytical review. *Child Adolesc Psychiatry Ment Health.* 2019;13(1):1-10. doi:10.1186/s13034-019-0287-y

6. 2018 demographics report: profile of the military community. Department of Defense; United States of America. 2018. https://download.militaryonesource.mil/12038/MOS/Reports/2018-demographics-report.pdf

7.   DeSimone D. 5 things you need to know about military families. United Service Organizations. August 15, 2018. Accessed May 23, 2022. https://www.uso.org/ stories/2277-5-things-to-know-about-military-families#:~:text=Military%20 families%20are%20made%20up,that%20creates%20a%20different%20lifestyle

8.   Department of Defense press briefing on military community and family policy family readiness programs, policies, and initiatives. US Department of Defense. October 29, 2020. Accessed May 24, 2022. https://www.defense.gov/News/ Transcripts/Transcript/Article/2399392/department-of-defense-press-briefing- on-military-community-and-family-policy-fa/

9.   DoD Instruction 6400.01, Family Advocacy Program (FAP). 2019. Accessed May 24, 2022. https://www.esd.whs.mil/Portals/54/Documents/DD/issuances/ dodi/640001p.pdf

10. Child Abuse Prevention and Treatment Act, as amended. US Department of Health and Human Services. 1992. Accessed May 24, 2022. https://www.ojp. gov/pdffiles1/Digitization/152157NCJRS.pdf

11. Schaeffer K. The changing face of America's veteran population. Pew Research Center. April 5, 2021. Accessed May 23, 2022. https://www.pewresearch.org/ fact-tank/2021/04/05/the-changing-face-of-americas-veteran-population/

12. The family advocacy program. Military One Source, Department of Defense. Updated August 23, 2020. Accessed March 12, 2022. https://www.militaryone- source.mil/family-relationships/family-life/preventing-abuse-neglect/the-family- advocacy-program/

13. Mitnick DM, Slep AMS, Heyman RE, Lively D, Perkins DF. The FAIR System for child maltreatment substantiation determinations: an evaluation of Alaska's statewide implementation. [Manuscript submitted for publication.]

14. Heyman RE, Snarr JD, Slep AMS, Baucom KJW, Linkh DJ. Self-reporting DSM-5/ICD-11 clinically significant intimate partner violence and child abuse: convergent and response process validity. *J Fam Psychol.* 2020;34(1):101-111. doi:10.1037/fam0000560

15. Slep AMS, Heyman RE. Child maltreatment and intimate partner violence in military families. In: Gewirtz AH, Youssef AM, Wadsworth SM, eds. *Parenting and Children's Resilience in Military Families.* Springer International Publishing; 2016:131-150.

16. The new parent support program. Military One Source, Department of Defense. Updated February 13, 2020. Accessed March 12, 2022. https://www.militaryo- nesource.mil/family-relationships/parenting-and-children/parenting-infants- and-toddlers/the-new-parent-support-program/

17. Olds DL, Henderson Jr CR, Chamberlin R, Tatelbaum R. Preventing child abuse and neglect: a randomized trial of nurse home visitation. *Pediatrics.* 1986;78 (1):65-78. doi:10.1542/peds.78.1.65

18. Recame MA. Childbirth education and parental support programs within the US military population. *Int J Childbirth Educ.* 2013;28(1):67-71. doi:10.1624/ 105812408X298381

19. Heyman RE, Slep AMS. Creating and field-testing diagnostic criteria for partner and child maltreatment. *J Fam Psychol.* 2006;20(3):397-408. doi:10.1037/0893- 3200.20.3.397

20. Heyman RE, Slep AMS. Reliability of family maltreatment diagnostic criteria: 41 site dissemination field trial. *J Fam Psychol.* 2009;23(6):905-910. doi:10.1037/ a0017011

21. Slep AMS, Heyman RE. Creating and field-testing child maltreatment definitions: improving the reliability of substantiation determinations. *Child Maltreat.* 2006;11(3):217-236. doi:10.1177/1077559506288878

22. Snarr JD, Heyman RE, Slep AMS, Malik J; United States Air Force Family Advocacy Program. Preventive impacts of reliable family maltreatment criteria. *J Consult Clin Psychol.* 2011;79(6):826-833. doi:10.1037/a0025994

23. Heyman RE, Collins PS, Slep AMS, Knickerbocker L. Evidence-based substantiation criteria: improving the reliability of field decisions of child maltreatment and partner abuse. *Prot Child.* 2010;25:35-46.

24. Heyman RE, Slep AMS, McCarroll J. Development of the Decision Tree Algorithm (DTA) and validity of the definitions: interview with Richard Heyman, PhD, and Amy Slep, PhD, Conducted by James McCarroll, PhD. *JFJF.* 2010;11(4):1-8.

25. Slep AMS, Foran HM, Heyman RE, Snarr JD; United States Air Force Family Advocacy Program. Risk factors for clinically significant intimate partner violence among active duty members. *J Marriage Fam.* 2011;73(2):486-501. doi:10.1111/j.1741-3737.2010.00820.x

26. Slep AMS, Heyman RE, Mitnick D, Lorber M, Nichols S, Perkins D. Fairly-decided maltreatment determinations significantly reduce recidivism? A quasi-experimental evaluation of a system-level intervention implementation. *Research Square.* 2021. doi:10.21203/rs.3.rs-185613/v1

27. Heyman RE, Slep AMS, Mitnick DM, et al. Evaluation of two approaches for responding to allegations of family maltreatment in the US Army: coordinated community response impacts and costs. *Mil Med.* 2021;1-8. doi:10.1093/milmed/usab115

28. Erlanger ACE, Heyman RE, Slep AMS. Creating and testing the reliability of a family maltreatment severity classification system. *J Interpers Violence.* 2022;37(7-8):1-20. doi:10.1177/0886260520961866

29. Slep AMS, Heyman RE, Snarr JD, Foran HM. Practical tools for assessing child maltreatment in clinical practice and public health. In: Foran HM, Beach S, Slep AMS, Heyman RE, Wamboldt M, eds. *Family Problems and Family Violence: Reliable Assessment and the ICD- 11.* York: Springer; 2012:159-184.

IMMIGRATION AND CHILD MALTREATMENT

Cathi Tillman, MSW, ACSW, LSW, Certificate: Harvard Program in Refugee Trauma

OBJECTIVES

After reading this chapter, the reader will be able to:

1. *Provide a well-integrated and interdisciplinary overview of child maltreatment from a transnational perspective that captures both the obvious and more nuanced concerns of immigrant children.*

2. *Discuss aspects of child maltreatment in multiple cultural contexts that provide effective points of prevention and intervention relating to mental health, for providers and policy makers alike.*

3. *Identify ways in which the discussion of child maltreatment through a transnational lens incorporates the universal rights and needs of children while considering healthy physical and emotional development.*

BACKGROUND AND SIGNIFICANCE

Children migrate from other countries to the United States due to a variety of "push" factors such as community and family violence, extreme poverty, lack of adequate parental care resulting in physical, emotional, and sexual trauma, and lack of access to basic needs and education.[1]

Child maltreatment is often intergenerational and normalized within the context of family and community life. This can obfuscate the connection between past events, past traumas, and their harmful consequences. A migrant child's ability to relate an accurate history of past experiences is often limited by their lack of emotional language and other barriers to seeking safety. Additionally, the wide range of circumstances under which children migrate across borders contributes to underreporting and the subsequent lack of helpful interventions or prevention strategies. As the complexities of maltreatment are considered through a transnational lens, direct service providers and policy makers can be better equipped to establish protocols that can prevent future harm while developing strategies to promote healing and healthy emotional growth.

Much of the current discussion and literature relating to child maltreatment is through a Western lens, using norms and expectations of parenting and enforcement of child welfare guidelines established in major industrialized countries.[2] This chapter is intended to broaden the conversation and understanding of child maltreatment to include the child's experience in their country of origin, the dynamics and experiences of transnational migration, and how providers and policy makers can approach the complicated challenges with more robust and better-integrated planning and implementation across community systems with multiple overlapping languages and cultures.

It should be noted that, for the purposes of this chapter, the population discussed will be described as "immigrant" or "migrating children" and will include children who enter the United States without authorization but who are typically eligible for immigration relief. The term "refugee" will not be used, since all refugees are immigrants, but not all immigrants qualify for refugee status.

WHERE DOES CHILD MALTREATMENT OCCUR IN MIGRANT POPULATIONS?

As children migrate across borders and encounter law enforcement and social service personnel, information regarding past experiences of maltreatment is often not consistently or accurately communicated. The reporting of past traumatic events can occur in the context of an intake or other type of general evaluation when a child is detained or treated at a clinic at United States borders. The narrative of the child's experience, however, is often compromised by the evaluator's intake protocol, which oftentimes does not factor in a child's difficulty in emotional expression or insight into their traumatic experiences. As border policies and practices are constantly shifting, the impact on staffing as well as inadequate support for interviewers and other personnel oftentimes results in a lack of appreciation for the complex traumas that a child presents at the time of an interview.[3]

Furthermore, there are corroborated reports that many children held in detention after entering the United States "without authorization" experience "deliberate and malicious withholding of needs, including the withholding of food, water, medical attention, and other basic necessities."[4] It is incumbent upon mental health care workers or advocates to ask about any maltreatment that might have occurred after entering the United States, including by representatives of the government while they were detained under the protections of the United States Customs and Border Protection Agency. It is advisable to consider these points of possible maltreatment for migrant children and to account for the impact of these experiences on their mental health and emotional development.

Limited data exist about the prevalence of child abuse in Central America; the greatest focus is on child sexual abuse, with the assumption that most victims are female and that the experience of sexual trauma is so culturally embedded that it is part of the overall "norm" of many communities. There are indications, however, that other forms of maltreatment are also underreported, due largely to the lack of formal reporting mechanisms in children's countries of origin. For example, the tracking of unaccompanied children who enter the United States without adult supervision or support generally takes place at the point of border entry, but it is difficult to evaluate the circumstances of children who, prior to migration, were abandoned by or separated from their caregivers, or who had an extensive history of disrupted attachment and overall lack of bonding with reliable, trustworthy adults.[5]

GENDER CONSIDERATIONS

Gender plays a significant role in the maltreatment of migrating children. Evidence across numerous studies indicates that females experience higher rates of sexual abuse than males, although male children are also known to be victims of sexual abuse, but it is reported to a lesser degree. Part of this appears due to the normalization of gender-based abuse as well as the cultural acceptance of certain varieties of child maltreatment.[6]

There are both clear and nuanced implications regarding gender when understanding child maltreatment from a transnational perspective. Gender-based violence is prevalent in communities across the globe, and the normalization of this type of abuse and maltreatment contributes to the overall lack of prevention and intervention strategies in many parts of the world. Increased visibility of LGBTQIA+ children coming across borders has also raised concerns about queer and trans children and adolescents being targets of family and community-based maltreatment. In this context, before, during, and upon settling into communities, immigrant children need protections and advocacy for physical and emotional safety as they navigate the complexities of sexual orientation and gender identity.[7] Ensuring these protections is often more challenging than for their peers born in the United States due to the language, cultural, and various social barriers facing migrant children. It is also important to consider that children may have previously experienced maltreatment based on gender or sexual orientation in their country of origin.

COMPLICATING FACTORS IN ASSESSING FOR CHILD MALTREATMENT WITH IMMIGRANT CHILDREN

Explanations for increased child arrivals include the persistence of Central American gang violence, pervasive economic strains now worsened by a global pandemic, climate change, limited work and educational opportunities, and the multiple interpersonal stressors that develop in the face of these realities. As children leave their home countries to seek safety and security in the United States, their unification or reunification with family members is often complicated and stressful for all involved. Understanding and identifying the risk of maltreatment by family members is complicated because of the radically different cultural norms that legitimize many forms of maltreatment, despite living in a new country that has—and enforces— different expectations of child safety.

It is not unusual for newly arrived immigrant children to move to other areas of the country, often to unite with adult family members who have sponsored them after crossing the border. However, when placement with an identified family is not successful, children might be placed into the custody of the local child welfare system. This can also occur if a family member is not identified, as in the case of "unaccompanied minor children." In these cases, information relating to past experiences becomes less consistent and available, yet it has significant bearing on the psychological needs of the child and the subsequent services that might be sought. As a result, opportunities for addressing past traumas are often overlooked or might be obscured by other, more immediate needs such as housing, school enrollment, and legal counsel. Furthermore, maltreatment is often normalized by children and family members alike, particularly when it does not fall within the constellation of assessments or supports (however limited) made available to the newly arrived children.

There are multiple concerns relating to a report of maltreatment for immigrant families under any circumstance. Many immigrant families face barriers that are generally unknown or misunderstood by the larger child welfare system, such as housing and job insecurity, language access, and overall challenges with navigating the complex child welfare systems. In addition to the limitations to services imposed by the (usually) overworked and underpaid status of staff in most child welfare systems, there is often a general lack of training and supervision for workers who encounter the migrant children that come into these systems. This places the child and family at additional risk for further harm on different levels and places more stress and despair on the workers who are tasked with the care of these individuals.[8]

It should also be noted that immigration enforcement and its consequences to families create an additional layer of complication and trauma for both children and their caretakers. When a parent is detained or deported, children are often placed in the foster care system if an alternate caretaker is not identified. Even though the detained or deported parent has not been charged with child maltreatment, there can be significant psychological impact on the child(ren) going into placement. Hence, it is important to understand how children can be considered victims of an enforcement system in the United States when United States-born or migrated children enter the foster care system after the detention or deportation of a custodial adult. The mental health consequences of this displacement are often overlooked and mired in the larger immigration policy discussions.[9]

CONCLUSION

Proposing realistic and relatively immediate recommendations for professionals and other community members working with migrant children who experience maltreatment is complicated but certainly not impossible. Children who are identified as or suspected of being the victims of maltreatment in any form, including abusive neglect, hold unique qualities, such as resilience, openness to learning, and other developmental capacities for growth. All adults involved in the lives of migrating children, including those who have experienced maltreatment, have the responsibility to explore opportunities for connection, stability, and reliability in the context of safe and caring relationships. Community providers have an ethical responsibility to advocate for direct services that are culturally sensitive, linguistically appropriate, and responsive to the complex behaviors and needs of children who have been maltreated.[10] Additionally, advocates, providers, and policymakers must consider how the structures of our international regulatory systems frequently dismiss or overlook how exploitative practices such as child labor and sex trafficking contribute to the vulnerabilities that children face across national borders as well as upon their arrival in the United States.

To this end, it is recommended that, at their many different points of contact with migrant children, professionals conduct interviews, formally or informally, to assess and document instances of maltreatment. Challenges are often revealed in this process, particularly when reports of maltreatment refer to incidents that occurred in the child's home country by a family member who did not migrate with the child. Child welfare professionals often struggle to assess how or if there is continued risk to the child and with how to initiate a process of healing and emotional grounding with assurances of future safety. It is important for all providers in systems working with immigrant children to become more familiar with the policies and experiences that impact immigrant children and their families, so oversight and healing can be provided in ways that are meaningful, culturally-informed, and trauma-informed, and that factor in the complex experiences that immigrant children have along their physical and emotional journeys to the United States.[2]

CASE STUDY

Case Study 13-1

Sonia came to the United States after fleeing domestic violence toward her and her 6-year-old child, Jorge, in her home country. Sonia and Jorge were briefly detained and separated after crossing into the country due to border policies at the time. When Sonia was finally allowed to settle in Philadelphia with Jorge, she was able to find a room in a house with 2 other migrant families whom she did not know, sharing a kitchen and bathroom.

Upon finding work in a factory, Sonia had no child care options and felt it safe to lock Jorge in the bedroom overnight while she worked. She instructed her son to stay in the room and sleep until she arrived home early in the morning. However, one evening, Jorge was able to open the door and leave, finding his way to the street. He was quickly discovered by a police officer and placed in custody. Sonia arrived home to find the police at her door, and she was arrested for abusive neglect. Jorge was removed from Sonia's care and placed in emergency foster care with a family that did not speak Spanish.

Discussion

Sonia and Jorge were referred to a local organization that provided pro bono family therapy for the Spanish speaking immigrant community. The therapy focused on a combination of Sonia's own experiences in her home country and perspectives on child rearing, with an integration of psychoeducation relating to healthy attachments, parent-child relationship fortification, and the impact of traumatic events on both her own emotional health and Jorge's. The therapist was able to advocate for the return of Jorge to Sonia's care, particularly since the repeated separation of the son from his mother created yet another layer of trauma in his young life. Sonia's parenting practices (including the factors that led up to the charge of abandonment and neglect) were addressed through a holistic lens. All the supports were provided by a bilingual, bicultural therapist who had extensive training in working with the transnational community. Sonia was also looped into a network of community-based organizations that were able to assist with secure housing, food security, and economic stability.

It is important to consider all elements of this scenario through a transnational lens, given that the lived experiences of migrant children occur on a life continuum that originates in their home countries, spans the experiences of home and community life, and exists across geographic spaces and entry into the United States. The experiences along this continuum shape a child's perspective and expectations of relationships with adults who interact with them on varying levels.[11]

Furthermore, when reviewing literature, as well as gathering insights and informal data points through storytelling and the therapy process with immigrant children, there is an aspect to the evidence of maltreatment that reflects the pervasive consequence of untreated trauma that becomes embedded in intergenerational patterns of abuse.[12] Parents or other caregivers might not consider their practices hurtful, although the parenting that is practiced can be driven by a lack of emotional grounding, cultural stigmatization of mental health concerns, and a profound lack of resources within the home country and even upon migration to the United States.

KEY POINTS

1. When addressing child maltreatment with children who have migrated from other countries, a transnational lens is a critical part of the evaluation and determination of therapeutic interventions.

2. The assessment of a child's holistic needs must begin at the point of leaving the home country and take place on a continuum through the arrival and settlement into the United States.

3. Attachment theory is a helpful theoretical foundation for understanding the mental health needs of immigrant children who have experienced maltreatment anywhere along the continuum of migration.

REFERENCES

1. Children on the run. UN Refugee Agency (UNHCR). Accessed July 1, 2022. https://www.unhcr.org/en-us/children-on-the-run.html

2. Schmidt S. Child maltreatment and child migration: abuse disclosures by central american and mexican unaccompanied migrant children. *J Migr Hum Secur.* 2022;10(1):77-92. doi:10.1177/23315024221078951

3. Fontes LA, Tishelman AC. Language competence in forensic interviews for suspected child sexual abuse. *Child Abuse Negl.* 2014;58:51-62. doi:10.1016/j.chiabu.2016.06.014

4. Sessions C. Widespread infringement of the civil rights and civil liberties of unaccompanied noncitizen children held in the custody of CBP. Kids in Need of Defense. 2022. https://supportkind.org/wp-content/uploads/2022/04/2022.04.6-FINAL-Public-CRCL-OIG-Complaint.pdf

5. Juang LP, Simpson JA, Lee RM, et al. Using attachment and relational perspectives to understand adaptation and resilience among immigrant and refugee youth. *Am Psychol.* 2018;73(6):797-811. doi:10.1037/amp0000286

6. Childhood cut short: sexual and gender-based violence against central american migrant and refugee children. Kids in Need of Defense. 2017. Accessed July 1, 2022. https://supportkind.org/wp-content/uploads/2017/06/Childhood-Cut-Short-KIND-SGBV-Report_June2017.pdf

7. Alessi EJ, Cheung S, Kahn S, Yu M. A scoping review of the experiences of violence and abuse among sexual and gender minority migrants across the migration trajectory. *Trauma Violence Abuse.* 2021;22(5):1139-1355. doi:10.1177/15248380211043892

8. How can child protection agencies support families and children who lack lawful immigration status? Casey Family Programs. 2020. Accessed July 1, 2022. https://www.casey.org/immigration-and-child-protection/

9. Policy statement: statement on the effects of deportation and forced separation on immigrants, their families, and communities. *Am J Community Psychol.* 2018; 62(1-2):3-12. doi:10.1002/ajcp.12256

10. Fontes LA. Child maltreatment services for culturally diverse families. In: Klika JB, Conte JR, eds. *The APSAC Handbook for Child Maltreatment.* 4th ed. Sage; 2017.

11. Shubin S, Lemke L. Children displaced across borders: charting new directions for research from interdisciplinary perspectives. *Child Geogr.* 2020;18(5):505-515. doi:10.1080/14733285.2020.1781061

12. Fortuna L, Londoño Tobón A, Leonor Anglero Y, Postlethwaite A, Porche MV, Rothe EM. Focusing on racial, historical and intergenerational trauma, and resilience: a paradigm to better serving children and families. *Child Adolesc Psychiatr Clin N Am.* 2022;31(2):237-250. doi:10.1016/j.chc.2021.11.004

RELIGION, CULTURE, AND ETHNICITY

Mitzy D. Flores, PhDc, MSN, RN, AHN-BC, CHSE, COI, Caritas Coach©,
    Introspective Hypnosis Practitioner

OBJECTIVES
After reading this chapter, the reader will be able to:

1. *Evaluate data pertaining to religion, culture, and ethnicity amongst children living in the United States.*

2. *Identify previous United States family units and the current family unit.*

3. *Understand various definitions of culture.*

4. *Identify strategies to promote cultural celebration.*

BACKGROUND AND SIGNIFICANCE

The population of the United States has grown by approximately 7.4% between 2010 and 2020, making for a total population of nearly 331 400 000 people in April of 2020.[1] Based on the results of the 2020 census, there was a significant increase in racial diversity over the course of the decade, both in the population as a whole and in children.[2]

Consequently, children are said to be at the leading edge of the nation's growing diversity. Results from the 2020 census also illustrated that 52.7% of the United States' population younger than 18 years old belonged to Black, Indigenous, and people of color (BIPOC) communities versus only 39.2% of the population who were older than 18 years of age.[1] Dr. Kenneth Johnson,[2] a professor of Sociology at the University of New Hampshire, notes that the greater diversity seen in the data, as it relates to children, is the result of 2 diverging trends; one trend being the increase in population of BIPOC children and the second being the decline in overall child population numbers in the United States. Johnson also notes that since 2010, the BIPOC child population increased by 11.8% (38 500 000) despite a modest decline in the number of non-Hispanic/Latinx Black children.[2] During the same timeframe, the non-Hispanic/Latinx White child population declined by 12.9% (34 000 000).[2] Hence, the child population in the United States has declined by 1.4% (1 100 000) between 2010 and 2020 because the child gain among other groups was not sufficient to offset the non-Hispanic/Latinx White and Black decline.[2]

Changes in child populations have also changed the living arrangements for children in the United States. Those arrangements have become more racially and ethnically diverse as the number of children living in interracial and interethnic households increased from 2008 to 2018.[3] Additionally, living in a multigenerational or mixed household was seen as a more common trend, reflecting continued child immigration to the United States.[3] This indicates that the nation's growing racial/ethnic diversity will likely increase interactions across racial boundaries in the workplace and community as well.[2]

AMERICAN FAMILY UNIT

The average family in the United States has commonly been illustrated as a nuclear family (ie, consisting of a husband, wife, and children).[4] The extended family is also acknowledged in United States culture, but typically those members live separately from the nuclear family. Though the nuclear family framework is still practiced in modern society, it is no longer identified as the only social expectation. Relationship status variations in 21st century societies, such as divorce, remarriage, cohabitation of couples, births outside of marriage, LGBTQIA+ families, and individuals choosing not to have children have become more common.[4] Regarding the size of the family unit in the United States, evidence suggests that the unit size has shifted to a preference for smaller family sizes.[5] However, Asian, Black, and Hispanic/Latinx families are more likely to live in multigenerational arrangements and have larger households than non-Hispanic/Latinx White Americans.[6]

On the other hand, United States family dynamics are governed by the influences of individualism,[4] the most prevalent notion being that a person is what they make of themself and who they choose to be. Therefore, the expectation is to keep adhering to an 18th century myth of the rugged individual, who is self-reliant and self-responsible to meet personal needs and wants. As an example, parents in the United States often emphasize a child's independence, accepting that, at times, it may differ from the family's preconceived expectation of them.[4] Likewise, United States educational systems, more often than not, teach children to think of themselves as "special" or "unique" during their formative years.[4] Ironically, children's narratives and unique perspectives regarding religion, culture, and ethnicity have been minimally explored, warranting a need for further research on the topic.

RELIGION

Children's voices are often absent from the historical record; most research regarding religion and children downplays the impact that the child's traditions have on them.[7] According to a 2019 survey analysis,[8] when it comes to religion, teenagers in the United States tend to share the religious affiliation of their parents or legal guardians and attend religious services at roughly the same rate. The latter may be due to the socialization norms provided by the caregivers to the child. The adult population in the United States is trending toward being less religious in recent decades, which is accredited largely to young adults being much less likely to identify with a religious group or partake in traditional religious practices than their elders.[8] Moreover, teenagers are split on their primary reason for attending religious services: 38% say they attend because their parents want them to, 35% say they attend because they want to, and roughly 26% say that they never attend religious services. Furthermore, the survey revealed that teenagers who did not identify with any religion were less likely to rely on adults (eg, parents, other family members) than their religious peers.[8]

An Early Childhood Longitudinal Study (ECLS)-Kindergarten Cohort[7] examined the effects of parents' religious attendance and how the religious environment in the household influenced a nationally representative sample of third graders. The study looked at the children's psychological adjustment, interpersonal skills, problem behaviors, and performance on standardized tests (eg, reading, math, and science). Researchers found that third graders' psychological adjustment and social competence were positively correlated with various religious factors.[7] However, students' performance on reading, math, and science tests were negatively associated with several forms of parental religiosity, including stricter views on religion and greater adherence to service worship.[7] In summary, the findings suggest that parental religiosity produces significant gains in social psychological development among third graders while potentially undermining academic performance, particularly in math and science.[7]

CULTURE AND ETHNICITY

"Culture" can be defined in many ways and is described differently across various disciplines; however, it is often noted as a complex, organic understanding of many factors related to the human experience. Culture affects the way children and their families behave, what they value, and their identities.[9] Therefore, it is recommended that early childhood educators partner with families, when possible, in order to understand, value, respect, and honor the individual cultures of the children in their classrooms.[9] Various definitions of culture are as follows[9]:

— The organized and common practices of particular communities

— A shared organization of ideas that includes the intellectual, moral, and aesthetic standards prevalent in a community and the meaning of communicative actions

— The complex processes of human social interaction and symbolic communication

— A set of activities by which different groups produce collective memories, knowledge, social relationships, and values within historically controlled relations of power

— An instrument people use as they attempt to survive within a particular social group

— A framework that guides and bounds life practices

— All that is done by people

— The ways and manners people use to see, perceive, represent, interpret, and assign value and meaning to the reality they live or experience

— The complex whole that includes knowledge, beliefs, art, morals, customs, and any other capabilities and habits acquired by mankind as a member of society

— Shared understanding, as well as the public customs and artifacts that embody these understandings

— Patterns, explicit and implicit, of and for behavior acquired and transmitted by symbols, constituting the distinctive achievement of human groups, including their embodiments in artifacts

— A historical construction by people that is always changing rather than an inert system in which people operate

As noted from the previous section, the United States' child population is more diverse than its total population.[1-4] Hence, one can argue that cultural appreciation and awareness contributes to the building of positive self-image for children. Moreover, this appreciation assists in the developing of a strong foundation of belonging and acceptance. Interventions and practices that foster these things include cultural celebrations such as music and art appreciation as well as language education. Nonetheless, cultural appreciation should not only focus on food, festivals, and fun, but also be allowed to have sacred, safe space to honor the diversity and complexity that encompasses its definition. Ultimately, those practices, within that safe, honored space, fosters a diverse social network while the child transitions into adulthood.[9]

Statistical data from the 2016 National Survey of Children Health (NSCH) echo similar sentiments. The data indicates that children's mental health and the built environment in neighborhood vary across racial/ethnic groups, with BIPOC groups, particularly American Indian children, being more likely to live in disadvantaged neighborhoods and to experience more mental health disorders.[10] Hence, the call to action is now about supporting cultural inclusivity, beginning at the playgrounds of children. One way for adults to embody cultural inclusivity is by actively practicing the framework of cultural humility.

Cultural humility is a concept developed by Dr. Melanie Tervalon and Dr. Jann Murray-Garcia, rooted in their experiences as medical doctors in the 1990s.[11] In its most basic understanding, the model has 3 tenets, conceptualized to address inconsistencies in health care practices (**Table 14-1-a; Table 14-1-b**). Nonetheless, the cultural humility framework is applicable within education as well, recognizing that similar power imbalances can exist in the classroom and activities outside the classroom, and, more broadly, within the structures of colleges and universities.

The 3 tenets include:

— *Lifelong Learning and Critical Self-Reflection.* The understanding that each person is a complex, multidimensional human, each with their own history, story, heritage, and point of view.

— *Recognize and Challenge Power Imbalances.* A desire to co-create solutions that balance out power, with people and groups who advocate for others.

— *Institutional Accountability.*

Table 14-1-a. Potential Strategies for Enhancing Cultural Competence in Organizations Serving Hispanic Clients*	
AREA OF OPERATION	STRATEGIES
Mission & Vision	— Develop a vision and mission statement that embraces diversity.
Organizational Culture	— Foster a culture of learning about Hispanic children and families. — Form collaborative partnerships with communities served by the organization. — Engage in needs assessments of communities served by the organization. — Provide ongoing workforce development and cultural competence staff trainings. — Create forums and other opportunities for ongoing dialogue for staff to reflect on what is and what is not working when serving Hispanic families. — Engage in self-assessment of cultural competence practices via self-ratings; collect feedback from Hispanic service users. — Work with consultants, such as culture-specific healers or cultural brokers, who have in-depth knowledge of the community or Hispanic culture.
Organizational Culture	— Create and implement systems of accountability for cultural competence standards. — Engage in advocacy for communities served by the organization.
General Practices	— Follow culturally-sensitive engagement and outreach practices, such as participation in local community events, home visits, and walk-in appointments. — Follow a culturally-sensitive communication style that emphasizes the Hispanic community's preference for personalized, in-person (rather than written mail and email) communication. — Provide translation services to all children and families who need them. — Plan and allow for extended family members at appointments and other agency events. — Use culturally-relevant screening and assessment tools that are translated into Spanish at the appropriate literacy level and have been validated with Hispanics (ideally, with members of the local Hispanic community).

(continued)

Table 14-1-a. Potential Strategies for Enhancing Cultural Competence in Organizations Serving Hispanic Clients* *(continued)*

Area of Operation	Strategies
General Practices	— Allow staff to engage in cultural immersion in the community.
Staffing Practices	— Recruit, mentor and promote bicultural and bilingual Hispanic staff at all levels.
	— Hire staff from the community and community health workers to help with engagement and outreach.
	— Recruit well trained, experienced translators to provide translation and interpretation services.
Physical environment & Resources	— Create a familiar, welcoming physical environment by depicting Hispanic families in promotional materials and displaying Hispanic décor and artwork.
	— Arrange reception and meeting areas to accommodate large, extended families.
	— Hire Spanish-speaking receptionists.
	— Provide materials in Spanish at the appropriate literacy level.

See also the National Center for Cultural Competence at Georgetown University (in Resources) for relevant self-assessment and practice tools

Sue, D.W. (2001). Multidimensional Facets of Cultural Competence. The Counseling Psychologist, 29(6), pp. 790-821.

Table 14-1-b. Potential Strategies for Enhancing Cultural Competence among Individual Staff Serving Hispanic Clients*

Areas of Individual Ability	Strategies
Awareness & Self-reflection	— Engage in self-reflection about one's culture and potential biases.
	— Identify one's preparedness to serve Hispanic populations.
	— Participate in cultural immersion experiences with Hispanic communities.
	— Participate in cultural competence trainings.
	— Be willing to learn and ask questions.
Knowledge	— Stay informed on scientific evidence relevant to the evaluation and treatment of Hispanic children and families.
	— Critically evaluate and determine the fit between an assessment or intervention and the cultural backgrounds of children and families.
	— Gain knowledge about the culture (ie, values, beliefs, and practices) and history of Hispanic children and families.
	— Guided by understanding of the Hispanic population as a whole, gain knowledge regarding the individual client on their values, beliefs and practices; views on health, disability and disease; family rituals, traditions and routines; role of authority figures within and outside of their family; religion and spirituality; acculturation level; use of traditional and spiritual healers; understanding of and desire for services.
Skills	— Develop relationship building and communication skills, including how to address family members and how to use and interpret nonverbal cues, that are syntonic with Hispanic norms.
	— If not Spanish-speaking, become skilled at working with a translator.

(continued)

Table 14-1-b. Potential Strategies for Enhancing Cultural Competence among Individual Staff Serving Hispanic Clients* *(continued)*	
AREAS OF INDIVIDUAL ABILITY	STRATEGIES
Skills	— Become skilled in engaging and working with family members in services.
	— Partner with traditional and spiritual leaders.
	— Try new strategies when traditional strategies do not work.
	— When unsure, ask questions and practice active listening.

*See also the National Center for Cultural and Linguistic Responsiveness (listed in Resources) for tools and resources that promote cultural competence at the staff level.

CULTURAL CELEBRATION PRACTICES

Oral History

Stories of cultural history can provide a curious view for a child that is learning their cultural heritage. Folklore that has been passed down through generations, such as stories, fables, and adventure tales, are likely to be saturated with rich vocabulary, customs, tradition, and cultural norms that children can learn to relate to. Examples of oral history activities for children may include exploring their family tree or exercises that include descriptions of landscapes in which there is an acknowledgment of the colors, sounds, tastes, and geographical landmarks. This, in return, may allow the child to imagine a world that they can immerse themselves in and belong to. Additionally, discussing family history with the child may also help facilitate the understanding of diversity. It is noted that having a better understanding of family can help children be confident in their identity.[12]

Language Appreciation

Language is an extremely powerful tool that can provide enhanced insight on family history, stories, and traditions.[12] Between the ages of 0 and 3 years old, the brains of children are uniquely suited to learn a second language, as the brain is in its most flexible stage. Additionally, bilingually exposed infants excel in detecting a switch in language as early as 6 months old. It is also suggested that children can learn a second language as easily as they learn their primary language. Learning a second language does not negatively impact the child's native language.[13] This indicates that children who are literate in multiple languages may be able to better comprehend the multi-layers of their heritage through various written and oral mediums.

Food

Cooking creates bonding opportunities between caregivers and children and allows for additional cultural conversations.[12] Discussing traditional recipes, ingredients, and food presentations can foster the child's curiosity about cultural practices and norms. It also leaves room for other stories that relate to food, such as the likes and dislikes of family members, deepening family bonds. Through food, children can learn empathy and tolerance as they learn the diversity that exists within various cultural meals. As the exploration of cultural gastronomy begins with children of all ages in a public setting, service providers, educators, and caregivers must assist in cultivating an atmosphere of safety and support. Food customs, colors, smells, and looks may be significantly different than the mainstream norms, and that may cause insecurity and increase vulnerability to the child that is introducing their dishes.

SUMMARY

Diversity in the United States is growing the most among those younger than 18 years old. Therefore, child-centered institutions, such as schools and health care provider settings, will be the first to serve this diverse population.[2] This growing population will need more multiracial and multiethnic communities that will enhance interracial relations, widen friendship networks, and prepare them for life in an increasingly diverse nation.[2] Children are affected by adult responses to diversity on multiple plains of their existence. For example, child populations with diverse linguistic and religious backgrounds can face discrimination in their school settings, while also experiencing microaggression and inequalities in other public spaces. Educators as well as service practitioners should therefore be versed in the social, political, and cultural environment they practice in to help that population promote a more equitable landscape of success.

CASE STUDY

Case Study 14-1

During the holiday season, a local public school pre-school educator wanted to invite her students and their families to an end of the year party. Additionally, the educator wanted all the pre-school sections of the school to be able to participate in the festivities. The educator acknowledged that the district she worked in serves underrepresented populations as well as culturally diverse individuals. The educator believed that a fun and creative approach would be to theme the celebration a "Global Extravaganza." The educator envisioned a kaleidoscope of activities and elicited the help of administration and local community members to help support all the moving parts of such an event.

Discussion

The educator created several activities for children and their respective families to participate in, each touching on different cultural domains. In order to involve oral histories in the celebration, she had students ask their parents to tell them a fairytale that may have originated within their cultural, ethnic, or religious background. She also asked the children and their parents to create a short list of traditional songs from their cultures. The children were able to participate in a show and tell on the night of the event, sharing the stories they learned from their parents with each other, while the music played throughout the celebration was a combination of the songs recommended by each family.

Other activities at the celebration included an arts station that allowed the children to color, make, and craft various ideas that represented different cultural, ethnic, and religious customs that belonged to various populations that attended the pre-school.

The party also involved a food component, with children and parents invited to bring their favorite dishes to share with the class. The parents wrote down short descriptions of their dishes and why they were important to the family unit. They were also asked to write down all of the ingredients in the dishes they brought so that individuals with food allergies or restrictions were able to discern what they could eat.

Both children and parents were invited to showcase their traditional regalia at the event.

In order to ensure that the children participating in the event felt safe, respected, and seen, the educator constantly checked in with the children to gauge whether or not they were enjoying the festivities. She also created a quieter and less stimulating area off to the side in case any child felt overwhelmed and wanted to step away (with appropriate supervision as needed). Parents and volunteers were reminded at the beginning of the event to be open and gentle when introducing new languages and customs to the children in attendance.

The next time class was held at the pre-school, the educator created an assignment that mimicked a debriefing so that the children were able to share how they felt about the multicultural festival.

KEY POINTS

1. The United States' growing racial/ethnic diversity will likely increase the interaction across racial/ethnic boundaries in the workplace and in communities.

2. There is no moral difference between children who are raised as religious and those raised secular or non-believing.

3. Cultural appreciation and awareness contribute to the building of positive self-image for children.

REFERENCES

1. Johnson K. New census reflects growing US population diversity, with children in the forefront. Carsey School of Public Policy. 2021. Accessed June 21, 2022. https://carsey.unh.edu/publication/new-census-reflects-growing-US-population-diversity

2. Census bureau releases new report on living arrangements of children. United States Census Bureau. Updated February 22, 2022. Accessed June 21, 2022. https://www.census.gov/newsroom/press-releases/2022/living-arrangements-of-chldren.html

3. Anderson LR, Hemez PF, Kreider RM. Household economic studies. United States Census Bureau. 2022. https://www.census.gov/content/dam/Census/library/publications/2022/demo/p70-174.pdf

4. American culture - family. Cultural Atlas. 2020. Accessed June 21, 2022. https://culturalatlas.sbs.com.au/american-culture/american-culture-family

5. Gao G. Americans' ideal family size is smaller than it used to be. Pew Research Center. 2015. Accessed June 21, 2022. https://www.pewresearch.org/fact-tank/2015/05/08/ideal-size-of-the-american-family/

6. Cohn D, Horowitz JM, Minkin R, Fry R, Hurst K. Financial issues top the list of reasons US adults live in multigenerational homes. Pew Research Center. 2022. Accessed June 21, 2022. https://www.pewresearch.org/social-trends/2022/03/24/the-demographics-of-multigenerational-households/

7. Bartkowski J, Xu X, Bartkowski S. Mixed blessing: the beneficial and detrimental effects of religion on child development among third-graders. *Religions.* 2019; 10(1):37. doi:10.3390/rel10010037

8. US teens take after their parents religiously, attend services together and enjoy family rituals. Pew Research Center. 2020. Accessed June 21, 2022. https://www.pewresearch.org/religion/2020/09/10/u-s-teens-take-after-their-parents-religiously-attend-services-together-and-enjoy-family-rituals/

9. Esquivel K, Elam E, Paris J, Tafoya M. The importance of culture. In: Northeast Wisconsin Technical College, eds. *Infant & Toddler Development.* Pressbooks; 2019. https://wtcs.pressbooks.pub/infanttoddlerdev/chapter/chapter-12-the-importance-of-culture/#:~:text=Culture%20is%E2%80%A6&text=A%20set%20of%20activities%20by,historically%20controlled%20relations%20of%20power

10. Shen Y. Race/ethnicity, built environment in neighborhood, and children's mental health in the US. *Int J Environ Health Res.* 2020;32(2):277-291. doi:10.1080/09603123.2020.1753663

11. Tervalon M, Murray-Garcia J. Cultural humility versus cultural competence: a critical distinction in defining physician training outcomes in multicultural education. *JHCPU.* 1998;9:117-125. doi:10.1353/hpu.2010.0233

12. Celebrate tradition and cultural awareness with young children. Southwest Human Development. 2018. Accessed June 21, 2022. https://www.swhd.org/celebrating-tradition-and-cultural-awareness-with-young-children/#:~:text=Cultural%20awareness%20and%20tradition%20play

13. Trautner T. Advantages of a bilingual brain. Michigan State University. 2019. Accessed June 21, 2022. https://www.canr.msu.edu/news/advantages_of_a_bilingual_brain

THE SCHOOL ENVIRONMENT AND THE IMPACTS OF EDUCATION WHEN THE TEACHER IS THE BULLY

Eileen F. Starr, PhD, LCSW
Adjoa D. Robinson, PhD, MSW

OBJECTIVES

After reading this chapter, the reader will be able to:

1. *Define teacher bullying.*

2. *Describe the effects of teacher bullying on academic and mental health outcomes among primary and secondary age students.*

3. *Discuss the long-term effects of teacher bullying.*

BACKGROUND AND SIGNIFICANCE

The research on bullying from primary to higher education and the long-term implications is extensive. However, there is only rudimentary research studying educator-on-student bullying. Further, victimization of students by teachers and teachers by students has long been recognized in the United States but is rarely reported.[1] The focus of teacher bullying in this chapter includes primary and secondary education, typically referred to as kindergarten through 12th grade (K-12). Teacher bullying is defined as "a teacher who uses his/her power to punish, manipulate, or disparage a student beyond what would be a reasonable disciplinary procedure."[1] It is "a pattern of conduct, rooted in a power differential, that threatens, harms, humiliates, induces fear, or causes students substantial emotional distress."[2] Historical examples of teacher bullying include having students stand in the corner with a "dunce cap," repeatedly slapping a student's outstretched hands with rulers, and using the "board of education" (ie, an elongated wooden paddle with holes used on a student's buttocks while bent over the principal's desk for a series of "whacks"). Another example of teacher bullying via humiliation is announcing a student's failing grade as they receive their assignment or test.

OUTCOMES OF TEACHER BULLYING

Brendgen & Poulin[3] suggest that students who are impacted by bullying experience a greater likelihood of lifelong mental health issues and negative psychosocial outcomes. Regardless of the way one is bullied, victims are at risk for several coexisting and short-term and long-term adjustment problems. These challenges include school difficulties, internalizing and externalizing behaviors, and compromised physical health.[4] There is a growing body of evidence that suggests victims of bullying are more likely than others to suffer from psychiatric disorders and poorer social relationships, as well as financial and work-related problems once they become adults.[5,6] Further, Brendgen & Poulin[3] note a link to victimization in school and being vulnerable to future victimization in the workplace. This type of chronic abuse throughout childhood is believed to significantly contribute to the development of depressive symptoms. The manifestation of these symptoms in the workplace may in turn generate negative reactions from colleagues, thus putting individuals at risk of repeated bullying in adulthood.[3] There are different types of bullying that include but are not limited to direct and social victimization. ***Direct victimization*** typically includes physical and verbal aggression, which is a type of emotional abuse with higher prevalence among male students. ***Social victimization*** involves manipulating social relationships in order to hurt the victim (eg, spreading rumors or social exclusion), which is typically more predominant among female students.[3] Unfortunately, identifying teacher-led bullying is challenging as most of the abuse is typically emotional or verbal, used with the intent to embarrass students in front of their peers. As a result, there is uncertainty for parents about how to address this due to a fear of making things worse for their child.

PREVALENCE

According to national data, the prevalence of purposefully targeted teacher-on-student bullying ranges from approximately 15% to as high as 30% of primary and secondary school students.[7] However, it is likely much higher than what the data suggests, due to the limited research involving the teacher as the bully.[7] The suspected higher prevalence of teacher-on-student bullying is evidenced by focus group interviews with over 200 public, private, and parochial students in which they identified at least one or more teachers who would be considered bullies.[8] Further, out of these students surveyed, 47% identified 3 or more teachers whom they considered to be bullies.

THEORETICAL PERSPECTIVES AS TO WHY TEACHERS BULLY

There are several theoretical perspectives to support the relationship between the teacher who bullies and the student victim. Further, there is compelling data indicating that teachers who bully were also victims of teacher bullying themselves as students.[1] Accordingly, these teacher bullies were more likely to utilize the same or similar strategies in their classroom.

THEORY OF SHAME

While shame is a natural emotion that everyone experiences, it can have strong negative impacts on a person's self-image. Notions of shame can make one feel as though they are a bad person, "less than" others, unlovable, or unworthy of happiness. When these feelings become overwhelming, they can become self-fulfilling prophecies. The theory of shame postulates that those subjected to physical abuse as children often live with a sense of guilt and humiliation, impacting their neuropsychobiological functioning.[9] As a result, with shame being such a powerful and complex emotion, it often surfaces when the sense of inadequacy becomes palpable. Internal factors can exacerbate these feelings of inadequacy that stem from historical and current family dynamics, personal values, or external professional pressures. When a teacher is the one experiencing this overwhelming sense of shame, they are vulnerable to externalizing blame, and in their position of power, this can morph into bullying behaviors. This results in increased susceptibility for psychopathology, which manifests as interpersonal relationship difficulties, including involvement in bullying.[10]

SOCIAL LEARNING THEORY

The social learning theory is another perspective supporting the relationship between the teacher bully and student victim. From the lens of the social learning theory, children who experience physical violence or live in violent households (including those who experience psychological and emotional abuse) learn that these family dynamics are a normal way of being treated or that violence is an acceptable way to respond to conflicts.[11] Further, since these maladaptive responses are learned behaviors, the same pattern often continues with others, especially those perceived as weaker.[12] Thus, a teacher bully who grew up in a violent household will respond with those same bullying behaviors towards the children in their care.

ECOLOGICAL PERSPECTIVE OF INDIVIDUAL DEVELOPMENT

A final theoretical perspective supporting the teacher bully and student victim dynamic is the ecological perspective of individual development. This framework postulates a transactional relationship between an individual and the nested environmental ecosystems that they exist within (for a more detailed explanation of the scales of an individual's environment, see Volume 1, Chapter 5: Social Determinants of Health). These interconnected environments interact with one another as well as the individual to influence the individual's adaptive and maladaptive behaviors.[10] For example, if a teacher humiliates a student in the classroom, the student may experience emotional distress and react either overtly or through internalizing their distress in relation to this treatment by their teacher. If members of the larger school environment (eg, other teachers, school administrators, parents) know about this humiliation but for one reason or another enable the teacher to continue bullying the student, the student may experience a variety of physical and mental health sequelae, such as decompensated self-esteem and self-worth, anxiety regarding the bullying teacher's class, and somatic complaints.[13] This may lead to attendance issues that worsen in severity and other maladaptive behaviors. Conversely, sanctions or professional development may result in a positive behavior change by the teacher towards the student, thus promoting adaptive behaviors/outcomes in the student.

Those who have experienced physical, emotional, verbal, or psychological abuse as children tend to struggle, resulting in difficulties with adapting, thus increasing the risk of becoming a perpetrator of similar abuse. Additionally, these individuals typically experience poor mental health outcomes throughout their lives.[14] Another tenant of the ecological theory of social development suggests those who experience childhood physical abuse also have increased challenges with social adaptation, increasing the risk of participation in peer bullying.[14]

THE ROLE OF THE SOCIAL WORKER

Training for clinical social workers, specifically those who work in schools, typically emphasizes being solution-focused and proactive in addressing bullying incidents. Social workers can use these skills to be an important member of an interdisciplinary team made up of administrators, faculty, and support staff. Together, they can develop and implement policies, training, and curriculum that promote a safe school environment for all. This can be accomplished through many different avenues, such as being a member of a committee, writing grants to obtain state or federal dollars, developing trainings, and enhancing practical resources for teachers to strengthen classroom management skills. Further, social workers can develop opportunities for teachers to recognize their sources of frustration and triggers with particular students in order to increase awareness of how negative interactions are detrimental to the students and the overall school environment.

THE CHALLENGES FOR TODAY'S EDUCATOR

Notwithstanding occasional negative interactions, most teachers sincerely care about the physical and emotional wellbeing, learning, success, and happiness of their students. This attitude is prevalent despite significant job stressors, being poorly compensated, sacrificing free time, and using their personal funds to provide supplies and resources for the classroom. Further, the considerable pressures and expectations for educators can be unrealistic at times.

UNINTENDED CONSEQUENCES OF FEDERAL POLICIES

The federal government ratified the 2015 Every Student Succeeds Act (ESSA),[15] which replaces the Bush Administration's 2002 No Child Left Behind Policy (NCLB). ESSA policies present as less retaliatory from the competitive and punitive-based NCLB policy; however, these federal policies continue to contribute to substantial pressures and stress as they will "punish" schools by way of decreasing federal/state funding for not meeting the acceptable minimum testing standards. For example, one of the expectations of ESSA is that every state is required to identify and submit the data to the Department of Education. This information includes the names of the lowest performing schools based on standardized testing outcomes, along with a plan to improve them. This system tends to blame and chastise educators and their administrators with the intent to incentivize teachers to work harder.[16] The sanctions imposed at both the federal and state level for the underperforming schools severely affect administrators, teachers, and students. Therefore, the existing pressures for teachers and administrators are exacerbated due to the burden of having to maintain or raise test scores year after year. Further, a state or school district can choose to continue the NCLB value-added assessment, basing teachers' salaries on student standardized testing outcomes.[15] As a result, teachers have increasingly more burdens and responsibilities, which impact classroom dynamics and student-teacher interactions.

INFLUENCE OF THE STUDENT-TEACHER RELATIONSHIP

There has been limited research on how student-teacher relationships can shield or exacerbate negative outcomes on affected students. Implications suggest that positive student-teacher relationships correlate with a decrease in challenging psychosocial outcomes.[17] If a student is a bully or a bullying victim, but also has a poor relationship(s) with the teacher(s), there is an increased risk of depression.[17] Further, students struggling with ongoing sadness or depression typically have a greater dependence on their teachers as compared to their non-depressed peers.[18] As a result, these particular students have an increased probability of being bullied by both peers and adults.[19]

The importance of student-teacher relationships cannot be overstated. They are meaningful for the emotional and relational connections that develop primarily due to their extended daily interactions.[20] Further, Settanni et al[21] suggests that positive student-teacher relationships have a correlation to higher academic achievement, increased self-esteem, adjustments to school and life challenges, higher resiliency, and social skill development. Other outcomes of positive student-teacher connections are a decrease in incidents of school absences or school avoidance as well as an increased motivation to learn.[21] Further, these encouraging mentorship relationships cause students to be less judgmental, thus demonstrating more empathy, and include positive influences on emotional regulation and social skills.[22]

WHEN IT IS THE TEACHER WHO IS THE CLASSROOM BULLY

According to the National School Climate Center,[23] large class sizes, students with cognitive limitations or behavioral challenges, and minority students are more likely to be in classrooms with a teacher who tends to be more oppressive and present with a tough demeanor. Despite the more vulnerable students having more exposure to teacher bullying, most students experience a "mean teacher" at some point in their primary, middle, or secondary schooling.[1]

Estimates range from 15% to 30% of students reporting physical, verbal, or sexual harassment by their teachers.[1] Teachers responding as having participated in bullying behaviors in their classrooms attribute the negative interactions to a myriad of issues. These issues range from personality conflicts, learning style differences, and students "testing" the teacher/classroom boundaries to burnout and personal or work-related stressors. However, when do "mean" behaviors cross the line and the teacher becomes the classroom bully?

To further support the data that indicate teachers can abuse the power dynamic in the classroom, an anonymous survey polling teachers indicated that almost half of those surveyed (48%) acknowledged having bullied a student.[1] Researchers hypothesized the rationale for teachers who bully include inconsistent or limited training on effective classroom management techniques and one-to-one disciplinary strategies. This is supported by teachers acknowledging feeling frustrated with the lack of access to resources or professional development seminars about classroom and student intervention strategies. Unfortunately, these professional development training opportunities for teachers remain inconsistent across schools, even within individual districts. Due to the variability of opportunities for teachers to grasp effective classroom management skills, learn strengths-based interventions, and gain strategies to increase positive outcomes for interacting with challenging students, this often leads to retaliation from the teacher to the student.

CHALLENGES TO ADDRESSING TEACHER BULLYING

It is difficult to effectively address teacher bullying in the classroom because parents, administrators, and school counselors typically manage conflicts, physical altercations, and emotional or verbal abuse between students. Negative interactions between students and teachers, especially psychological abuses, are far less likely to be reported by the student victim when the teacher is the perpetrator. It is of great consequence to note that when negative student-teacher relationships exist, there is the consideration of a power differential between the teacher and student. The result of a negative dynamic between a teacher and their student is connected to higher levels of student-to-student victimization and increased bystander effect (ie, when the presence of others discourages an individual from intervening in a situation against a bully or during an assault or other crime).[24]

These are important considerations due to the influence of positive as well as negative student-teacher relationships on a student's social-emotional and psychological wellbeing. Notably, mixed messages about what makes an effective teacher remain ubiquitous. Some teachers use profanity or intimidation via body language (eg, posturing, lack of respect for a student's personal space) as a way to exert authority. Administrators and teaching colleagues often perceive students as respecting these teachers, thereby teacher bullies are considered to be effective educators and are not to be challenged. Unfortunately, what is actually communicated by these teachers is not mutual respect, courtesy, or an appreciation for others, but rather coerciveness and intimidation. More often than not, students will do whatever they need to do in an effort to not "rock the boat" for fear of retaliation.[25] When students fear teachers, it impacts their ability to effectively learn, comprehend, and retain information.[1] This analysis is supported by the outcomes of negative student-teacher relationships as evidenced by the substantiated reports of teachers who berate students, verbalize expectations of the students having undesirable outcomes for their future lives, and the correlation to increased student involvement in bullying-related and aggressive behaviors.[26]

IMPLICATIONS FOR STUDENTS

Surprisingly, there is limited data on the destructiveness of the teacher as the bully. McEvoy[2] notes that students who are on the receiving end of a teacher's hostility are in a situation often consistent with a violent domestic or interpersonal relationship wherein the abuser is considered all-powerful. The student often feels trapped in a classroom environment where they bear the brunt of the teacher's antagonistic behaviors day-in and day-out. This type of abuse may be less likely to be reported because students fear the teacher retaliating via graded assignments and classroom behavior.[27]

THE INFLUENCE OF TEACHER INTERVENTION

Student-to-student bullying-related behaviors involve both active bullying and passive bullying. That is, actively participating in the bullying of others, such as assisting in restraining a victim, or passive bullying, such as the encouragement of the bullying by provoking a confrontation. As previously noted, research consistently demonstrates that the quality of student-teacher relationships has a significant influence on interpersonal interactions between students. This is especially influential in elementary school grades (ie, K-5).[27]

TEACHER INDIFFERENCE OR VICARIOUS TRAUMA?

The consequences of an educator either not interceding or directly mistreating and harassing students has collateral negative effects in the classroom, making the task of effective classroom management an uphill battle.[1] Per Twemlow et al,[1] in order for students to maintain control, they have to see fair and consistent discipline along with clear expectations for themselves and their peers. If there is unpredictability (eg, overly harsh treatment of one student while enabling or not responding to another student's inappropriate behavior), students will often feel that teachers are unreliable and unfair, and thereby they become adversaries who are not to be recognized as trustworthy or safe.

The role of the teacher in modeling appropriate behaviors, creating a safe learning space, and dealing both immediately and effectively with bullying when it occurs cannot be understated. How teachers set classroom norms and whether they engage in bullying students sets the tone for the classroom and larger school community. The data in various studies indicate that without a consistent and sustained approach to managing bullying, both between students and the manner in which teachers interact with students, it will continue to be an issue. Further, when the teacher engages in bullying, either directly or indirectly, this will have a deleterious effect on maintaining classroom dynamics and even undermine the larger educational systems' attempts to incorporate anti-bullying efforts.[28]

CULTURAL IMPLICATIONS

Students subjected to ongoing harassment, intimidation, isolation, and abuse at school have greater incidence of poor emotional regulation and psychological wellbeing, which can continue throughout their lives. Mostly absent from the research is the bullying and harassment of marginalized populations. Language such as the "invasion of illegal aliens," or the 2022 Texas Republican Party Platform declaring "homosexuality an abnormal life choice," from the larger society can also be propagated by teachers and school staff. Such language and beliefs can render the bullying of BIPOC, sexual, and religious minorities acceptable or can lead teachers to "look the other way" when such bullying occurs, leaving students feeling invisible, undeserving of being protected, and excluded, in addition to potentially experiencing emotional and verbal abuse and violence.[29,30] Teachers who are offenders or teacher bystanders who are reticent to intervene when they witness or have knowledge of students engaging in the victimization of their peers intensifies the victim's traumatization. Further, teachers' conscious or unconscious biases play a substantial role in enabling actions that specifically target students based on race, culture, ethnicity, sexual orientation (actual or perceived), or religious affiliation. As a result, minority students often have more severe trauma, with effects that can be lifelong.

CONSIDERATIONS

Most students will internalize feelings and emotions if they are targeted by a teacher, and there are many variables related to their hesitancy to disclose. Some of these variables include but are not limited to embarrassment (especially with adolescents), fear of retribution from the teacher, and worries about being believed. As noted earlier, BIPOC and special needs students are more likely to be victimized than their peers. Interestingly, academically high-performing students are at greater risk for being victimized by teachers who struggle with insecurities when feeling intimidated or challenged by these students.[1]

SOMATIC COMPLAINTS

As a result of ambiguity to disclose, a child manifests internal struggles differently than an adult. Awareness by caregivers, family, friends, coaches, and other concerned adults of moderate or significant fluctuations in managing emotions, academic changes, or behavioral changes is essential. Further, students who previously enjoyed attending school but share they no longer wish to have a tendency to report an increase in vague somatic complaints such as stomach aches, headaches, and general malaise.

TEACHER COMPLAINTS

It is not atypical that, on occasion, students will complain about "having a mean teacher." Naturally, these complaints may be a result of a personality conflict, a teacher having higher expectations for their students, or having more structure and boundaries in the classroom. Nevertheless, caregivers asking open-ended questions (eg, "[student name] has come home upset and preoccupied since school began; I'm wondering if you have noticed any dynamics with them in the classroom that I should be aware of?") that come from a place of curiosity when inquiring about the child's relationship with their teacher or if other students have the same feelings will assist in making the student feel less reticent to express their feelings.

If the student does share their feelings, listen for clues or buzzwords such as "they yell a lot," "they make me feel bad about myself," or other indications that the student is being singled out via humiliation or belittlement.

BEHAVIORAL AND ACADEMIC CHANGES

Children, particularly primary school students who are being victimized by their teacher, will exhibit emotional dysregulation via angry outbursts, clinginess, mood shifts, and isolation prior to leaving or coming home from school. Further, they also may present self-deprecating thoughts about themselves, their intelligence, or the quality of their school assignments or homework. This is especially concerning if the student typically produces passing to excellent grades or if there is a significant change in grades. Younger children, primarily due to their cognitive/developmental level, have a limited capacity to concretely disclose "my teacher is abusing me," especially when the abuse is emotional or verbal in nature. They may also have an increase in vague somatic complaints related to stomach pain, headaches, gastrointestinal distress, insomnia, or hypersomnia.

IMPORTANCE OF COMMUNICATION AND ADVOCACY

Caregivers and concerned loved ones often vacillate on how to best address suspected teacher bullying. Encouraging the student to construct a timeline of when the incidents began, dates of subsequent occurrences, and who was present or involved (even as bystanders) will aid in effectively addressing the victimization.

Depending on the severity of the bullying, scheduling a time to meet with the teacher to discuss their perspective will be beneficial because this makes them aware of the issue and the impact on the student's social, emotional, and behavioral functioning. It will also be helpful to ask if other students are having similar experiences. Following the chain of command to rectify the situation is essential to mitigate the emotional damage to the student and potentially peers who are being bullied by the teacher. If going up the chain of command is proving ineffective or the school administration is not satisfactorily effective in addressing the situation, other considerations, such as requesting a classroom change or even a transfer to a different school, may be an option in the short-term in order to provide some relief for the student until the issue can be resolved. Interventions are essential due to the long-term risks and implications discussed earlier associated with being victimized in school, especially by people in positions of power.

CASE STUDY

Case Study 15-1

An eighth grade male student was verbally and emotionally abused by a peer who was using racial slurs, profanity, and epithets. Other peers did not directly engage, but per the student's report, they "stood by and laughed." The student reported that he unsuccessfully attempted to acquire help from his teacher, noting, "I told him that other people were laughing, and it made me feel bad, but what really bothered me was that when I told him [the teacher], he just shrugged and he said, 'Yeah, okay.'"

Discussion

Teachers who are indifferent to witnessing such abuse, exacerbated by the use of racial slurs and encouraged by other students (as evidenced by the victim report), give the impression that they are approving of the bullying via their inaction (ie, bystander effect).[1]

KEY POINTS

1. Teacher bullying is an intentional pattern of behavior that causes harm—verbal, physical, emotional, or social.

2. Teacher bullying is underresearched and underreported but widely experienced, resulting in short- and long-term negative emotional, psychological, and academic outcomes.

3. The theory of shame, social learning theory, and the ecological perspective of individual development can help explain why teachers bully and the mechanisms by which teacher bullying affects student outcomes.

4. Minority status students are particularly vulnerable to teacher bullying as the school and classroom reflect dominant cultural biases and structural inequities.

5. Social workers have a critical role to play as members of interdisciplinary teams. As proactive and solution-focused advocates, they can promote, develop, and implement interventions and policies that support safe school environments.

REFERENCES

1. Twemlow SW, Fonagy P, Sacco FC, Brethour JR. Teachers who bully students: a hidden trauma. *Int J Soc Psychiatry.* 2006;52(3):187-198. doi:10.1177/0020764006067234

2. McEvoy A. Abuse of power. Learning for Justice. August 28, 2014. Accessed June 27, 2022. https://www.learningforjustice.org/magazine/fall-2014/abuse-of-power

3. Brendgen M, Poulin F. Continued bullying victimization from childhood to young adulthood: a longitudinal study of mediating and protective factors. *J Abnorm Child Psychol.* 2018;46(1):27-39. doi:10.1007/s10802-017-0314-5

4. Vaillancourt T, Brittain HL, McDougall P, Duku E. Longitudinal links between childhood peer victimization, internalizing and externalizing problems, and academic functioning: developmental cascades. *J Abnorm Child Psychol.* 2013;41(8):1203-1215. doi:10.1007/s10802-013-9781-5

5. Copeland WE, Wolke D, Angold A, Costello EJ. Adult psychiatric outcomes of bullying and being bullied by peers in childhood and adolescence. *JAMA Psychiatry.* 2013;70(4):419-426. doi:10.1001/jamapsychiatry.2013.504

6. Wolke D, Copeland WE, Angold A, Costello EJ. Impact of bullying in childhood on adult health, wealth, crime and social outcomes. *Psychol Sci.* 2013;24(10):1958-1970. doi:10.1177/0956797613481608

7. Morin A. The truth about how many people are bullied at school and at work. Verywell Family. April 19, 2019. Accessed June 27, 2022. https://www.verywell-family.com/bullying-statistics-to-know-4589438

8. Zerillo C, Osterman KF. Teacher perceptions of teacher bullying. *Improv Sch.* 2011;14(3):239-257. doi:10.1177/1365480211419586

9. Annerbäck EM, Sahlqvist L, Svedin CG, Wingren G, Gustafsson PA. Child physical abuse and concurrence of other types of child abuse in Sweden-Associations with health and risk behaviors. *Child Abuse Negl.* 2012;36(7-8):585-595. doi:10.1016/j.chiabu.2012.05.006

10. Yen CF, Ko CH, Liu TL, Hu HF. Physical child abuse and teacher harassment and their effects on mental health problems amongst adolescent bully-victims in Taiwan. *Child Psychiatry Hum Dev.* 2015;46(5):683-692. doi:10.1007/s10578-014-0510-2

11. Ephraim R. Albert bandura. *Arch Ment Health.* 2015;16(2):151-153.

12. Baldry AC. Bullying in schools and exposure to domestic violence. *Child Abuse Negl.* 2003;27(7):713-732. doi:10.1016/s0145-2134(03)00114-5

13. Demol K, Verschueren K, Salmivalli C, Colpin H. Perceived teacher responses to bullying influence students' social cognitions. *Front Psychol.* 2020;11:592582. doi:10.3389/fpsyg.2020.592582

14. Duke NN, Pettingell SL, McMorris BJ, Borowsky IW. Adolescent violence perpetration: associations with multiple types of adverse childhood experiences. *Pediatrics.* 2010;125(4):e778-786. doi:10.1542/peds.2009-0597

15. Every Student Succeeds Act, HR Rep No. 114-354, US Cong, (2015). Accessed May 22, 2022. http://www.congress.gov/

16. Resseger J. Federally mandated standardized testing: if nothing is done to change a bad public policy, it never goes away. National Education Policy Center. February 22, 2022. Accessed May 18, 2022. https://nepc.colorado.edu/blog/federally-mandated

17. Huang FL, Lewis C, Cohen DR, Prewett S, Herman K. Bullying involvement, teacher–student relationships, and psychosocial outcomes. *Sch Psychol Q.* 2018; 33(2):223-234. doi:10.1037/spq0000249

18. Henricsson L, Rydell AM. Elementary school children with behavior problems: teacher-child relations and self-perception. A prospective study. *Merrill-Palmer Q.* 2004;50(2):111-138. doi:10.1353/mpq.2004.0012

19. Troop-Gordon W, Kopp J. Teacher–child relationship quality and children's peer victimization and aggressive behavior in late childhood. *Soc Dev.* 2011;20(3):536-561. doi:10.1111/j.1467-9507.2011.00604.x

20. Fraire M, Longobardi C, Prino LE, Sclavo E, Settanni M. Examining the student-teacher relationship scale in the italian context: a factorial validity study. *Electron J Res Educ Psychol.* 2013;11(3):851-882. doi:10.14204/ejrep.31.13068

21. Settanni M, Longobardi C, Sclavo E, Fraire M, Prino LE. Development and psychometric analysis of the student–teacher relationship scale – short form. *Front Psychol.* 2015;6:898. doi:10.3389/fpsyg.2015.00898

22. Zins J, Greenberg M, Weissberg R, Minke K, Bear G. Promoting social and emotional competence in children: strategies and programs that work. In: Bar-On R, Maree JG, Elias MJ, eds. *Educating People to Be Emotionally Intelligent.* Praeger Publishers/Greenwood Publishing Group; 2007.

23. The school climate improvement process: essential elements. National School Climate Center. 2012. Accessed May 19, 2022. https://schoolclimate.org/services/measuring-school-climate-csci/

24. Juvonen J, Galván A. Peer influence in involuntary social groups: lessons from research on bullying. In: Prinstein MJ, Dodge KA, eds. *Understanding Peer Influence in Children and Adolescents*. The Guilford Press; 2008:225-244.

25. Devine J. *Maximum Security: The Culture of Violence in Inner-City Schools.* University of Chicago Press; 1997. Accessed June 29, 2022. https://press.uchicago.edu/ucp/books/book/chicago/M/bo3683561.html

26. Longobardi C, Iotti NO, Jungert T, Settanni M. Student-teacher relationships and bullying: the role of student social status. *J Adolesc.* 2018;63:1-10. doi:10.1016/j.adolescence.2017.12.001

27. Wang C, Swearer SM, Lembeck P, Collins A, Berry B. Teachers matter: an examination of student-teacher relationships, attitudes toward bullying, and bullying behavior. *J Appl Sch Psychol.* 2015;31(3):219-238. doi:10.1080/15377903.2015.1056923

28. James DJ, Lawlor M, Flynn A, Murphy N, Courtney P, Henry B. One school's experience of engaging with a comprehensive anti-bullying programme in the Irish context: adolescent and teacher perspectives. *Pastor Care Educ.* 2006;24(4):39-48. doi:10.1111/j.1468-0122.2006.00389.x

29. Republican Party of Texas. Platform and Resolutions as Amended and Adopted by the 2022 State Convention of the Republican Party of Texas. Accessed June 19, 2022. https://texasgop.org/wp-content/uploads/2022/07/2022-RPT-Platform.pdf

30. Subramanian M. *Bullying: The Ultimate Teen Guide, Volume 38.* Rowman & Littlefield; 2014.

BULLYING AND CYBERBULLYING

Eileen M. Alexy, PhD, RN, APN, PMHCNS-BC
Paul Thomas Clements, PhD, RN, ANEF, DF-IAFN, DF-AFN

OBJECTIVES
After reading this chapter, the reader will be able to:

1. *Define bullying and cyberbullying.*

2. *Evaluate the health, psychosocial, social, behavioral, and academic impacts of bullying and cyberbullying.*

3. *Employ various prevention, educational, and clinical interventions for bullying and cyberbullying.*

BACKGROUND AND SIGNIFICANCE

Bullying is a form of child maltreatment that is typically pervasive and, unfortunately, ever-present in the lives of some children. Bullying can take on many forms. Children often feel lost within the perceived position of helplessness and hopelessness that envelops them as a result of bullying, which often seems like an inescapable black hole of anxiety and fear and has a crushing impact on their psychosocial growth and development. When adults respond quickly and consistently to bullying behavior, they convey that it is not acceptable, and they can assist children in regaining power and control over their lives.[1]

Bullying has historically had many different manifestations, views, stereotypes, and even names. Some views, including those of parents and teachers, have considered things such as "teasing"[2] to be a "rite of passage"[3] or something that they tell children will stop as bullies age and "grow out of it."[4] However, as research and reporting reflect, bullying is not a simple developmental "phase," and often, as those bullies progress in age, physical stature, and "popularity," the bullying typically continues to expand and escalate. Ultimately, this can result in significant emotional and developmental trauma,[5,6] and, unfortunately, as seen in current statistics, an increased risk for suicide and other forms of self-harm.[7] Subsequently, it is important to understand what bullying is, and what it is not.

Dan Olweus is generally recognized for creating the seminal definition of bullying, one that continues to be primarily used today to operationally represent the actions of bullies and those who are being bullied. Specifically, his definition is, "A person is bullied when he or she is exposed, repeatedly and over time, to negative actions on the part of one or more other persons, and he or she has difficulty defending himself or herself."[8,9]

This definition includes 3 necessary components:

1. Bullying is aggressive behavior that involves unwanted, negative actions.

2. Bullying involves a pattern of behavior ***repeated over time***.

3. Bullying involves an imbalance of power or strength.

In his writings, Dr. Olweus is very clear that bullying is peer abuse that should not be tolerated under any circumstances. Today, an increasing number of states have adopted laws against bullying.

PREVALENCE

In a comprehensive overview of current bullying prevention research conducted by governmental and higher education agencies, specifically, the National Bullying Prevention Center and the National Center for Education Statistics, it was reported that[10,11]:

— 1 out of every 5 (20.2%) students report being bullied.

— A higher percentage of male than female students report being physically bullied (6% versus 4%), whereas a higher percentage of female than male students report being the subjects of rumors (18% versus 9%) and being excluded from activities on purpose (7% versus 4%).

— 41% of students who report being bullied at school indicated that they think the bullying would happen again.

— Of those students who report being bullied, 13% were made fun of, called names, or insulted; 13% were the subject of rumors; 5% were pushed, shoved, tripped, or spit on; and 5% were excluded from activities on purpose.

— A slightly higher portion of female than male students report being bullied at school (24% versus 17%).

— Bullied students report that bullying occurred in the following places:

  — the hallway or stairwell at school (43%)

  — inside the classroom (42%)

  — in the cafeteria (27%)

  — outside on school grounds (22%)

  — online or by text (15%)

  — in the bathroom or locker room (12%)

  — on the school bus (8%)

— The reasons for being bullied reported most often by students include: physical appearance, race/ethnicity, gender, disability, religion, or sexual orientation.

— 46% of bullied students report notifying an adult at school about the incident.

Additionally, statistics for a very vulnerable group (ie, those between the ages of 9 and 12 years) indicate the following[11,12]:

— 1 in 5 (20.9%) have been cyberbullied, cyberbullied others, or witnessed cyberbullying of others.

— 49.8% said they experienced bullying at school, and 14.5% shared they experienced bullying online.

— 13% reported experiencing bullying at school and online, while only 1% reported being bullied solely online.

The low number of online bullying statistics among 9 to 12-year-olds is rational, because, technically, most social media platforms require children to be 13 years old to use their services.[13]

Prevalence rates vary based on how the frequency and duration of bullying are operationally defined.[9,14,15] However, regardless of this variance in prevalence across studies, bullying and cyberbullying remain substantial issues confronting children and adolescents today.

TYPES OF BULLYING

Bullying can take on many forms. In addition to understanding the prevalence and impact that bullying has on the targeted student victims, it is also important to recognize the characteristics of students who bully, which may help prevent bullying and allow for early intervention. A single student who bullies can have a wide-ranging impact on the students they bully, students who observe that bullying, and the overall climate of the school and community.[8,16] Olweus[8,12] claims that there are 3 interrelated reasons as to why students bully:

— They have strong needs for power and (negative) dominance.

— They find satisfaction in causing injury and suffering to other students.

— They are often rewarded in some way for their behavior with material or psychological rewards.

As part of the Revised Olweus Bullying Questionnaire,[9,17-19] students are asked if they have been bullied in any of these 9 ways:

1. Verbal bullying, including derogatory comments and bad names

2. Bullying through social exclusion or isolation

3. Physical bullying such as hitting, kicking, shoving, or spitting

4. Bullying through lies and false rumors

5. Having money or other things taken or damaged by students who bully

6. Being threatened or being forced to do things by students who bully

7. Racial bullying

8. Cyberbullying (via cellular phone or internet)

9. Sexual bullying

SEXUAL BULLYING

Sexual bullying is a form of bullying that occurs when a student or a group of students intend to harass, hurt, offend, or intimidate others through comments, gestures, attention, and actions that are sexual in nature. Such activities can lead to sexual harassment and potential sexual assault. Sexual bullying comprises some alarming actions and comments, such as[20,21]:

— Making sexual jokes, comments, or gestures

— Participating in catcalling or harassment of someone

— Engaging in slut-shaming, public shaming, or cyberbullying that is sexual in nature

— Spreading sexual rumors (in person, by text, or via social media)

— Posting sexual comments, pictures, or videos (eg, social media sites)

— Taking and forwarding sexually explicit text messages and inappropriate pictures/videos via text or email

— Grabbing someone's clothing or brushing up against them in a purposefully sexual way

— Touching, grabbing, or pinching someone in a deliberately sexual way

— Sending sexually explicit text messages and pictures/videos via text message, also known as sexting, or pressuring someone to participate in sexting to show commitment or love

— Impersonating other people online and making sexual comments or offers on their behalf

— Making comments about someone's gender identity, sexual orientation, or sexual activity

— Sharing inappropriate sexual videos or pictures

— Spreading sexual rumors or gossip in person, by text, or online

— Writing sexual comments about someone in blogs, on bathroom stalls, or in other public places

Often, sexual bullying is not reported to adults. To address sexual bullying, it needs to be defined, regular discussions are required, and reporting needs to be made safe by using various methods. One way to make reporting safe is to allow anonymous reporting. If the student does feel comfortable telling the clinician directly, the clinician should listen, be empathetic, and believe the student. Some students just want an adult to be aware of the situation that they are experiencing. If the actions they are experiencing are not unlawful, a clinician can allow them to be engaged in how the situation is handled. This empowers them to speak up when they encounter or see something that is not right without drawing attention or fear of reprisal to themselves.[19]

CYBERBULLYING: UNIQUE CHARACTERISTICS

In a 2018 survey conducted by the Pew Research Center,[22] 59% of adolescents in the United States reported that they had directly experienced at least 1 type of cyberbullying. Cyberbullying is bullying through email, instant messaging (IMing), chat room exchanges, website posts, or digital messages or images sent via electronic communication devices such as a cellular phone, personal digital assistant (PDA),[23] or other digital technology. Cyberbullying has some unique characteristics that are different from traditional bullying, and they are as follows[24]:

—*Anonymity:* As bad as the bully on the playground may be, he or she can be readily identified and potentially avoided. On the other hand, the child who cyberbullies is often anonymous. The victim is left wondering who the cyberbully is, which can cause a great deal of stress.

—*Accessibility:* Most children use traditional ways of bullying to terrorize their victim at school, on the bus, or walking to or from school. Although bullying can happen elsewhere in the community, there is usually a standard, repeated period of time during which these children have access to their victims. Children who cyberbully can wreak havoc any time of the day or night.

—*Punitive Fears:* Victims of cyberbullying often do not report it because of: (1) fear of retribution from their tormentors, and (2) fear that their computer or phone privileges will be taken away. Often, adults' responses to cyberbullying are to remove the technology from a victim, which in the child's eyes can be seen as punishment.

—*Bystanders:* Most traditional bullying episodes occur in the presence of other people who assume the role of bystanders or witnesses. The phenomenon of being a bystander in the cyberworld is different in that bystanders may receive and forward emails, view web pages, or forward images sent to cell phones. The number of bystanders in the cyberworld can reach into the millions.

— ***Disinhibition:*** The anonymity afforded by the internet can lead children to engage in behaviors that they might not do face-to-face. Ironically, it is their very anonymity that allows some individuals to bully at all.

COMMON FORMS OF CYBERBULLYING

Cyberbullying can take many forms, but some of the most common are[23-25]:

— ***Cyberstalking:*** Repeatedly sending messages that include threats of harm or are highly intimidating, or engaging in other online activities that make a person afraid for their safety (note, clinicians should be mindful that depending on the content of the message, it may be illegal and need to be reported to law enforcement).

— ***Online Harassment:*** Repeatedly sending offensive, rude, and insulting messages.

— ***Flaming:*** Online "fighting" using electronic messages with angry, vulgar language.

— ***Excluding:*** Cruelly and deliberately rejecting someone from an online group.

— ***Denigrating:*** Distributing information about another that is derogatory and untrue through posting it on a web page, sending it to others through email, texting, or instant messaging, or posting or sending digitally altered photos of someone.

— ***Impersonating:*** Breaking into an email or social networking account (also called "fraping," or Facebook raping) and using that person's online identity to delete information or send or post vicious or embarrassing material to/about others.

— ***Masquerading:*** Creating a fake identity to harass someone anonymously. Similar to impersonating, the bully can use the fake identity to send or post malicious messages to the victim and others.

— ***Outing:*** Sharing someone's secrets or embarrassing information without their consent (including actual or presumed sexual orientation, which may or may not be accurate).

— ***Trickery/Hoodwinking:*** Like outing, the bully uses deception to gain trust and then mislead someone into revealing secrets or embarrassing information and posting or forwarding it to others online.

— ***Doxxing:*** Involves revealing someone's personally identifiable details (eg, home address, school, work) so that others can engage in harassing, shaming, or causing harm to people with whom they disagree.

— ***Swatting:*** A form of doxxing whereby the public release of information and reporting or prank-calling false emergencies instigates a law enforcement response (usually to someone's home).

— ***Internet Polling:*** Creating and posting or texting an online survey with embarrassing or denigrating questions and publishing the results.

— ***Happy Slapping:*** Publishing a video that displays someone being physically hurt or humiliated.

— ***Online Grooming:*** An individual targets a child and gradually gains their trust to ultimately prepare him/her for abuse.

As digital technology and electronic devices continue to emerge, so do the means of cyberbullying and harassment. Social media platforms that include online gaming can provide a rich environment for cyberbullying.[26] Multiplayer online games, which can be played on a computer, game console, handheld system, cell phone, or tablet, permit players to engage with people they know in person and others they meet in a digital environment.[27] Although teamwork and sociability are common in multiplayer online games, forms of cyberbullying, such as denigrating and harassment are also common.[28]

The next frontier for bullying is in the "metaverse." The metaverse is a fully realized digital world that exists beyond the analog one in which people live.[29] In these extended reality (XR) environments, and through various equipment, people can experience all 5 senses. This allows individuals to see, hear, shout, strike, or grope a person in virtual reality.[30] Strategies to combat such behaviors are continuing to be developed.

BYSTANDER EFFECT

The bystander effect occurs when the presence of others discourages an individual from intervening in an emergency, against a bully, or during an assault or other crime. The greater the number of bystanders, the less likely it is for any one of them to provide help to a person in distress. People are more likely to take action in a crisis when there are few or no other witnesses present.[31] Children and adolescents who are bullied often feel even more alone because there are witnesses who do nothing. When no one intervenes, the person being targeted may feel that bystanders do not care or may agree with what is happening.

Someone who witnesses bullying, either in person or online, is a bystander. Friends, students, peers, teachers, school staff, parents, coaches, and other child- and adolescent-serving adults can be bystanders. With cyberbullying, even strangers can be bystanders.[32,33] There are many reasons why a bystander may not interject, even if they believe that bullying is wrong, including fear of retaliation or of becoming the target of bullying themselves. They might worry that getting involved could have negative social consequences.[31] These consequences of bullying affect the bystanders, the victims, and the perpetrators. These various roles are described by Dan Olweus in "The Bullying Circle" (**Figure 16-1**).[34]

EFFECTS OF BULLYING AND CYBERBULLYING

Bullying can affect the current and future health of both the bullies and the students who are victims of bullying. For victims of bullying, physical health issues, such as sleep difficulties and physical injuries, may be immediate and, depending on their nature, may last a lifetime. Emotional issues, such as anxiety, depression, loneliness, low self-esteem, and self-harm, may be present both in the short-term and later in life.[35]

There is a strong association between bullying and suicide-related behaviors, but this relationship is often mediated by other factors, including depression, violent behavior, and substance abuse.[11,36] Students who report frequently bullying others and students who report being frequently bullied are at increased risk for suicide-related behavior.[37-39] In a 2019 globally conducted study[40] on bullying victimization and suicide attempts among adolescents aged 12 to 15 years from 48 countries, data were collected and analyzed from 134 229 participants. The overall prevalence of a past 12 months suicide attempt was 10.7% (with boys reporting a 10% risk level and girls 11.2%). Overall, 18.7%, 6.0%, 3.5%, and 2.2% of adolescents were bullied 1 to 2, 3 to 5, 6 to 19, and 20 to 30 days in the past 30 days, respectively. In the overall sample that included boys and girls, compared with those who were not bullied in the past 30 days, those who were bullied for 1 to 2, 3 to 5, 6 to 19, and 20 to 30 days respectively had 2.39, 3.65, 4.89, and 5.51 times higher odds for suicide attempts. Although few studies investigate the relationship between suicide risk and students who are bystanders or witnesses to bullying, two studies found an increased risk to these students.[41,42] Students who are both bullied and engage in bullying behavior are the highest risk group for adverse outcomes.[11] The false notion that suicide is a

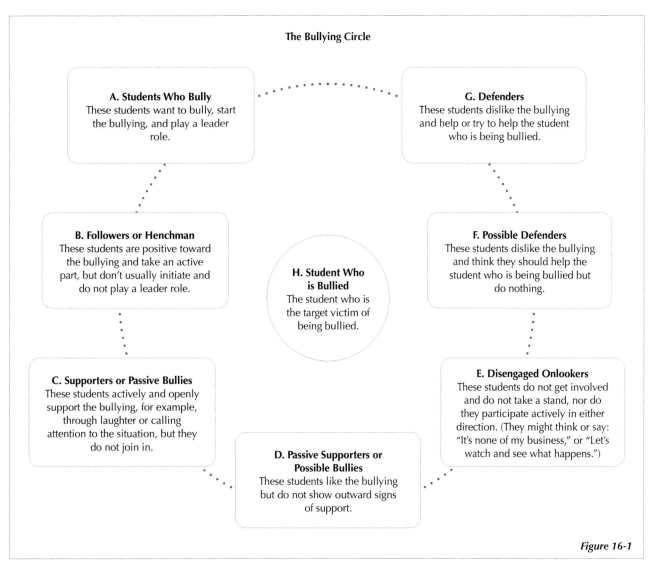

Figure 16-1. The Bullying Circle, as described by Dan Olweus.

"natural response" to being bullied has the dangerous potential to normalize the response, and thus, create copycat behavior among children and adolescents.[37-39]

Currently, investigators are examining the mediating roles of resilience and self-esteem to combat anxiety and depressive symptoms from bullying victimization.[43,44] Not surprisingly, those students with higher self-esteem who experience bullying report fewer depressive symptoms than their counterparts with decreased self-esteem.[44] Similarly, those students who are bullied but possess higher resilience display less anxiety and depressive symptomatology than their colleagues.[43]

Bullying experiences can also affect social and behavioral interactions. Student victims of bullying may have lower academic achievement and drop out of school or activities to avoid being bullied.[45] The most egregious scenario for victims of bullying is to retaliate against their bullies and bystanders through actions, such as a school shooting.[46] Research found that between 60% to 71% of school shooters were victims of bullying that they described as "severe" or "tormenting."[47]

Students who perpetrate bullying are also at a high risk for dropping out of school and developing behavioral difficulties such as truancy, vandalism, fighting, early sexual activity, and substance use disorders.[45] These behaviors can extend into adulthood and lead to abusive actions with romantic partners and children.[45] Such problematic behaviors may lead to involvement with the juvenile or criminal justice systems.

Prevention and Intervention
How Children Can Confront Bullying

An "upstander" is someone who acts when they witness bullying. Even one person's support can make a big difference for someone who is being bullied. When children and adolescents who are being bullied are defended and supported by their peers, they are less anxious and depressed than those who are not. The following are some of the many things that bystanders to bullying can do to become upstanders[33]:

— Question the bullying behavior. Simple things like changing the subject or questioning the behavior can shift the focus.

— Use humor to say something funny and redirect the conversation.

— Intervene as a group to show there are several people who do not agree with the bullying; there is strength in numbers.

— Walk with the person who is the target of bullying to help diffuse potential bullying interactions.

— Reach out privately to check in with the person who was bullied to let them know they do not agree with it and that they care. It makes a difference.

Additionally, STOMP recommends approaches for children to change the culture regarding being a bystander.[32] Specifically, whether knowing the victim or not, there are things that a bystander can safely do to support the victim[31-33]:

— Do not laugh

— Do not encourage the bully in any way

— Do not participate

— Stay at a safe distance and help the target get away

— Do not become an "audience" for the bully

— Reach out in friendship

— Help the victim in any way you can

— Support the victim in private

— If you notice someone being isolated from others, invite them to join you

— Include the victim in some of your activities

— Tell an adult

Every school and every community has more children who care than those who bully. One excellent resource is the educational video "Be Someone's Hero," (available in both English[48] and Spanish[49]) which discusses the school-aged community issues of bullying and active approaches toward culture change among children.

There are a variety of strategies that can be beneficial to the child who is being bullied, including[48,50]:

— Look directly at the kid engaging in bullying and tell him or her to stop in a calm, clear voice.

— Try to laugh it off. This works best if joking is easy for the child. It could catch the kid who is bullying off guard.

— If speaking up seems too hard or not safe, walk away and stay away. Do not fight back. Find an adult to stop the bullying on the spot.

There are things the child can do to stay safe in the future, too.

— Talk to an adult they trust. Do not keep their feelings inside. Telling someone can help them feel less alone. An adult can help them make a plan to stop the bullying.

— Stay away from places where bullying happens.

— Stay near adults and other kids. Most bullying happens when adults are not around.

The US Department of Health and Human Services additionally created an educational video, "What To Do If You've Been Bullied,"[51] which provides foundational guidance and methods for support.

Federal Laws

Although no federal law directly addresses bullying, in some cases, bullying overlaps with discriminatory harassment when it is based on race, national origin, color, sex (including sexual orientation and gender identity), age, disability, or religion. Federally-funded schools (including colleges and universities) have an obligation to resolve harassment on these bases.[52]

No matter what label is used (eg, bullying, hazing, teasing), schools are obligated by these laws to address the conduct when it meets all 3 of the criteria below[52]:

— Unwelcome and objectively offensive, such as derogatory language, intimidation, threats, physical contact, or physical violence

— Creates a hostile environment at school (ie, it is sufficiently serious that it interferes with or limits a student's ability to participate in or benefit from the services, activities, or opportunities offered by a school)

— Based on a student's race, color, national origin, sex, disability, or religion

  — Sex includes sexual orientation, gender identity, and intersex traits. Sex also includes sex-based stereotypes and sexual harassment.

  — National origin harassment can include harassment because a student speaks another language.

Further, federal civil rights laws cover harassment of LGBTQIA+ children and adolescents. The US Department of Education and US Department of Justice have clarified that Title IX's prohibition against sex discrimination includes discrimination on the basis of sexual orientation and gender identity. The two aforementioned agencies have developed a resource, "Confronting Anti-LGBTQI+ Harassment in Schools,"[53] to help students, parents, and educators understand their rights and actions to take.

When the bullying situation is not adequately resolved, the following should be considered:

— Filing a formal grievance with the school district.

— Contacting the US Department of Education's Office for Civil Rights[54] and the US Department of Justice's Civil Rights Division for help.[55]

Case Study

Case Study 16-1

At the beginning of the season, a cheerleader who was upset that another teammate was named captain starts a social media page about the captain that was both derogatory and insulting. The link to this social media site was then distributed throughout the school, and people were encouraged to comment on all the things this adolescent did wrong throughout the season. As time went on, more and more negative and offensive posts and pictures accumulated on the site.

Discussion

If involved in this case, a clinician would complete a comprehensive initial assessment of the physical and mental health of the targeted adolescent. This assessment can highlight potential consequences of cyberbullying, such as physical bullying, anxiety, depression, non-suicidal self-injury, and suicidal behaviors. The clinician should discuss and maintain an open dialogue and encourage the targeted adolescent to refrain from monitoring the online content, as this can cause increased distress. The clinician needs to reinforce that these actions are not the adolescent's fault; nobody deserves to be bullied. The targeted adolescent's response to such a violation cannot be reactive. The clinician should provide support and encourage the adolescent not to respond or retaliate against the bullies, as this only empowers them. Additionally, with the permission of the adolescent, the clinician should discuss the situation with child and adolescent-serving adults (eg, parents, teachers, counselors, coaches). A point of emphasis in this discussion is not to deny the targeted adolescent access to technology. A further benefit of sharing the situation with community-based child and adolescent-serving adults is that their organizations have antibullying and behavioral policies to address a duty of care to those who attend and engage in their programs.

With aid from a child and adolescent-serving adult, the targeted adolescent can disrupt this cyberbullying by reporting the account to the social media platform. Almost all social media platforms have a process for disabling fake or impersonating profiles. When reporting the account, it is important to keep a copy of information by printing out or taking screen shots of the fake profile. This can be useful if the harassment continues, and the targeted adolescent needs to work with the social media site or law enforcement to resolve the issue. Finally, because the information is now in the public domain, reassessing and providing ongoing support to the targeted adolescent is most essential to prevent the development of negative consequences.

KEY POINTS

1. Bullying has the potential to negatively affect everyone involved – the bully, victim, and bystander.

2. Cyberbullying can be as harmful as physical bullying.

3. Silence and ignoring it are not acceptable responses to bullying.

ADDITIONAL RESOURCES

— **US Department of Health and Human Services:** https://www.stopbullying. gov

— **Bullying Resources for Educators and Parents:** https://teach.com/online-ed/counseling-degrees/online-masters-school-counseling/bullying-resources/

— **Resources for Educators and Families:** https://www.cfchildren.org/resources/bullying-prevention-resources/

— **PACER's National Bullying Prevention Center:** https://www.pacer.org/bullying/info/

— **Cyberbullying Research Center:** https://cyberbullying.org/

REFERENCES

1. Prevention: learn how to identify bullying and stand up to it safely. Stop Bullying. 2022. https://www.stopbullying.gov

2. Lee AMI. The difference between teasing and bullying. Understood. 2022. https://www.understood.org/en/articles/difference-between-teasing-and-bullying

3. Wolke D, Lereya ST. Long-term effects of bullying. *Arch Dis Child.* 2015; 100(9):879-885. doi:10.1136/archdischild-2014-306667

4. Storch E, Blanton N. Once a bully, always a bully? Tips to address adult bullying behavior. Baylor College of Medicine. 2018. https://blogs.bcm.edu/2018/01/30/once-a-bully-always-a-bully-tips-to-address-adult-bullying-behavior/

5. Hinduja S, Patchin JW. Cyberbullying: identification, prevention, and response. Cyberbullying Research Center. 2014. https://cyberbullying.org/Cyberbullying-Identification-Prevention-Response.pdf

6. Bullying, cyberbullying, and suicide statistics. Megan Meier Foundation. 2021. https://static1.squarespace.com/static/5b33ed96372b964a1d83073a/t/60d619f d4d52ae0ca2c07a3e/1624644094476/Updated+Statistics+2021.pdf

7. John A, Glendenning AC, Marchant A, et al. Self-harm, suicidal behaviours, and cyberbullying in children and young people: systematic review. *J Med Internet Res.* 2018;20(4):e129. doi:10.2196/jmir.9044

8. Olweus D. Bullying in schools: facts and intervention. *Kriminalistik.* 2010;64(6): 28-32.

9. Olweus D. The Revised Olweus Bully/Victim Questionnaire for students. 1996. doi:1037/t09634-000

10. Bullying at school and electronic bullying. National Center for Education Statistics. 2021. https://nces.ed.gov/programs/coe/indicator/a10

11. Bullying statistics by the numbers: rates of incidence. PACER's National Bullying Prevention Center. 2020. https://www.pacer.org/bullying/info/stats.asp

12. Patchin JW, Hinduja S. Tween cyberbullying in 2020. Cyberbullying Research Center and Cartoon Network. 2020. https://i.cartoonnetwork.com/stop-bullying/pdfs/CN_Stop_Bullying_Cyber_Bullying_Report_9.30.20.pdf

13. Canales K. Silicon Valley says kids over the age of 13 can handle the big, bad world of social media. Experts say that's the result of a 'problematic' 1990s internet law. Business Insider. 2022. https://www.businessinsider.com/why-you-must-be-13-facebook-instagram-problematic-law-coppa-2022-1

14. Leymann H. The content and development of mobbing at work. *Eur J Work Org Psychol.* 1996;5(2):165-184. doi:10.1080/ 13594329608414853

15. Kowalski RM, Giumetti GW, Schroeder AN, Lattanner MR. Bullying in the digital age: a critical review and meta-analysis of cyberbullying research among youth. *Psychol Bull.* 2014;140(4):1073-1137. doi:10.1037/a0035618

16. Hazeldon Foundation. Recognizing bullying. 2016. https://www.violenceprevention-works.org/public/recognizing_bullying.page

17. Kyriakides L, Kaloyirou C, Lindsay G. An analysis of the Revised Olweus Bully/Victim Questionnaire using the Rasch measurement model. *Brit J Edu Psychol.* 2006;76:781-801. doi:10.1348/000709905X53499

18. Olweus D, Limber SP, Riese J, Urbanski J, Solberg ME, Breivik K. The Olweus bullying prevention program (obpp): development and consolidation. In: Smith PK, Norman JOH, eds. *The Wiley Blackwell Handbook of Bullying: A Comprehensive and International Review of Research and Intervention.* John Wiley & Sons Ltd.; 2021:410-429.

19. Olweus D, Limber SP, Breivik K. Addressing specific forms of bullying: a large-scale evaluation of the Olweus Bullying Prevention Program. *Intern J Bully Prev.* 2019;1(1):1-15. doi:10.1007/s42380-019-00009-7

20. Sexual harassment and sexual bullying. The Nemours Foundation. 2021. https://kidshealth.org/en/teens/harassment.html

21. Gordon S. What is sexual bullying and why do kids engage in it? Verywell Family. Updated May 11, 2021. Accessed 2022. https://www.verywellfamily.com/what-is-sexual-bullying-and-why-do-kids-engage-in-it-460499#citation-3

22. A majority of teens have experienced some form of cyberbullying. Pew Research Center. 2018. https://www.pewresearch.org/internet/2018/09/27/a-majority-of-teens-have-experienced-some-form-of-cyberbullying/

23. Kowalski RM, Limber SP, Agatston PW. *Cyber Bullying: Bullying in the Digital Age*. John Wiley & Sons; 2008:224.

24. Hazeldon Foundation. What is cyber bullying? 2016. https://www.violence preventionworks.org/public/cyber_bullying.page

25. Kowalski RM, Toth A. Cyberbullying among youth with and without disabilities. *J Child Adoles Trauma*. 2018;11(1):7-15. doi:10.1007/s40653-017-0139-y

26. Rover C. Why games are the new social platform. September 27, 2022. https://www.alistdaily.com/digital/why-games-are-the-new-social-platform/

27. Cyberbullying and online gaming. Stopbullying.gov. https://www.stopbullying.gov/cyberbullying/cyberbullying-online-gaming

28. Hilvert-Bruce Z, Neill JT. I'm just trolling: the role of normative beliefs in aggressive behaviour in online gaming. *Comput Hum Behav*. 2020;102:303-311. doi:10.1016/j.chb.2019.09.003

29. Herrman J, Browning K. Are we in the metaverse yet? *The New York Times*. July 10, 2021. Accessed 2022. https://www.nytimes.com/2021/07/10/style/met-averse-virtual-worlds.html

30. Frenkel S, Browning K. The metaverse's dark side: here come harassment and assaults. *The New York Times*. December 30, 2021. Accessed 2022. https://www.nytimes.com/2021/12/30/technology/metaverse-harassment-assaults.html

31. Bystander effect. Psychology Today. Accessed 2022. https://www.psychology-today.com/us/basics/bystander-effect

32. Bullying bystanders... become upstanders. STOMP Out Bullying. Accessed 2022. https://www.stompoutbullying.org/bullying-bystanders-become-upstanders

33. Bystanders to bullying. stopbullying.gov. Updated October 23, 2018. Accessed 2022. https://www.stopbullying.gov/prevention/bystanders-to-bullying

34. Olweus D. Peer harassment: a critical analysis and some important issues. In: Juvonen J, Graham S, eds. *Peer Harassment in School*. Guilford Publications; 2001:3-20.

35. Fact sheet: prevent bullying. Centers for Disease Control and Prevention. 2018. https://www.cdc.gov/violenceprevention/pdf/bullying-factsheet508.pdf

36. Reed KP, Cooper RL, Nugent WR, Russell K. Cyberbullying: a literature review of its relationship to adolescent depression and current intervention strategies. *J Human Behav Soc Environ*. 2015;26(1):37-45. doi:10.1080/10911359.2015.1059165

37. Armitage R. Bullying in children: impact on child health. *BMJ Paedetri Open*. 2021;5(1):e000939. March 11, 2021. doi:10.1136/bmjpo-2020-000939 https://www.ncbi.nlm.nih.gov/pmc/articles/PMC7957129/

38. How does bullying affect health and well-being? Eunice Kennedy Shriver National Institute of Child Health and Human Development. Updated January 31, 2017. https://www.nichd.nih.gov/health/topics/bullying/conditioninfo/health

39. The relationship between bullying and suicide: what we know and what it means for schools. Centers for Disease Control and Prevention. 2014. https://www.cdc.gov/violenceprevention/pdf/bullying-definitions-final-a.pdf

40. Koyanagi A, Oh H, Carvalho AF, et al. Bullying victimization and suicide attempt among adolescents aged 12-15 years from 48 countries. *J Am Acad Child Adolesc Psychiatry.* 2019;58(9):907-918.e4. doi:10.1016/j.jaac.2018.10.018

41. Duan S, Duan Z, Li R, et al. Bullying victimization, bullying witnessing, bullying perpetration and T suicide risk among adolescents: a serial mediation analysis. *J Affective Disorders.* 2020;273:274-279. doi:10.1016/j.jad.2020.03.143

42. Holt MK, Vivolo-Kantor AM, Polanin JR, et al. Bullying and suicidal ideation and behaviors: a meta-analysis. *Pediatrics.* 2015;135(2):e496-e509. doi:10.1542/peds.2014-1864

43. Anderson JR, Mayes TL, Fuller A, Hughes JL, Minhajuddin A, Trivedi MH. Experiencing bullying's impact on adolescent depression and anxiety: mediating role of adolescent resilience. *J Affective Disorders.* 2022;310:477-483. doi:10.1016/j.jad.2022.04.003

44. Zhong M, Huang X, Huebner ES, Tian L. Association between bullying victimization and depressive symptoms in children: the mediating role of self-esteem. *J Affective Disorders.* 2021;294:322-328. doi:10.1016/j.jad.2021.07.016

45. Hazeldon Foundation. How bullying affects children. 2016. https://www.violencepreventionworks.org/public/bullying_effects.page

46. Rivara F, Le Menestrel S, eds. *Preventing Bullying Through Science, Policy, and Practice.* National Academies Press (US); 2016.

47. Dowdell EB, Freitas E, Owens A, Greenle MM. School shooters: patterns of adverse childhood experiences, bullying, and social media. *J Pediatric Health Care.* 2022;36(4):339-346. doi:10.1016/j.pedhc.2021.12.004

48. *Be Someone's Hero.* Centers for Disease Control and Prevention; 2017. https://www.youtube.com/watch?v=64LNwrd0fHg .

49. *Be Someone's Hero.* Centers for Disease Control and Prevention; 2018. https://www.youtube.com/watch?v=Vfv_jbXCsYs

50. What kids can do. Stopbullying.gov. https://www.stopbullying.gov/kids/what-you-can-do

51. *What to do if you have been bullied.* US Department of Health and Human Services; 2019. https://www.youtube.com/watch?v=uynUWJ_hhBk

52. Federal laws. Stopbullying.gov. Updated October 6, 2021. https://www.stopbullying.gov/resources/laws/federal

53. Confronting anti-LGBTQI+ harassment in schools: a resource for students and families. US Department of Education Office for Civil Rights. 2021. https://www2.ed.gov/about/offices/list/ocr/docs/ocr-factsheet-tix-202106.pdf

54. How to file a discrimination complaint with the Office for Civil Rights. US Department of Education Office for Civil Rights. 2021. https://www2.ed.gov/about/offices/list/ocr/docs/howto.html?src=rt

55. Contact the Department of Justice to report a civil rights violation. US Department of Justice Civil Rights Division. https://civilrights.justice.gov/report/

56. Bikin-kita N. The bullying circle from a bystander to a defender. bBrave. https://bbrave.org.mt/2019/04/03/the-bullying-circle/

57. Salmivalli C, Lagerspetz K, Bjorkqvist K, Osterman K, Kaukiainen A. Bullying as a group process: participant roles and their relations to social status within the group. *Agress Behav.* 1996;22(1):1-15. doi:10.1002/(SICI)1098-2337(1996)22:1<1::AID-AB1>3.0.CO;2-T

Chapter 17

SIBLING-ON-SIBLING ABUSE

Jeannette B. Wyatt, PhD, LCSW

OBJECTIVES

After reading this chapter, the reader will be able to:

1. *Identify the significance of sibling relations.*

2. *Recognize the effects of sibling-on-sibling abuse across different realms of functioning.*

3. *Demonstrate awareness of interventions in cases of sibling-on-sibling abuse.*

BACKGROUND AND SIGNIFICANCE

Sibling-on-sibling abuse is the most common form of intrafamily abuse and crosses all categories of child abuse, including physical, sexual, psychological, and neglect.[1] The traumatic effects of such abuse are congruent with abuse stemming from other perpetrators; however, sibling-on-sibling abuse is often minimized by parents and professionals.[2] In addition, the relational dynamics within families and between siblings can make things even more complex. Norms of secrecy and loyalty, as well as dynamics of intimacy and trust, often lead to victims feeling conflicted, further disempowered, and potentially silenced. Sibling incest, for instance, is one type of sibling-on-sibling abuse that is often unacknowledged in the family and underreported by victims.[3]

WHAT IS SPECIAL ABOUT SIBLINGS

The relational dynamics between siblings are substantial and unique because they share experiences, perspectives, norms, and values from the same family system. Siblings are potentially important companions, supports, and confidants as they can serve as close friends, role models, mentors, and mediators for one another during development.[4] These relationships are often taken for granted and go unrecognized for their pivotal role in development, but nonetheless, they serve as a foundational and important influence. Sibling relationships fulfill unique, dynamic needs according to theories of personality and human functioning. These include providing foundational attachment[5]; fulfilling the self-object needs identified in self-psychology of idealizing and twinship[6]; contributing to an influential subsystem within the family[4]; serving as mechanisms for learning behaviors, beliefs, and relationship skills[7]; and facilitating evaluation of the self as part of social comparison processes.[7]

Sibling relations can serve as foundational attachment relations,[8] analogous to parents, especially with the propensity for siblings to raise other siblings either due to parents working or being unable to raise their children because of their own stresses or dysfunctions.[9] This elevates the influence of one sibling onto another and can even heighten the possibility of sibling abuse, as the authority of the abusing sibling is informally validated within the family.[9] As foundational attachment experiences,[8] abusive sibling relations can have a detrimental effect on the development of internal capabilities for self-regulation, constructive relational patterns, and overall security for developmental challenges.

The experiences of siblings can also differ greatly, even within the same household. Individual differences belong to each sibling, including their temperament, personality dynamics, intellectual ability, and social skills, along with variations in their relations with others such as their parents or other family members. Furthermore, separation by age leads to different developmental tasks, challenges, and abilities, with each individual sibling developing their own interests, capabilities, and relationships with the external environment. These differences can lead to differences in power, authority, and independence.

THE PROBLEM AND ITS CAUSES

According to the National Survey of Children's Exposure to Violence,[10] 33% of children and 14% of adolescents have reported being victimized by a sibling. Additionally, the analysis found that being abused by a sibling may also increase one's vulnerability to peer victimization.[10] The types of abuse by siblings varies and can include bullying, coercion, emotional abuse, neglect, physical harm, and sexual abuse. Sexual abuse can be particularly challenging as it is sometimes viewed as behavior evolving from curiosity and lack of malice, depending on the age of the offending child.[2]

The development of abuse perpetrators is a complex issue that is not easily understood. Sibling-on-sibling abuse can develop from systemic, relational, or individual factors.[11] Abusive behaviors can stem from learned experiences, both by witnessing aggressive behaviors or being abused themselves; inadequate dynamic capabilities for self-regulation that result from faulty attachment relations; and may develop as displacement strategies for current stress. In addition, sibling-on-sibling abuse can reflect family dynamics as siblings who experience different treatment from parents may react to it via competitive and even abusive relations with each other. Furthermore, norms of power and authority between siblings can be enabled by dynamics associated with gender and age, along with the absence of parental supervision.[11]

EFFECTS OF SIBLING-ON-SIBLING ABUSE

Sibling-on-sibling abuse often constitutes the first trauma experience, which may result in trauma reactions and the view of oneself as worthless.[12] Sibling-on-sibling abuse can also lead to powerlessness and longstanding emotional distress, as the sibling(s) that is(are) abused may lack skills for internal regulation of emotions and behaviors, and lack support because of parental deficits.[9,12] Sibling abuse can lead to increased mental health challenges and behavioral difficulties such as aggression and poor interpersonal skills.[1] This type of abuse can also lead to post-traumatic stress symptoms (PTSS) and post-traumatic stress disorder (PTSD), depending on the baseline functioning, as well as reactions to the trauma of abuse. Children with attachment deficits, either emanating from sibling abuse or as a precursor to it, are more likely to develop PTSS.[13] In addition, victims can experience loss or fear of rejection by other family members for reporting such abuse. The sibling subsystem can influence dynamics in the family system and be influenced by it.[11] Sibling abuse constitutes a crisis for the entire family and can challenge internal family dynamics, secure subsystem relations, and put members of the family into various stages of crisis reaction.

The effects of trauma on children can vary across realms of functioning, including developmental, behavioral, cognitive, emotional, physical, and interpersonal functioning. These outcomes also differ depending on the developmental stage of the child. A 2021 review[14] found that the research on trauma responses to child maltreatment is lacking in uniform terminology and theory and necessitates a complex framework to understand the various effects and mediating factors, including the psychosocial environment. In addition, the focus of responding professionals is often on physical safety rather than the potential emotional repercussions of abuse between siblings, in part because they are often conceptualized as equals.[2]

DEVELOPMENT

Children who have experienced maltreatment and trauma are more likely to have their normative trajectory of development challenged. Trauma can result in developmental fixation wherein progression halts or results in regression to earlier stages of development.[3] Such regression can lead to changes across areas of functioning, including clinginess, more infantile play, heightened anxiety, disrupted sleep or bedwetting, poor impulse control, or tantrums. Progression in development, particularly with executive functions that help regulate the self, can be thwarted.

EMOTIONAL FUNCTIONING

Emotionally, victims of abuse have a greater likelihood of experiencing depression, anger, and anxiety.[15] Direct grief processes about the sibling relationship itself can lead to internalizing disorders, especially since sibling relations are often a mainstay of childhood relational support.[4] Internalized distortions about one's own worth can increase vulnerability to depression. Concerns about safety and security propel ongoing apprehension, both consciously and unconsciously in terms of the neurobiological attunement to impending threat.[14] In addition, victims of sibling abuse are ambivalent about disclosing their abuse, in part because abusive relations may be all they know, or the family norms may instill denial and secrecy. Children can experience great distress in disclosing abuse to parents or caregivers and may be met with varying levels of validation in that process, further exacerbating the detrimental effects of the sibling abuse.[16]

BEHAVIOR

In behavioral functioning, there is an association between sibling abuse and the development of externalizing behaviors, such as conduct disorders, substance abuse,[17] and victims' increased engagement with aggressive behavior.[15] Older children may displace anger and by doing so may mimic abusive behavior from the home into peer relations. As stated earlier, younger children are vulnerable to regressive behaviors[3] such as clinging, bedwetting, infantile play, and fantasy. Depending on the level of depression and internalized shame, children may withdraw from interactions and activities and become more isolated in order to protect themselves. Trauma reactions can be difficult to differentiate from other disorders, such as ADHD, with difficulties in attention, impulse control, and self-regulation.[18] Adolescents who have experienced or witnessed family violence are more likely to misuse substances or engage in problem gambling.[19] Childhood maltreatment is also associated with avoidant coping and eating disorders.[20]

COGNITIVE FUNCTIONING

Victims of abuse are more vulnerable to ongoing thoughts of potential harm and dissociation in reaction to such trauma.[14] Victims may also have cognitive distortions, both about their own worth and about expectations for secure and stable relationships. Someone who has experienced abuse may not only feel devalued within that experience, but often see themselves as less worthy of loving relations in general. Additionally, perpetrators sometimes use coercion and victim blaming to rationalize their own abusive actions, and those distortions can become internalized by the victim. Sexual abuse may also lead to distortions about healthy sexuality and sexual behaviors in addition to self-esteem, and in fact, can lead to sexually offending behaviors.[21] Trauma and the resulting depression can challenge normal capabilities of attention span and memory,[18] and may thereby adversely influence academic functioning.

PHYSICAL EFFECTS

Physically, the effects of trauma cover a spectrum of injuries from small bruises to broken bones to fatal wounds. In addition, trauma literature highlights that being abused may activate the sympathetic nervous system, thereby increasing levels of cortisol and continually activating the fight, flight, freeze response.[14] This influences one's ability to engage in rational problem solving, develop coherent, explicit memories, and regulate one's own impulses and emotions. As Rueness et al[22] report, adolescents who are sexually abused are more likely to report traumatic stress reactions, including dissociation, depression, and problems with their physical health.

INTERPERSONAL FUNCTIONING

Abuse experiences can significantly alter interpersonal functioning. The effects from abusive relationships can carry over to other relations,[8] thereby leading to expectations of further abuse along with a diminished sense of self and empowerment within those relationships. As Caffaro & Conn-Caffaro[3] report, sexual coercion among siblings continues to have an effect on adult relationships. Trauma reactions can lead to reenactments and associations in the implicit memory of those victimized, creating destructive relational patterns and defensive functioning even within positive relationships. Attachment insecurity is also directly related to heightened trauma symptoms.[13] Within the family, dynamics from one subsystem can be a protective factor or adversely influence the quality of relations in other subsystems.[4]

ASSESSMENT

Assessment of sibling-on-sibling abuse can be complicated. The victim needs to be assessed first and foremost for safety, serious injury, and the effects of trauma as outlined above. An important distinction may be whether the abusive experience was a singular incident or a pattern within the sibling relationship over a period of time. The type of abuse is also important, especially as it relates to the effects of such abuse on various realms of functioning. In addition, the family system needs to be evaluated, particularly for the ability to provide safety for the victim, but also regarding the dynamics that both led to the abuse and that may emanate from it. This evaluation includes an assessment of parents/caregivers as well as other siblings. Lastly, the offending child needs to be assessed for potential removal for safety reasons as well as evaluated regarding the family dynamics that may have led to their abuse. Overarching issues of safety, secrecy, loyalty, and loss may also be pertinent.

INTERVENTIONS

There are a variety of interventions for sibling-on-sibling abuse that may be carried out by professionals from various disciplines and in different types of practice settings depending on the training and expertise of the professional and the focus of the setting.

MANDATED REPORTING

First and foremost is the helping professional's role as a mandated reporter. Federal and state statutes provide explicit guidelines about who is a mandated reporter and therefore is required to report suspected abuse or neglect. It is important to know that as a mandated reporter, the role is not to determine whether abuse or neglect did or did not occur, but rather to report suspicions. The responsibility for investigation falls to child welfare professionals. If a provider is unsure about the need for mandated reporting, supervision or legal counsel in their agency or a call to child welfare professionals should be utilized. Professionals can be ambivalent about reporting, as they may not know all of the facts, be worried about repercussions for the child, offending sibling, or family, and anxious about how it may influence the helping relationship. However, the child's safety and acting in a timely manner to stop and prevent any potential abuse is of paramount importance.

CRISIS INTERVENTION

Crisis intervention aims to re-establish equilibrium and safety after a traumatic experience. A tripartite assessment determines the nature of the crisis, individual factors involved, and factors in the immediate support system.[23] Collins & Collins[24] outline a developmental and ecological approach to crisis intervention that focuses on the individual, their development, and contextual factors. As with most approaches in crisis work, the initial work includes engaging a client with support and empathy. It is important to focus on establishing safety, de-escalating tensions, stabilizing the environment, and attending to practical needs. With children, this often means establishing or re-establishing an adult protective shield. Ongoing assessment of the effects of the crisis, facilitating appropriate expression, and then problem solving helps to ensure safety along with the mobilization of further support.[24] This work may include immediate steps for soothing and emotional expression or referral for further support and treatment.[23,24]

COLLABORATION AND ADVOCACY

Intervention with sibling-on-sibling abuse often necessitates collaborative work with other professionals and caregivers. Helping professionals should focus on protecting the child from further harm and assisting them in navigating the various processes (eg, court) that may be involved.[23]

Initial interventions from first responders provide assessment information and manage immediate safety concerns. Health care providers in various settings may also be involved in the evaluation and treatment of the victim.

Collaborative work with child welfare professionals is important regarding mandated reporting and to further ensure the safety of the child victim. Protective and investigative processes may constitute another crisis for the child or family with corresponding loss issues.[23] Legal proceedings have the potential for re-traumatization, anxiety, grief, and other emotional reactions.[23]

School personnel are important partners in the assessment of concerns and as supports for ongoing functioning. Community-based social service and mental health providers may be involved in interventions if they are already providing services or as follow up to child welfare recommendations or treatment needs.

Lastly, extended family or other caregivers can provide valuable input in assessment and provide ongoing support.

POLICY AND ADVOCACY

Policy development, professional training, and advocacy are needed with sibling-on-sibling abuse.[25,26] Professionals need to be aware of the potential abuse dynamic between siblings.[16] Child welfare professionals need help enhancing the uniformity of assessment and documentation standards, attention to non-abused children in abusive families, and methods of assessing needs for all family members.[25] Policy development should occur at all levels, beginning with definitions, which sometimes do not include intrasibling maltreatment.[16,26]

TREATMENT INTERVENTIONS

Sibling-on-sibling abuse requires multifaceted approaches as both assessment and treatment are aimed at separate individuals, their dynamics with each other, and issues with parents and in the family. Assessment should occur throughout intervention, particularly to assess the client's level of distress, their capabilities, and the need for pragmatic problem solving. This assessment highlights the need to identify target problems, establish goals in a collaborative manner, and empower victims whenever possible. Further, flexibility of intervention methods is required and should include the involvement of collateral contacts. Reflexivity by providers about their abilities to provide care and their potential experience of vicarious trauma is needed and emphasizes the important role of professional peer consultation and supervision.

As with any patient, treatment options should be determined based on the patient's presenting problems and how they are manifested, their acuity, and their abilities and preferences. Treatment options should also consider the professional's area of expertise, setting, and timeframe. Focusing on the therapeutic alliance is pivotal, as it not only provides safety for the patient, but it also allows for a corrective relationship and safe holding environment for their work. Interventions informed by research and practice wisdom should be prioritized when evaluating a patient's ability to partake in such methods. Cognitive behavioral therapy (CBT) has a strong legacy of research, for instance, but if a client is in a state of hyperarousal from their trauma, they may not be able to engage in the rational and methodical methods of such interventions. With these considerations, and in addition to those already reviewed, trauma-focused cognitive behavioral therapy (TF-CBT) targets skill development with siblings themselves, attachment-based approaches, and family therapy. Special attention is also given to play therapy, especially for clients younger than 10 years. More detailed information on specific interventions can be found in the first section of this volume.

SKILL DEVELOPMENT INTERVENTIONS

Interventions focused on skill development could technically fall under the umbrella of CBT and dialectical behavioral therapies, but they may be provided in various settings for children, such as schools, and be guided by professionals from education and social service disciplines in a group format. Tucker & Finkelhor[27] conducted a systematic review of interventions for conflict and aggression between siblings. They found that effective programs included those that targeted skill development in children, as well as parent education on how to mediate conflict between siblings. The programs that focused on helping children directly, which included developing social skills and relationship management abilities, were most effective in addressing aggression between siblings and preventing it through positive relationship qualities. Parent training was most effective for those families with younger sibling groups.

FAMILY THERAPY

Sibling-on-sibling abuse necessitates the assessment of family dynamics and, potentially, direct treatment of the family.[10] The dynamics of families with physical and sexual abuse are more likely to include dysfunction in impulse control, problem solving, constructive coping, and communication as well as increased stress and substance abuse.[28] These dynamics are often manifested by parental withdrawal due to emotional distress or parental control due to disempowerment and lack of skill. In addition, abusive behaviors between parents can be emulated by sibling subsystems.[27] Marital discord, rigidity, enmeshment, and other family system dysfunctions directly affect sibling relations.[7] As a result of these dynamics, ways of interaction become learned within the family system, and they can either perpetuate the abusive dynamic or defend against it, often at an unconscious level.[28] See Chapter 6: Alternatives for Families: A Cognitive Behavioral Treatment Approach for Family Conflict and Harsh Physical Parenting regarding family interventions.

PREVENTION

Prevention efforts are needed to protect against sibling-on-sibling abuse. Prevention methods can increase recognition and help offset adverse effects,[19] especially since victims are more at risk for developing PTSD from future traumatic events.[29] Sibling-on-sibling abuse is often invalidated by professionals who focus on the positive aspects of keeping siblings together and minimize the harm, especially of sexual abuse.[2] Training for professionals should highlight characteristics of siblings such as age and gender, as well as the quality of relations between them.[17]

SUMMARY

The problem of sibling-on-sibling abuse is longstanding and pervasive. As outlined above, practice in this area involves the careful assessment of trauma and individual and family capabilities, a range of interventions from crisis to collaboration and advocacy to direct treatment methods, and reflexivity on the part of helping professionals. The care and empathy for victims of such abuse can be emotionally taxing, change our world view, trigger our own traumatic vulnerabilities, and lead to difficulties in our work. Forensic interviewers, for instance, were shown to have higher levels of burnout and secondary stress.[30] As such, helping professionals need to attend to their own needs for care, recognize the signs of chronic stress or vicarious traumatization, and utilize supports such as supervision.[23]

CASE STUDY

Case Study 17-1

Jeffrey, who was 12 years old, and Anna, who was 7 years old, were siblings in the same household with their biological parents. Anna reported to her parents that she and Jeffrey "played house." When their parents inquired about this further, Anna reported that this was "acting like a Mommy and Daddy" and involved touching each other's "private parts" while "cuddling" in their parents' bed. At the time of the incident, the parents were out of the house, and Jeffrey was watching his sister. Jeffrey reported that they were just playing, and he had heard about this type of fondling from peers and wanted to know what it was like.

Discussion

In order to do an assessment in this case, further questions should include how often this has occurred, whether this behavior developed from sexual curiosity or from exploitation, the effects of the incident(s) on either child, family dynamics, the parents' responses to the situation, and a plan for safety as well as who to call as a mandated reporter. The advantages of such follow up questions regarding the family involved in this case are as follows:

— The number of times such incidences occurred can help distinguish between 'curiosity' and an ongoing threat/pattern.

— The degree of exploitation that was involved in those incidents can help identify the dynamics of abuse. For instance, asking the younger child how she was approached, what was said, and how she responded and felt, can help determine the power exerted by the older sibling.

— Dysfunctions in the family dynamics, such as substance abuse, lack of parental supervision, and other experiences of sexual abuse (with these children, others, or the parents themselves) would lead to more concern about risks.

— Exploring the interest of the 12-year-old and distinguishing between curiosity versus desire/attraction, would help identify risks for him as a perpetrator. For example: What did you hear from your friends? What part were you curious about? What did you think might happen? How did this affect you?

Such a comprehensive assessment is needed to contextualize the family dynamics and the propensity of the 12-year-old to be a perpetrator.

KEY POINTS

1. Sibling-on-sibling abuse is one the most pervasive forms of family violence, and can include physical, emotional, and sexual abuse, as well as neglect and coercion.

2. The exact causes of this abuse are unknown but could include characteristics in the individual offender or within the family system.

3. The effects of abuse can include manifestations across all realms of functioning.

4. Treatment includes general approaches in crisis intervention, collaborations, policy, advocacy, and specific therapeutic approaches such as TF-CBT, skill development, attachment-based therapy, and family systems therapy.

ADDITIONAL RESOURCES

— American Academy of Child and Adolescent Psychiatry: www.aacap.org

— American Humane Association: http://www.americanhumane.org/children/stop-child-abuse/advocacy/federal-legislative-updates.html

— Administration for Children and Families: www.acf.dhhs.gov

— Association for Children's Mental Health: www.acmh-mi.org

— Association for Play Therapy: www.iapt.org

— Center for Children's Law and Policy: http://www.cclp.org/

— Childhelp: National Child Abuse Hotline: https://childhelphotline.org/

— Child Trauma Academy: http://childtrauma.org

— Child Welfare: www.childwelfare.com

— Child Welfare Information Gateway: www.childwelfare.gov

— International Society for Traumatic Stress Studies: http://www.istss.org

— National Association of Counsel for Children: http://www.naccchildlaw. org/?page=Policy_Guide

— National Child Traumatic Stress Network: https://www.nctsn.org/

— Society of Clinical Child and Adolescent Psychology, Evidence-Based Therapies: https://effectivechildtherapy.org/therapies/

— Trauma Center at Justice Resource Institute: http://www.traumacenter.org/

— US Department of Health & Human Services, Administration for Children and Families, Administration on Children, Youth and Families, Children's Bureau. *Child Maltreatment 2020*. 2022. https://www.acf.hhs.gov/cb/data-research/child-maltreatment

REFERENCES

1. Perkins NH, Meyers A. The manifestation of physical and emotional sibling abuse across the lifespan and the need for social work intervention. *J Fam Soc Work*. 2020;23(4):338-356. doi:10.1080/10522158.2020.1799894

2. Yates P. "It's just the abuse that needs to stop": professional framing of sibling relationships in a grounded theory study of social worker decision making following sibling sexual behavior. *J Child Sex Abus*. 2020;29(2):222-245. doi:10. 1080/10538712.2019.1692399

3. Caffaro JV, Conn-Caffaro A. Treating sibling abuse families. *Aggress Violent Behav*. 2005:10:604-623. doi:10.1016/j.avb.2004.12.001

4. Geerts-Perry AT, Riggs SA, Kaminski PL, Murrell A. Psychological well-being and family functioning in middle childhood: the unique role of sibling relational dynamics. *J Fam Issues*. 2021;42(12):2965-2985. doi:10.1177/0192513X21993191

5. Shepherd D, Geodeke S, Landon J, Taylor S, Williams J. The impact of sibling relationships on later-life psychological and subjective well-being. *J Adult Dev* 2021;28:76-86. doi:10.1037/14776-004

6. Hart C. "I am you and you are me": a self psychology perspective on sibling relationships. *Psychoanal Soc Work*. 2021;28(1):64-85. doi:10.1080/15228878.2 020.1861470

7. Whiteman SD, McHale SM, Soli A. Theoretical perspectives on sibling relationships. *J Fam Theory Rev*. 2011;3(2):124-139. doi:10.1111/j.1756-2589.2011. 00087.x

8. Caffaro J. Treating adult survivors of sibling sexual abuse: a relational strengths-based approach. *J Fam Viol*. 2017;32:543-552. doi:10.1007/s10896-016-9877-0

9. Meyers A. *Sibling Abuse: understanding developmental consequences through object relations, family systems, and resiliency theories*. Dissertation. Hunter College; 2011.

10. Tucker CJ, Finkelhor D, Turner H, Shattuck AM. Family dynamics and young children's sibling victimization. *J Fam Psychol.* 2014;28(5):625-633. doi:10.1037/fam0000016

11. Williams JS, Riggs SA, Kaminski PL. A typology of childhood sibling subsystems that may emerge in abusive family systems. *Fam J.* 2016;24(4):378-384. doi:10.1177/1066480716663182

12. Meyers AB. Notes from the field: understand why sibling abuse remains under the radar and pathways to outing. *Fac Works: Soc Work.* 2015;18(2).

13. Lim BH, Hodges MH, Lilly MM. The differential effects of insecure attachment on post-traumatic stress: a systematic review of extant findings and explanatory mechanisms. *Trauma Violence Abuse.* 2020;21(5):1044-1060. doi:10.1177/1524838018815136

14. Katz C, Tsur N, Nicolet R, Carmel N, Klebanov B. Children's responses to maltreatment: key conclusions from a systematic literature review. *Trauma Violence Abuse.* 2021;22(5):1155-1168. doi:10.1177/1524838020908851

15. Renner LM, Schwab-Reese LM, Coppola EC, Boel-Studt S. The contribution of interpersonal violence victimization types to psychological distress among youth. *Child Abuse Negl.* 2020;106. doi:10.1016/j.chiabu.2020.104493

16. Meyers A. A call to child welfare: protect children from sibling abuse. *Qual Soc Work.* 2014;13(5):654-670. doi:10.1177/1473325014527332

17. Waid JD, Tanana MJ, Vanderloo MJ, Voit R, Kothari BH. The role of siblings in the development of externalizing behaviors during childhood and adolescence: a scoping review. *J Fam Soc Work.* 2020;23(4):318-337. doi:10.1080/10522158.2020.1799893

18. Llorens M, Barba M, Torralbas J, et al. Stress-related biomarkers and cognitive functioning in adolescents with ADHD: effect of childhood maltreatment. *J Psychiatr Res.* 2022;149:217-225. doi:10.1016/j.jpsychires.2022.02.041

19. Li W, O'Brien JE, Zhu Y, Chen Q. Violence, addictive behaviors, and trauma among adolescents in China. *J Fam Viol.* 2021;36:709-720.

20. Rosenbaum DL, White KS, Artime TM. Coping with childhood maltreatment: avoidance and eating disorder symptoms. *J Health Psychol.* 2021;26(14):2832-2840. doi:10.1177/1359105320937068

21. McDonald C, Martinez K. Victims' retrospective explanations of sibling sexual violence. *J Child Sex Abus.* 2017;26(7):874-888. doi:10.1080/10538712.2017.1354953

22. Rueness J, Augusti E, Strom IF, Wentzel-Larsen T, Myhre MC. Adolescent abuse victims displayed physical health complaints and trauma symptoms during post disclosure interviews. *Acta Paediatr.* 2020;109(11):2409-2415. doi:10.1111/apa.15244

23. Webb N. *Social Work Practice with Children.* 4th ed. The Guilford Press; 2019.

24. Collins BG, Collins TM. *Crisis and Trauma: Developmental-ecological Intervention.* Houghton Mifflin Publishers; 2005.

25. Renner LM, Driessen MC. Siblings who are exposed to child maltreatment: practice reported by county children's supervisors. *J Public Child Welf.* 2019;13(5):491-511. doi:10.1080/15548732.2018.1514350

26. Perkins NH, O'Connor MK. Physical and emotional sibling violence: a necessary role for social work. *Soc Work.* 2016;61(1):91-93. doi:10.1093/sw/swv048

27. Tucker CJ, Finkelhor D. The state of interventions for sibling conflict and aggression. *Trauma Violence Abuse*. 2017;18(4):396-406. doi:10.1177/1524 838015622438

28. Haskins C. Treating sibling incest using a family systems approach. *J Ment Health Couns*. 2003;25(4):337-351. doi:10.17744/mehc.25.4.r0vm1whayctmlmww

29. Gould F, Harvey PD, Hodgins G, et al. Prior trauma-related experiences predict the development of posttraumatic stress disorder after a new traumatic event. *Depress Anxiety*. 2021;38(1):40-47. doi:10.1002/da.23084

30. Starcher D, Stolzenberg SN. Burnout and secondary trauma among forensic interviewers. *Child Fam Soc Work*. 2020;25(4):924-934.

Chapter 18

SUBSTANCE USE IN ADOLESCENTS

Savannah Dettman, MA, LCMHCA

OBJECTIVES

After reading this chapter, the reader will be able to:

1.   *Understand the risk factors and common patterns of adolescent substance use.*

2.   *Determine the appropriate action based on adolescent presentation.*

3.   *Tailor services to meet adolescents' developmental needs.*

BACKGROUND AND SIGNIFICANCE

Adolescence is often conceptualized in 3 phases: early adolescence (ie, between the ages of 10 and 14), mid-adolescence (ie, between the ages of 15 and 16), and late adolescence (ie, between the ages of 17 and 18). This chapter will consider those stages of adolescence, as well as emerging adults (ie, between the ages of 18 and 21), to better understand substance use in this population. It should be noted, however, that these substages of adolescence vary by culture,[1] and this chapter may better reflect patterns that align more closely to individualistic cultures. Additionally, these stages are based on chronological age, which may not adequately represent an adolescent's experience.[1]

COMMON PATTERNS OF SUBSTANCE USE

Substance use is often initiated in adolescence or before 25 years of age.[2-7] Initiation and progression of substance use are influenced by a variety of risk factors, which may change over the individual's lifetime, including[2-5,8-14]:

— Maltreatment

— Exposure to violence

— Family dynamics

— Parental substance abuse and mental health concerns

— Low socioeconomic status

— Genetic predisposition

— Co-occurring mental health conditions

— Exposure to stress and trauma

— Belonging to a minority group

— Lack of perceived risk

— Peer group influence

— Influence of mass media and idolized entertainment figures

— Gender

In the years before this book was published, there has been an increase in the substances that are available to adolescents, substance potency, and the ways in which substances are administered.[7,14,15] The most used substances are influenced by availability, peer group, culture, and perception of risk.[2,5,7,10,11,14] It is critical that providers are continuously being educated on new psychoactive substances and synthetic drugs,[10] as well as norms and trends in their community. Data show that alcohol, cannabis, and nicotine remain the most common psychoactive substances used by adolescents.[7,10,14] Vaping has become the most popular method for consuming nicotine and continues to rise in popularity for cannabis.[2,5,10] According to the 2020 National Survey on Drug Use and Health,[2] the most common substances used by adolescents—after alcohol, cannabis, and nicotine—are prescription drugs, inhalants, and hallucinogens. Prescription drugs, over-the-counter drugs, and inhalants are especially important to assess for, as they are often the most readily accessible.[2]

Furthermore, the use of multiple substances is more common than the use of a single substance.[12,14] This is especially true for older adolescents, particularly individuals who are entering college, as this environment tends to promote substance-using behaviors. The intensity and frequency of substance use may also increase in older subgroups,[9] as heavy episodic drinking peaks worldwide between 20 to 24 years of age,[10] and the age group with the highest reported substance use disorders in the United States, for both alcohol and illicit drugs, is young adults aged 18 to 25 years.[2]

DELIVERING DEVELOPMENTALLY APPROPRIATE SERVICES

Recommendations for developmentally appropriate services extend to all parts of the treatment process, including screening, assessment, and intervention, with client engagement being a key component of successful treatment.[9,16] Providers can encourage engagement by respecting adolescents' confidentiality.[9,17,18] Adolescents and their caregivers must be informed about the nature of confidentiality, the importance of private communication for the therapeutic process, and situations in which confidentiality does not apply.[9,18] An additional recommendation to increase engagement is hiring younger, more diverse, and bilingual staff members, as they are perceived as more relatable, can better meet the needs of the community, and raise the retention rates in clients of color.[17,19] It is also recommended that any staff members who are delivering adolescent services be specifically trained to meet their unique needs.[7]

Another key consideration in providing developmentally appropriate care is language choice.[18] Providers must find a balance as they engage with members of this transitional age period, speaking to adolescents with respect while also considering their level of understanding. Jargon and stigmatizing language should be avoided.[17] For example, labeling substance use as "bad" may contribute to a child's internalization of "I am bad." Psychoeducation should be fact-based rather than opinion-based. Providers must be knowledgeable of adolescent culture[17] and should incorporate language used by adolescents and relatable anecdotes when appropriate.

Other considerations include adolescent-friendly décor,[17] flexibility in the way services are provided,[19] and ensuring that adolescents are provided with choices in order to promote autonomy.[13,17] Additionally, providers should consider administering screening and other components of treatment electronically, if this functionality is available.[5,16-18,20] Further, providers must be aware of local laws as they pertain to adolescent services. For example, more than 1/2 of the United States allow minors to receive services for substance use without parental consent.[9]

SCREENING: IS THE SUBSTANCE USE NORMATIVE OR PATHOLOGICAL?

In some contexts and cultures, adolescent exploration of substances may be considered normative. When adults use substances, the pathological or problematic nature is determined by a variety of criteria and whether the use interferes with functioning. Screening tools are generally used as a first step to determine if a problem is present that would warrant further exploration through an assessment. A few validated screening tools unique to adolescent substance use include CRAFFT,[5,6,9,20] Brief Screener for Tobacco, Alcohol, and Other Drugs (BSTAD),[5,6,12] and Screening to Brief Intervention (S2BI).[5,6,9,12] Routine screening is recommended in primary care settings whether there is direct suspicion or evidence of substance use present or not.[7] Although adolescents could be using substances in a non-pathological manner, according to Welsh & Hadland,[9] "there is no known safe dose of psychoactive substances on the developing adolescent brain." This statement suggests that adolescent substance use merits some level of action, regardless of screening results. If substance use is present, but problematic use is not indicated, then the plan of action could include a brief intervention with periodic follow up to monitor any progression. If the screening does indicate problematic substance use, further assessment is necessary.

CONSIDERATIONS FOR ASSESSMENT AND DIAGNOSIS

Assessment is a process that helps determine the severity of substance use, as well as which services are most appropriate for treatment.[5,6] Adolescents most commonly receive outpatient services,[9] which range from one hour of individual therapy per week to several hours of group and individual therapy combined. The World Health Organization (WHO) recommends avoiding institutionalization.[3] Residential treatment is costly and does not necessarily produce better treatment outcomes as it can cause disruptions in the adolescent's life, which can then perpetuate the problem through feelings of isolation and betrayal.[21] Though the need for detoxification and residential services is rare among adolescents,[9] there is a time and place in which it may be appropriate. Adolescents with a particularly significant risk for overdose, suicide, or homicide may benefit from this higher level of care, especially if they lack community support or have unsafe family environments.[6,9,21] It is recommended that adolescents be placed in the lowest level of care that is clinically appropriate, as it is always possible to increase the level of care or try a new treatment approach if the individual does not show improvement.[22]

Providers must gather detailed information on patterns of substance use (eg, how often the adolescent engages in the behavior, the amount consumed in a typical occurrence, the context in which substances are used). It is particularly important to gather information on the function of the substance use, so that treatment can help replace the benefits with a safer activity that provides similar outcomes. One tactic for information gathering is to ask adolescents about general substance use behavior in their peer group prior to asking them about their own use. This progression can ease the adolescent into sharing and increase their level of comfort. In addition to assessing patterns of use, a biopsychosocial assessment inquiring about a variety of influencing factors helps develop a more complete conceptualization of the individual and their needs.[6] Assessors must develop an understanding of the child's risk and protective factors, as this combination plays a critical role in the adolescent's likelihood of continued use and progression to more problematic use.[10,14,18] Assessment should also extend to include the caregivers' needs, as they may benefit from parenting classes or treatment of their own.[13]

According to the *Diagnostic and Statistical Manual of Mental Disorders, 5th Edition* (DSM-5),[23] an individual meets the criteria for a mild substance use disorder when they have 2 to 3 of the following symptoms:

— Use of the substance in greater frequencies or more often than intended

— Unsuccessful efforts to stop using the substance

— A large amount of time spent using the substance

— Cravings for the substance

— Failure to fulfill responsibilities

— Interpersonal difficulties or social consequences due to substance use

— Decrease in activities due to substance use

— Use of the substance in hazardous situations

— Use of the substance despite its impact on physical or psychological conditions

— Increase in tolerance for the substance

— Experiences of withdrawal

It has been argued, however, that the DSM-5 criteria for substance use disorders is not developmentally appropriate.[24,25] Some suggest that parts of the criteria do not readily apply to adolescents, while other criteria are met easily without consideration of developmental context. It is recommended that diagnosis is avoided whenever possible, provided that the adolescent is still able to receive services in the absence of a diagnosis.

TREATMENT AND INTERVENTIONS

Most research for adolescent substance use focuses on family therapy, motivational interventions, and behavioral therapy. Treatment outcomes are often measured by treatment completion, reduction in substance use, and rates of relapse following treatment.[9] Relapse is a common occurrence, however, so this could require a shift in how success is defined.[5,9] A more appropriate goal may be optimizing safety among adolescents using substances.[9] It is important that providers and caregivers have realistic expectations, and that they do not assume that change will occur instantly.[9]

FAMILY THERAPY

Family therapy is the gold standard treatment method for adolescent substance use, especially for families with younger adolescents and those with high-risk behaviors.[9,16,20,22,24,26] Lack of family involvement and negative family perceptions, such as the belief that substance use is the adolescent's problem alone, are barriers to treatment.[19,20] Family therapy aims to increase family involvement and improve family dynamics, helping the child feel supported, thus increasing their level of motivation.[3,9,19] Family therapy also views substance use in the context of the family system, which helps lessen the stigma of substance use. Of note, a unique struggle of family therapy in this context is balancing the adolescent's need for autonomy with the structure and parental involvement that is often helpful in recovery.[7]

Several approaches to family therapy have been specifically designed or validated for adolescent substance use. These include multidimensional family therapy (MDFT), multisystemic family therapy (MST), brief strategic family therapy (BSFT), and functional family therapy (FFT).[9,20-22] These approaches are all flexible in nature, having the ability to individualize treatment based on family needs. MDFT and MST focus on strengthening family and community support, while BSFT and FFT focus more intensely on family functioning alone.[6,22] MDFT is a manualized approach available in several languages with positive results in decreasing externalizing behaviors.[16,22] MST may be most ideal for severe cases requiring crisis support, as it provides in-home services with 24/7 support and a unique goal of keeping adolescents in their home and community.[27] BSFT is known for addressing cultural factors related to engagement, and it is favored when parental substance use is also present.[22] Lastly, FFT is a behavioral approach known for its cultural sensitivity and use in several countries.[22]

Motivational Interventions

Adolescents are often mandated to attend treatment for substance use. The lack of agency in this decision is associated with low motivation for change, which is a barrier to treatment outcomes.[9,19,20] Motivational interviewing (MI) and motivational enhancement therapy (MET) address this barrier directly and have been validated for use in individual and group settings.[16,26,28,29] MI is also favored as a brief intervention among adolescents who are not seeking treatment,[15] which can be provided by a variety of professionals that engage with this population (eg, medical, behavioral health, criminal justice, school staff).[6,9,28,29] MI is person-centered, allowing for the adolescent's freedom of choice to be respected.[20,28] This approach aligns with the recommendations for developmentally appropriate services as it supports autonomy,[13] does not shame or judge the adolescent,[18] and opens the door for honest communication[9] regarding the adolescent's decisions and behaviors. Honest communication gives adolescents the opportunity to make decisions for themselves, which is more likely to lead to sustainable change. This approach also has an emphasis on the exploration of values, which aligns with the adolescent's primary developmental task of identity versus role confusion.

Behavioral Therapy

Behavioral approaches aim to change thoughts, feelings, and actions based on reinforcement theory.[6] Common behavioral approaches for adolescent substance use include cognitive behavioral therapy (CBT) and adolescent community reinforcement approach (A-CRA). Although CBT was originally designed for adults, it has been validated for use with adolescents as well.[16,24,26] CBT focuses on behavior change by examining antecedents and developing coping skills and self-regulation tools.[6,20] A-CRA uses ideas from CBT, while also incorporating components of motivational intervention and family therapy.[9] The goal is to enhance protective factors in the community and teach the adolescent strategies for coping, healthy communication, and problem solving.[6,9] Compared to CBT, A-CRA may be more appropriate in high-risk situations in which an ecological model is preferred.

Though not a therapeutic approach, contingency management (CM) is a behavioral strategy that can be used in combination with a variety of therapies.[16,20] Adolescents' choices often reflect rewards, even with the knowledge of present risk.[30] CM uses low-cost incentives to increase desired behavior and treatment outcomes,[6] presenting a reward that differs from the natural rewards associated with substance use (eg, peer acceptance, euphoria). Studies have shown mixed results though, with some individuals maintaining treatment gains and others relapsing when the positive reinforcement is taken away.[9] However, CM may still be a strategy worth implementing to increase treatment engagement, as relapse is a common phenomenon with all evidence-based practices.

Pharmacotherapy

Medication-assisted therapy for substance use disorders, though widely accepted in the adult population, has not been well studied or implemented for adolescents.[6,9] WHO recommends non-pharmacological approaches to be the priority.[3] However, unique circumstances may warrant consultation with a specialist and the use of medication.[18] It is critical that "risks and benefits [of pharmacotherapy are] weighed against the risks of continued substance use."[9] Cases in which adolescents are using lethal substances with a high risk for overdose may be a good fit for medication management.[9]

Therapeutic Themes and Developmental Considerations

Regardless of the chosen intervention, a common thread of therapeutic themes exists within adolescent approaches. Such themes, including goal setting, concept of self, emotional regulation, and community support, require adaptations based on the adolescent's developmental presentation.

GOAL SETTING

It is important to consider the development of the individual while setting goals. As individuals go through the later stages of adolescence, they gain greater capacity to conceptualize, plan, and act on future-oriented goals.[1] This suggests that younger adolescents may require goals that are focused on the present or near future. In developing treatment goals, it is important to collaborate with the adolescent to help foster their autonomy.

CONCEPT OF SELF

Therapy involves the exploration of self, which aligns with the typical developmental task of adolescents and emerging adults discovering who they are.[1] In CBT, this may include an exploration of thoughts and feelings, while MI focuses more on values. As adolescents form their identity, they may struggle with low self-esteem. Addressing self-stigma, a common treatment barrier,[31] may be especially important for early adolescents, as they report greater fluctuations of self-esteem than older adolescents do.[1] Additionally, it is important to explore the thoughts, feelings, and external contributions associated with low self-esteem.

Peer acceptance is another prevalent phenomenon influencing adolescent behavior and concept of self. Though present in all subgroups of adolescents, it is most influential in the earlier stages.[1,30] If adolescents explore and develop a healthy sense of self, it is possible that they may become more comfortable with individuality and less influenced by their peers.

EMOTIONAL REGULATION

Adolescents tend to be more vulnerable to stress,[1,2,4] experience more rapid fluctuation in emotions,[1] and express their emotions with actions more frequently than words, which may be especially true for early adolescents and males.[30] Although emotional regulation improves with age, a large facet of adolescent intervention for all substages is the promotion of socioemotional learning and coping skills.[4] The development of coping skills should be created in response to the individual's presentation, triggers, and interests. For example, feelings of instability and uncertainty may be more prevalent in emerging adults,[1] so they may respond well to mindfulness and acceptance practices. Furthermore, an adolescent who enjoys reading may benefit from incorporating the activity as a skill to use when overwhelmed.

COMMUNITY SUPPORT

Community support is a common emphasis of treatment and aftercare. Traditionally, this involves a setting in which people can relate to and support one another,[6,9] of which Alcoholics Anonymous (AA) and Narcotics Anonymous (NA) are the most common. Universality is a factor that makes these groups appealing; however, AA and NA are most often composed of adults,[20] potentially inhibiting adolescent ability to relate to other members. Despite these considerations, mutual self-help groups are beneficial for some adolescents when prescreened by a trusted adult.[6,9] Due to the high association between parental addiction and adolescent substance use, "Alateen" may be an appropriate self-help group for adolescents to attend, as it provides support for those impacted by parental substance use.

Fostering community support for adolescents may require some level of creativity. Risk taking as a natural part of adolescence does not have to be eliminated, but rather healthy risk-taking behaviors can be supported.[30] Research has shown the importance of increasing fun in recovery, which can take the form of encouraging the adolescent to try new clubs or activities.[9] A large component of an adolescent's community involves their school life. Some research suggests enrolling adolescents in recovery schools.[9] These schools, however, are not always accessible, and there is risk of social deviance and isolation by removing adolescents from their already-formed social circles. Similarly, there are several collegiate recovery programs for adolescents contemplating college. Recovery schools and collegiate recovery programs may be most appropriate when adolescents are motivated to attend.

SUMMARY

Substance use is influenced by a variety of factors and is often initiated in adolescence.[2-7] Alcohol, cannabis, and nicotine are the most common substances used,[7,10,14] with the risk for polysubstance use and greater frequency and intensity of substance use increasing in older adolescence.[9,12,14] Due to the impact of substances on adolescent development,[9] low and high severity use merit some level of response, ranging from brief intervention with periodic follow up to outpatient services or residential treatment. Treatment typically includes family therapy, motivational interventions, or behavioral therapy, with common themes of goal setting, concept of self, emotional regulation, and community support. Treatment should be individualized, reflecting the severity of the adolescent's substance use, their unique risk factors and interests, and their developmental presentation.

CASE STUDY

Case Study 18-1

Joshua McAbee was a White, 15-year-old boy brought for services at an agency providing mental health and substance misuse services after his father came home early from work and found that Joshua and several friends had skipped school to smoke marijuana at Joshua's house. Joshua's father was worried that his son was going down a "bad path" and stated that he had noticed that Joshua's grades were slipping. Joshua stated that "it's not a big deal" and "all [his] friends do it." Joshua reported that he had not used any other illicit substances, and his father confirmed that his son had taken a home drug test and only marijuana was detected. Joshua reported low use, typically social, although it had increased over the preceding few weeks compared to what it was when he started about 6 months ago. Joshua reported using marijuana to relax and fit in.

Discussion

An initial assessment session was performed to inform treatment recommendations. The goals of this assessment were to determine the pattern and severity of Joshua's marijuana use, as well as the presence of other notable mental health symptoms and risk and resilience factors (eg, the presence of community support, the state of the family environment) that could impact treatment. This assessment included a clinical interview, the CRAFFT, and several other general mental health screening instruments designed for adolescents. Joshua was found to have no significant mental health concerns or suicidal ideation needing to be addressed immediately, though he did appear to have mild anxiety and occasional behavioral problems at home (eg, refusal to do chores or homework). Joshua was assigned a younger male therapist to promote rapport and client engagement. Given the current low level of severity, sessions were scheduled to last one hour, once per week, following the guideline that clients receive the lowest appropriate level of care. Treatment included routine progress monitoring checks to determine if this level of care was appropriately meeting the family's needs and if alterations were needed. Sessions included both Joshua and his father, although each session did not necessarily include both individuals in the room at the same time, so as to allow Joshua to more openly discuss issues with his therapist. Therapy focused on providing accurate psychoeducation (eg, neither exaggerating nor minimizing the impacts of marijuana and other substance use), using motivational interviewing to help Joshua find intrinsic reasons for lowering use, and coping skills training him to develop more healthy means of coping with his anxiety. Family sessions additionally focused on increasing family cohesion, and Joshua's father was taught parent management techniques shown to reduce adolescent substance misuse and other behavioral problems. These include increased parental monitoring of the adolescent along with age-appropriate rewards and discipline, such as allowing the adolescent to earn back privileges that may have been lost due to the initial substance misuse.

KEY POINTS

1. Whenever possible, it is recommended to avoid diagnosis and provide the least restrictive level of care, encouraging the adolescent to stay in their community.

2. Several evidence-based practices are available for adolescent substance use, with family therapy being the gold standard.

3. Services should be individualized based on the adolescent's developmental needs, presenting risk and protective factors, and interests.

REFERENCES

1. Salmela-Aro K. Stages of adolescence. In: Brown BB, Prinstein MJ, eds. *Encyclopedia of Adolescence.* Academic Press; 2011:360-368.

2. Substance Abuse and Mental Health Services Administration. *Key Substance Use and Mental Health Indicators in the United States: Results from the 2020 National Survey on Drug Use and Health.* Center for Behavioral Health Statistics and Quality; 2021. Accessed May 17, 2022. https://www.samhsa.gov/data/sites/default/files/reports/rpt35325/NSDUHFFRPDFWHTMLFiles2020/2020NSDUHFFR1PDFW102121.pdf

3. Adolescent mental health. World Health Organization. Updated November 17, 2021. Accessed March 9, 2022. https://www.who.int/news-room/fact-sheets/detail/adolescent-mental-health

4. Guidelines on mental health promotive and preventive interventions for adolescents: helping adolescents thrive. World Health Organization. 2020. Accessed May 17, 2022. https://apps.who.int/iris/bitstream/handle/10665/336864/9789240011854-eng.pdf

5. Gray KM, Squeglia LM. Research review: what have we learned about adolescent substance use? *J Child Psychol Psychiatry.* 2018;59(6):618-627. doi:10.1111/jcpp.12783

6. Screening and treatment of substance use disorders among adolescents. Substance Abuse and Mental Health Services Administration. 2021. Accessed May 19, 2022. https://store.samhsa.gov/sites/default/files/SAMHSA_Digital_Download/PEP20-06-04-008.pdf

7. Levy S. Youth and the opioid epidemic. *Pediatrics.* 2019;143(2). doi:10.1542/peds.2018-2752

8. Benedini KM, Fagan AA. From child maltreatment to adolescent substance use: different pathways for males and females? *Fem Criminol.* 2018;15(2):147-173. doi:10.1177/1557085118810426

9. Welsh JW, Hadland SE. *Treating Adolescent Substance Use: A Clinician's Guide.* Springer; 2019.

10. World drug report 2021. United Nations; Office on Drugs and Crime. 2021. Accessed March 9, 2022. https://www.unodc.org/unodc/en/data-and-analysis/wdr2021.html

11. Global status report on alcohol and health 2018. World Health Organization. 2018. Accessed March 9, 2022. https://apps.who.int/iris/bitstream/handle/10665/274603/9789241565639-eng.pdf?ua=1&ua=1

12. Halladay J, Woock R, El-Khechen H, et al. Patterns of substance use among adolescents: a systematic review. *Drug Alcohol Depend.* 2020;1:216:108222. doi:10.1016/j.drugalcdep.2020.108222

13. Helping adolescents thrive toolkit: strategies to promote and protect adolescent mental health and reduce self-harm and other risk behaviours. World Health Organization and the United Nations Children's Fund. 2021. Accessed May 17, 2022. https://www.who.int/publications/i/item/9789240025554

14. World Drug Report 2018. United Nations. 2021. Accessed March 9, 2022. https://www.unodc.org/wdr2018/prelaunch/WDR18_Booklet_4_YOUTH.pdf

15. Kulak JA, Griswold KS. Adolescent substance use and misuse: recognition and management. *Am Fam Physician.* 2019;99(11):689-696.

16. Hogue A, Henderson CE, Becker SJ, Knight DK. Evidence base on outpatient behavioral treatments for adolescent substance use, 2014-2017: outcomes, treatment delivery, and promising horizons. *J Clin Child Adolesc Psychol.* 2018;47(4):499-526. doi:10.1080/15374416.2018.1466307

17. Hawke LD, Mehra K, Settipani C, et al. What makes mental health and substance use services youth friendly? A scoping review of literature. *BMC Health Serv Res.* 2019;19(257). doi:10.1186/s12913-019-4066-5

18. mhGAP intervention guide for mental, neurological and substance use disorders in non-specialized health settings. World Health Organization. 2016. https://www.who.int/publications/i/item/9789241549790

19. Acevedo A, Harvey N, Kamanu M, Tendulkar S, Fleary S. Barriers, facilitators, and disparities in retention for adolescents in treatment for substance use disorders: a qualitative study with treatment providers. *Subst Abuse Treat Prev Policy.* 2020;15(1):42. doi:10.1186/s13011-020-00284-4

20. Winters KC, Botzet AM, Stinchfield R, et al. Adolescent substance abuse treatment: a review of evidence-based research. In: Leukefeld CG, Gullotta TP, eds. *Adolescent Substance Abuse: Evidence-Based Approaches to Prevention and Treatment.* 2nd ed. Springer; 2018:141-171.

21. Liddle HA, Dakof GA, Rowe CL, et al. Multidimensional family therapy as a community-based alternative to residential treatment for adolescents with substance use and co-occurring mental health disorders. *J Subst Abuse Treat.* 2018;90:47-56. doi:10.1016/j.jsat.2018.04.011

22. Substance use disorder treatment and family therapy: treatment improvement protocol 39. Substance Abuse and Mental Health Services Administration. 2020. Accessed May 17, 2022. https://store.samhsa.gov/sites/default/files/SAM-HSA_Digital_Download/PEP20-02-02-012-508%20PDF.pdf

23. American Psychiatric Association. *Diagnostic and Statistical Manual of Mental Disorders.* 5th ed. American Psychiatric Association; 2013.

24. Hernandez L, Lavigne A, Wood M, Weirs RW. Moderators and mediators of treatment for youth with substance abuse. In: Maric M, Prins PJM, Ollendick TH, eds. *Moderators and Mediators of Youth Treatment Outcomes.* Oxford University Press; 2015:174-209.

25. De Micheli D, Andrade ALM, Galduróz JC. Limitations of DSM-5 diagnostic criteria for substance use disorder in adolescents: what have we learned after using these criteria for several years? *Braz J Psychiatry.* 2021;43(4):349-350. doi:10.1590/1516-4446-2020-1151

26. Steele DW, Becker SJ, Danko KJ, et al. Interventions for substance use disorders in adolescents: a systematic review. Agency for Healthcare Research and Quality. 2020. doi:10.23970/AHRQEPCCER225

27. Littell JH, Pigott TD, Nilsen KH, Green SJ, Montgomery OLK. Multisystemic therapy for social, emotional, and behavioural problems in youth aged 10 to 17: an updated systematic review and meta-analysis. *Campbell Syst Rev.* 2021;17(4). doi:10.1002/cl2.1158

28. Enhancing motivation for change in substance use disorder treatment: treatment improvement protocol 35. Substance Abuse and Mental Health Services Administration. 2019. Accessed May 17, 2022. https://store.samhsa.gov/sites/default/files/d7/priv/tip35_final_508_compliant_-_02252020_0.pdf

29. Steele DW, Becker SJ, Danko KJ, et al. Brief behavioral interventions for substance use in adolescence: a meta-analysis. *Pediatrics.* 2020;146(4). doi:10.1542/peds. 2020-0351

30. Adolescent development explained. US Department of Health and Human Services; Office of Population Affairs. 2018. Accessed May 17, 2022. https:// opa.hhs.gov/sites/default/files/2021-03/adolescent-development-explained-download.pdf

31. Vatanasin D, Dallas JC. Factors predicting self-stigma among youths receiving substance abuse treatment. *Pac Rim Int J Nurs Res.* 2022;26(1):78-89.

THE CHILD MALTREATMENT TO DELINQUENCY PATHWAY: *TRAUMA, MENTAL HEALTH, AND JUVENILE OFFENDING*

Christopher A. Mallett, PhD, Esq, LISW-S

OBJECTIVES

After reading this chapter, the reader will be able to:

1. Explain the pathways from child maltreatment to juvenile delinquency and how they differ depending on gender and maltreatment type.

2. Identify which effective trauma and mental health screening or assessment tools and interventions can be used by social service and juvenile justice system professionals to improve outcomes.

3. Describe how juvenile courts and detention/incarceration facilities can improve outcomes for child offenders with maltreatment victimization histories.

BACKGROUND AND SIGNIFICANCE

The maltreatment of children includes a number of difficult and painful experiences—physical abuse, sexual abuse, psychological abuse, and neglect. Those who are harmed in this way have a range of reactions and outcomes to this victimization. Some children are highly resilient and recover quickly, whereas some show immediate dysfunction, and some develop related behavioral, mental health, and trauma-induced problems. Of concern here are the children whose victimizations increase their risk for offending behaviors, delinquency, and formal juvenile court involvement. This pathway is challenging to discern because of the multiple risk and protective factors involved. Such a connection to the juvenile court system is commonly referred to as the child maltreatment to juvenile delinquency pathway.

The maltreatment to delinquency pathway has many facets, as maltreatment is one risk, among many, that increases the odds of a young person becoming formally involved with the juvenile courts. Other child-related risks include other traumas (eg, witnessing violence, bullying), mental health problems, and substance abuse.[1-3] Family-related risks include low parental involvement, inconsistent parenting, parent criminality, and parent-child separation.[4] School-related risks include academic problems, special education disabilities (eg, learning disabilities, social-emotional issues), truancy, negative or deviant peers, exclusionary school discipline (ie, suspensions and expulsions), and frequent school transitions; many of these school problems disproportionately impact students of color and those who are part of the LGBTQIA+ community.[5,6] Community or neighborhood-related risks include high levels of unemployment, unsafe neighborhoods, and residential instability, which disproportionately impact families of color.[7,8]

There are also a number of child and adolescent demographic factors that predict formal juvenile court involvement, especially when it comes to more serious forms of delinquent behaviors, including[9,10]:

— *The juvenile's age.* Adolescents are more likely to have court involvement.

— *Gender.* Males are more likely to have court involvement.

— *Race.* People of color are more likely to have court involvement.

— *Socioeconomic status.* Those living in poor households are more likely to have court involvement.

Because of the experience of multiple child and adolescent problems and risks, many of which also are linked to maltreatment, predicting juvenile delinquency outcomes is difficult, but possible.[4] It is important to understand the prevalence of this maltreatment to delinquency pathway.

CHILD WELFARE

Since the 1990s, the number of identified adolescent maltreatment victims has fallen from approximately 1000000 to 656000 annually in the United States.[11] These are the reported and substantiated maltreatment cases, with a majority being for neglect (ranging from 58% to 80%, depending on the year), followed by physical (17% to 27%), sexual (9% to 17%), and psychological abuse (4% to 7%).[11] These maltreatment rates have decreased because of changes in child protection agencies' report investigations and the response alternatives from these investigations.[11] Most experts do not believe that maltreatment victimizations have actually substantially decreased over this time period, but rather this decrease is due to the child protection agencies' administrative policies that have tightened investigation criteria, causing fewer children to come under agency supervision. Of the reported and substantiated maltreatment, those who are disproportionately affected are children under the age of 10 and Black, Hispanic, and American Indian children.[12]

Children of color are disproportionately involved with children's services even though rates of family maltreatment do not differ significantly by race.[11,13] The discrimination and bias across communities, law enforcement, and other involved stakeholder groups might explain this group's disproportionate involvement with children's services.[14] The higher likelihood of being involved with children's services, along with being disproportionally impacted by poverty and the history of residential segregation by race, may also explain the racial and ethnic gap across other negative life outcomes, including delinquency, crime engagement, and incarceration.[15]

JUVENILE JUSTICE

The United States juvenile courts handled over 722000 delinquency cases in 2019 with over 48000 children and adolescents held in locked facilities on any given day. Most of these delinquency cases (83%) involved high school-aged adolescents, with those aged 16 and 17 accounting for 48% of all juvenile cases.[16] For those who are adjudicated and formally involved with the juvenile courts, a majority recidivate and reenter the system numerous times.[17] Avoiding formal supervision with the juvenile courts is important because diversion and prevention efforts is effective for most child and adolescent offenders. The juvenile justice system is difficult for minors to disentangle from once involved, and delinquency increases the risk for involvement with the adult criminal justice system.[18] Involvement with juvenile courts, detention, and incarceration disproportionately impact certain groups of adolescents—those with trauma backgrounds and subsequent mental health difficulties, people of color, and members of the LGBTQIA+ community.[19]

Many of the children and adolescents involved with the juvenile courts have maltreatment histories estimated to be between 26% and 60% of those who are formally adjudicated delinquents.[20,21] A large proportion of those in the juvenile justice system have been maltreated, but a majority of children and adolescents that have been maltreated do not go on to be involved in the juvenile justice system.[22] Those who have been victims of abuse simply make up a significant percentage of the juvenile justice population.[23]

FROM CHILD MALTREATMENT TO JUVENILE DELINQUENCY

Those who have experienced childhood maltreatment are more likely to engage in offending and delinquent behaviors compared to those who have not been maltreated. Due to significant differences among the measurement of offending outcomes—arrest, conviction, delinquency, and whether official records or child self-reports were used—the link between certain maltreatment types and delinquency may be underestimated.[24]

In the late 1980s, maltreated children and adolescents were identified as having a significantly greater chance of being arrested (typically a year younger) than non-maltreated offenders.[25] Additionally, these maltreated children and adolescents were more likely to be formally supervised by the juvenile court for more serious offending behaviors.[9,26] Neglect is more often associated with being a risk factor for delinquency, as are living in poverty and having a single-parent household.[23,27,28] However, regardless of the presence or absence of all other risk factors, any type of childhood maltreatment is shown to have an impact on outcomes in a child's later childhood and adolescence.[24,26] Children and adolescents who have been neglected or physically abused are more likely to be arrested for a violent crime,[29] possibly because these maltreatment experiences are linked to other antisocial behaviors.[30] One review concluded that sexual abuse and neglect, but not physical abuse, are strongly associated with eventual involvement in violent crime.[31]

While complicated, the experience of repeated or recurring maltreatment directly impacts offending behavior in children and adolescents. Repeat victimization predicts the initiation, continuation, and severity of delinquent acts.[32] More extensive maltreatment is also associated with chronic and violent offending behaviors, especially when compared to non-maltreated children and adolescents.[31,33,34] In addition, those who are maltreated in their later childhood and early adolescent years[35] are at even higher risk of committing violent and delinquent acts.[2,19,32,35]

SERIOUS OFFENDING IN CHILDHOOD AND ADOLESCENCE

The evidence, as noted, reveals another disconcerting outcome: many of these maltreatment experiences are linked to repetitive serious offending in childhood and adolescence—both in regards to person and property crimes. Maltreatment is associated with serious offending even when other risk factors for these adolescent behaviors are present. In other words, the maltreatment victimization itself, more so than other risks, may be more directly linked to more serious offending. This is problematic because it is adolescents who commit and repeat more serious offenses that are much more likely to be placed into juvenile detention or child incarceration facilities. These detention and incarceration placement experiences are detrimental for the adolescents and are found to be part of the recidivism problem because of the punitive environment and new learned behaviors from peers.[18]

MENTAL HEALTH AND SUBSTANCE ABUSE PROBLEMS

Mental health and substance abuse problems are often an outcome of child and adolescent maltreatment. Depression and post-traumatic stress disorder (PTSD) can come from physical abuse,[36] anxiety difficulties and related problems are often outcomes of neglect, and sexual abuse is associated with both anxiety difficulties and PTSD.[37] In turn, there is increasing evidence that these, and other mental health difficulties are linked to subsequent offending behavior and delinquency, though the link may be direct or indirect through subsequent or interceding problems.[38] In addition, childhood depressive disorders and aggressive behaviors are strongly associated with delinquency.[1,39]

Within juvenile court detention and incarceration facilities, 2/3 of males and 3/4 of females meet criteria for at least one mental health disorder.[40] An overview of the mental health difficulties experienced can be seen in **Table 19-1**.

Table 19-1. Mental Health Problems of Incarcerated Youth[2]	
Depressive disorders	Between 13% and 30%
Psychotic disorders	Between 5% and 10%
Anxiety disorders	Up to 25%
Attention-deficit/hyperactivity disorder (ADHD)	Up to 20%
Disruptive behavior disorders	Between 30% and 70%
Substance use disorders	Between 25% and 65%

GENDER DIFFERENCES

There are differential pathways to the juvenile courts for boys and girls below the age of 18.[41] Though the explanations for the increase since the mid-1990s in female delinquency is not clear, of the child and adolescent offenders arrested and court-supervised, more females have reported having maltreatment histories than males.[42] It is not yet understood if maltreatment impacts are greater for females than for males, but it is strongly hypothesized. One possibility is that females who commit violent acts are likely to have had a history of violence committed against them.[43] In addition, females who had experienced child abuse have been found more likely to commit an offense (often violent), experience arrest, and be involved with the juvenile court.[44] This may be particularly true for victims of sexual abuse.[45] However, males with maltreatment histories are also at risk for violent offending behaviors, though at differing rates.[43,46] Research on gender differentiation and delinquency still has found that maltreatment is a more important, and potentially stronger link, for females than for males, though the explication to understand this is ongoing.[47]

ASSESSMENT AND INTERVENTION

Juvenile courts are in a precarious situation, as they are working with a population with a significant number of maltreatment victims. The first intervention stage to addressing this issue is to decrease the number of children and adolescents in the community who are abused or neglected, whereby fewer victims will fall into the pathway to delinquency. While efforts to decrease maltreatment should be vigorously pursued to keep children and adolescents safe from these victimizations—including new parent and family support groups, home visiting programs, parent education, early child and family screening and treatment, child care opportunities, and improved public education—it is not assumed that these efforts will eliminate future maltreatment.[4,48,49]

The persistence of child maltreatment reports over the decades have led the juvenile courts to work with a certain disproportionate number of juvenile offenders who have victimization histories. The next intervention stage is the prevention of delinquency. Prevention is an opportunity for schools, child care agencies, and the juvenile justice system to use evidence-based programming and diversion alternatives to lessen the risk of first contacts with the system. Typically, adolescents who have a first contact with the system (one-time arrests) do not have a second contact, falling in at 54% of males and 70% of females.[9] So by implementing prevention programs, formal court involvement can be eliminated entirely for many of these first-time offenders. However, the focus should be on those adolescents who repeat their offending and are at higher risk for adjudication, where either court-mandated interventions were not effective or underlying issues were not addressed. There are steps that the juvenile courts are pursuing and can expand upon in directly addressing the maltreatment to delinquency link, including assessment, treatment, and improving the outcomes for serious child and adolescent offenders.

EXPANDING ASSESSMENT AND TREATMENT

Imposing only punitive or negative consequences for child and adolescent offenders is unlikely to change the pattern of delinquency or other risk-taking behaviors. Juvenile courts can be more effective in identifying and understanding the impact of maltreatment and related mental health problems on these behaviors.[4,49] However, many courts lack the resources or the prioritization to perform significant assessments of the children and adolescents (and families thereof) who become involved. Historically, court personnel have struggled to judge juvenile offenders in terms of their dangerousness, blame, risk for future offending, and level of benefit from various interventions.

At numerous points within the juvenile courts—diversion, offense charge, and detention—court professionals make these judgments, sometimes based only on professional experience and intuition. It is well known that uncovering maltreatment histories are often difficult to do through the use of interviews or family reports.[50]

Standardized assessments are able to provide assistance in identifying past social and family histories, mental health concerns, and other related problems. Two of these assessments are the Massachusetts Youth Screening Instrument (MAYSI-2) and the Youth Level of Service/Case Management Inventory (Y-LSI). The MAYSI-2 is a 52-item standardized instrument with 7 subscales used to identify mental health needs of children and adolescents, and the Y-LSI is a 42-item checklist with 8 subscales: offense history, family circumstances/parenting, education, peer relations, substance abuse, leisure/recreation, personality/behavior, and attitudes/orientation.[51] There are also trauma screenings available that can identify young people with maltreatment histories including: the Traumatic Events Screening Inventory, which is a structured clinical interview used to assess the child and parent reports of past or ongoing traumatic events including maltreatment; the Child Welfare Trauma Screening Tool that assesses trauma and mental health needs; and the Trauma Symptom Checklist for Children, which is a self-report symptom inventory that identifies behavioral and mental health disorders resulting from maltreatment and includes measures to assess for chronic traumatic stress.[52]

Once children and adolescents with maltreatment histories and related problems are properly identified, evidence-based interventions can be provided by the juvenile court or other community-based providers. Overall, cognitive-behavioral treatments have been found to be significantly helpful for traumatized children and adolescents.[29] Specifically, the interventions with the most evidence include the Cognitive Behavioral Intervention for Trauma in Schools, Trauma Affect Regulation: A Guide for Education and Therapy, Seeking Safety, Trauma-Focused Cognitive Behavioral Therapy, and Skills Training in Affective and Interpersonal Regulation. In addition, the Trauma Recovery and Empowerment Model is effective for female adolescents, an important consideration because of the differential gender impact of maltreatment on delinquency. Most of these interventions include a number of the following components: psychoeducation sessions, emotional regulation, cognitive processing, family or caregiver involvement, a strengths-based approach, and personal empowerment training.[53-56]

IMPROVING JUVENILE JUSTICE SYSTEM EFFECTIVENESS

When children and adolescents, both with and without maltreatment histories, are formally involved with the juvenile courts, it is important to identify which interventions, programs, or services are most effective. Since most juvenile courts are underfunded and struggle with having sufficient disposition options beyond probation supervision and detention facility placement, knowing what works and what does not is essential in more wisely investing the funds available. While substantial evidence of effective programs and services for child and adolescent offenders does exist, there is often a disconnect between what is known and what juvenile courts provide. Implementing a risk-needs-responsivity model could address this gap. This approach uses a guiding principle to match services to level of risk, ensuring as much as possible that children and adolescents are funneled into the most appropriate level of service.

Using standardized assessments for court-involved children and adolescents helps accurately direct decision making in order to lessen this disconnect. Providing a continuum of supervision and evidence-based rehabilitative programming—group counseling, mentoring, cognitive-behavioral techniques, and social skill building— allows the courts to match the client risks and needs to appropriate dispositions, including community-based services from other child and adolescent-caring systems. Utilizing these rehabilitative services is effective at improving outcomes and decreasing recidivism.[4]

Some effective juvenile court initiatives include: training personnel on how to work with children and adolescents who have mental health, substance use, and trauma-related problems; establishing a greater range of system and individual level interventions; improved reentry and aftercare options for children and adolescents leaving locked facilities; and the use of case management programming.[57] Programs that address child and adolescent mental health and substance abuse difficulties should include: treatment that occurs with the family (at home, if possible); is built around family and community strengths; is comprehensive and integrated; is gender and culturally specific; and allows flexibility in treatment type (eg, behavior, cognitive, parent training).[58] The Office of Juvenile Justice and Delinquency Prevention has recognized the Blueprints for Violence Prevention and established their own Model Programs Guide that identifies evidence-based delinquency prevention programs.[4]

CASE STUDY

Case Study 19-1

James was a 14-year-old White male. He lived at home with his mother and visited his father regularly. His father lived with a woman who was an alcoholic, and his mother had been in a relationship with a man named Don for the past 6 years. For 3 of those 6 years, Don had physically abused James and his mother, almost strangling James' mother to death on 2 occasions. James and his mother moved to a women's shelter 4 months ago, where James began mental health treatment.

As a result of his situation, James developed nightmares, was afraid to sleep alone, and constantly called his parents when separated from them. He also had trouble at school; James had a reputation among his teachers and peers for cursing at others, starting arguments, and seldom completing his academic work. Last week, he stabbed a classmate in the arm with a pen after they started arguing. James was arrested by the school resource officer and referred to the local juvenile court, per the school's policy.

Discussion

The juvenile court processed James as a juvenile delinquent and assigned a probation officer. Neither the school nor the court was aware of James' home life or mental health issues before the probation officer completed the court's investigation. Had school professionals intervened with James when they first noted his troubled behavior, they may have been able to refer him to services that would have helped him navigate the difficulties he was facing and keep him out of the juvenile courts system. There is still the possibility that, after the completion of the court investigation, James may be referred to group therapy, cognitive-behavioral therapy, a mentorship program, or some other service that can keep him from further court involvement.

KEY POINTS

1. Children and adolescents who are maltreatment victims are disproportionately involved with the juvenile justice system, adjudicated delinquent, and placed into locked facilities.

2. The maltreatment to delinquency pathway is complicated and differentiates depending on gender and abuse type.

3. There are effective strategies and interventions the juvenile justice system can use to improve outcomes for child and adolescent offenders with maltreatment backgrounds.

REFERENCES

1. Developmental Services Group. Risk factors for delinquency: literature review. Office of Juvenile Justice and Delinquency Prevention, Office of Justice Programs, US Department of Justice. 2015.

2. Teplin LA, Welty LJ, Abram KM, et al. Psychiatric disorders of youth after detention. Office of Juvenile Justice and Delinquency Prevention, Office of Justice Programs, US Department of Justice. 2015. https://ojjdp.ojp.gov/sites/g/files/xyckuh176/files/pubs/246824.pdf

3. Kinscherff RT. Distinguishing and assessing treatment needs and amenability to rehabilitation. In: Heilbrun K, DeMatteo D, Goldstein NES, eds. *APA Handbook of Psychology and Juvenile Justice.* American Psychological Association; 2016:385-404.

4. OJJDP model programs guide. Office of Juvenile Justice and Delinquency Prevention. 2018. Accessed 2022. https://ojjdp.ojp.gov/model-programs-guide/home

5. Morgan E, Salomon N, Plotkin M, Cohen R. *The school discipline consensus report: Strategies from the field to keep students engaged in school and out of the juvenile justice system.* The Council of State Governments Justice Center; 2014.

6. Mallett CA. *The School to Prison Pipeline: A Comprehensive Assessment.* Springer Publishing; 2016.

7. Congressional Research Service. Demographic and social characteristics of persons in poverty: 2018. Congressional Research Service. 2020. https://crsreports.congress.gov/product/pdf/R/R46294

8. Economic Policy Institute. Economic indicators: state unemployment by race and ethnicity. Economic Policy Institute. November 2021. https://www.epi.org/indicators/state-unemployment-race-ethnicity-2021q3/

9. Mallett C, Tedor M. *Juvenile Delinquency: Pathways and Prevention.* SAGE Publications; 2019.

10. Mulder E, Brand E, Bullens R, van Marle H. Risk factors for overall recidivism and severity of recidivism in serious juvenile offenders. *Intl J Offender Ther Comp Criminol.* 2011;55(1):118-135. doi:10.1177/0306624X09356683

11. US Department of Health and Human Services. *Child maltreatment 2019.* Administration for Children and Families, Children's Bureau. 2021. Updated June 27, 2023. https://www.acf.hhs.gov/cb/report/child-maltreatment-2019

12. National Child Abuse and Neglect Data System (NCANDS). Administration for Children and Families, US Department of Health and Human Services. 2020.

13. US Department of Health and Human Services. Child welfare practice to address racial disproportionality and disparity. Administration for Children and

Families, Children's Bureau. 2021. https://www.childwelfare.gov/resources/child-welfare-practice-address-racial-disproportionality-and-disparity/

14. Kang H, Burton DL. Effects of racial discrimination, childhood trauma, and trauma symptoms on juvenile delinquency in African American incarcerated youth. *J Aggress Maltreat Trauma.* 2014;23(10):1109-1125. doi:10.1080/10926771.2014.968272

15. Rovner J. Racial disparities in youth incarceration persist. The Sentencing Project. February 2021. https://www.sentencingproject.org/app/uploads/2022/08/Racial-Disparities-in-Youth-Incarceration-Persist.pdf

16. Hockenberry S. Delinquency cases in juvenile court, 2019. Office of Juvenile Justice and Delinquency Prevention, Office of Justice Programs, US Department of Justice. February 2022. https://ojjdp.ojp.gov/publications/delinquency-cases-2019.pdf

17. Cohen M, Feyerherm W, Spinney E, Stephenson R, Yeide M. *Disproportionate minority contact in the US juvenile justice system: A review of the DMC literature, 2001 to 2010.* Development Services Group; 2014.

18. Petrosino A, Turpin-Petrosino C, Guckenburg S. Formal system processing of juveniles: effects on delinquency. 2010;6(1):1-88. doi:10.4073/csr.2010.1

19. Yun J, Fukushima-Tedor M, Mallett C, Quinn L, Quinn M. Explaining trauma and crime by gender and sexual orientation among youth: findings from the Add Health national longitudinal study. *Crime Delinquency.* 2021;68(5):814-839. doi:10.1177/0011128721999342

20. Skinner-Osei P, Mangan L, Liggett M, Kerrigan M, Levenson JS. Justice-involved youth and trauma informed interventions. *Justice Pol J.* 2019;16(2):1-25.

21. Mallett C, Stoddard-Dare P. Maltreated children who are adjudicated delinquent: an at-risk profile. *Intl J Child Fam Welfare.* 2009;12(4):134-144.

22. Bender K. Why do some maltreated youth become juvenile offenders? A call for further investigation and adaptation of youth services. *Children Youth Serv Rev.* 2009;32:466-473. doi:10.1016/j.childyouth.2009.10.022

23. Yun I, Ball JD, Lim H. Disentangling the relationship between child maltreatment and violent delinquency: using a nationally representative sample. *J Interp Viol.* 2011;26(1):88-110. doi:10.1177/0886260510362886

24. Lemmon JH. The effects of maltreatment recurrence and child welfare on dimensions of delinquency. *Crim J Rev.* 2006;31(1):5-32. doi:10.1177/0734016806287945

25. Jung H, Herrenkohl T, Lee J, Hemphill S, Heerde J, Skinner M. Gendered pathways from child abuse to adult crime through internalizing and externalizing behaviors in childhood and adolescence. *J Interpers Viol.* 2017;32(18):2724-2750. doi:10.1177/0886260515596146

26. National Children's Advocacy Center. Child maltreatment and links to later criminality: a bibliography. 2020. https://calio.org/wp-content/uploads/2020/08/child-mal-criminality-bib.pdf

27. Anjum R, Bano Z. Child maltreatment as pathway to delinquency. *J Pakistan Psych.* 2019;16(4):16-31.

28. Egeland B, Yates T, Appleyard K, van Dulmen M. The long-term consequences of maltreatment in the early years: a developmental pathway model to antisocial behavior. *Children's Services: Soc Pol Res Prac.* 2002;5(4):249-260. doi:10.1207/S15326918CS0504_2

29. Steketee M, Aussems C, Marshall IH. Exploring the impact of child maltreatment and interparental violence on violent delinquency in an international sample. *J Interpersonal Viol.* 2019;36(13-14):7319-7349. doi:10.1177/0886260518823291

30. Widom CS. Understanding child maltreatment and juvenile delinquency: the research. Office of Juvenile Justice and Delinquency Prevention, Office of Justice Programs, US Department of Justice. 2010. https://www.ojp.gov/ncjrs/virtual-library/abstracts/understanding-child-maltreatment-and-juvenile-delinquency-research

31. You S, Lim S. Developmental pathways from abusive parenting to delinquency: the mediating role of depression and aggression. *Child Abuse Negl.* 2015;46:152-162. doi:10.1016/j.chiabu.2015.05.009

32. Stewart A, Livingston M, Dennison S. Transitions and turning points: examining the links between child maltreatment and juvenile offending. *Child Abuse Negl.* 2008;32:51-66. doi:10.1016/j.chiabu.2007.04.011

33. Smith CA, Ireland TO, Thornberry TP. Adolescent maltreatment and its impact on young adult antisocial behavior. *Child Abuse Negl.* 2005;29:1099-1119. doi:10.1016/j.chiabu.2005.02.011

34. Loughran T, Mulvey E, Schubert C, Fagan J, Piquero A, Losoya S. Estimating a dose-response relationship between length of stay and future recidivism in serious juvenile offenders. *Criminology.* 2009;47(3):699-740. doi:10.1111/j.1745-9125.2009.00165.x

35. Kinscherff R. A primer for mental health practitioners working with youth involved in the juvenile justice system. National Center for Mental Health and Juvenile Justice. 2012. https://www.air.org/sites/default/files/A-Primer-for-Mental-Health-Practitioners-JJ-System-2012.pdf

36. Turner HA, Finkelhor D, Ormrod R. The effect of lifetime victimization on the mental health of children and adolescents. *Soc Sci Med.* 2006;62:13-27. doi:10.1016/j.socscimed.2005.05.030

37. Heilbrun K, Lee R, Cottle CC. Risk factors and intervention outcomes: meta-analyses of juvenile offending. In: Heilbrun K, Goldstein NES, Redding RE, eds. *Juvenile Delinquency: Prevention, Assessment, and Treatment.* Oxford University Press; 2005:111-133.

38. Mallett, C. *Linking Disorders to Delinquency: Treating High-risk Youth in our Juvenile Justice System.* Lynne Rienner Publishers; 2013.

39. Underwood LA, Washington A. Mental illness and juvenile offenders. *Int J Environ Res Public Health.* 2016;13(2):228-241. doi:10.3390/ijerph13020228

40. Watts JS. Gender, child maltreatment, and delinquency. *Victims and Offenders; An Intl J Evidence-based Rsch, Policy, and Practice.* 2019;2:165-182. doi:10.1080/15564886.2018.1557091

41. Zahn MA, Agnew R, Fishbein D, et al. Girls study group: causes and correlates of girls' delinquency. Office of Juvenile Justice and Delinquency Prevention, Office of Justice Programs, US Department of Justice. 2010. https://www.ojp.gov/pdffiles1/ojjdp/226358.pdf

42. Huizanga D, Miller S. Girls study group: Developmental sequences of girls' delinquent behavior. Office of Juvenile Justice and Delinquency Prevention, Office of Justice Programs, US Department of Justice. 2013. https://ojjdp.ojp.gov/library/publications/developmental-sequences-girls-delinquent-behavior-0

43. Zahn MA, Hawkins SR, Chiancone J, Whitworth A. The girls study group: charting the way to delinquency prevention for girls. Office of Juvenile Justice

and Delinquency Prevention, Office of Justice Programs, US Department of Justice. 2008. https://www.ojp.gov/pdffiles1/ojjdp/223434.pdf

44. Pasko L, Chesney-Lind M. Under lock and key: trauma, marginalization, and girls' juvenile justice involvement. *Just Res Policy*. 2010;12(2):25-49. doi:10.3818/JRP.12.2.2010.25

45. Lantos H, Wilkinson A, Winslow H, McDaniel T. Describing associations between child maltreatment frequency and the frequency and timing of subsequent delinquent or criminal behaviors across development: variation by sex, sexual orientation, and race. *BMC Public Health*. 2019;19:1306-1314. doi:10.1186/s12889-019-7655-7

46. Brumbaugh S, Hardison Walters JL, Winterfield LA. Girls study group: Understanding and responding to girls' delinquency: suitability of assessment instruments for delinquent girls. Office of Juvenile Justice and Delinquency Prevention, Office of Justice Programs, US Department of Justice. 2010. https://juvenilecouncil.ojp.gov/sites/g/files/xyckuh301/files/media/document/gsg_assessment_instruments_bulletin.pdf

47. Child Welfare Information Gateway. Preventing child abuse and neglect. US Department of Health and Human Services. Administration for Children and Families, Children's Bureau. 2018. https://www.childwelfare.gov/resources/preventing-child-abuse-and-neglect/

48. Stagner MW, Lansing J. Progress toward a prevention perspective. *Future Child*. 2009;19(2):19-38. doi:10.1353/foc.0.0036

49. Buffington K, Dierkhising CB, Marsh SC. Ten things every juvenile court judge should know about trauma and delinquency. National Council of Juvenile and Family Court Judges. 2010. https://www.ncjfcj.org/wp-content/uploads/2012/02/trauma-bulletin_0.pdf

50. Mulvey M, Iselin AR. Improving professional judgments of risk and amenability in juvenile justice. *Future Child*. 2008;18(2):35-57. doi:10.1353/foc.0.0012

51. Grisso T, Barnum R, Fletcher KE, Cauffman E, Peuschold D. Massachusetts Youth Screen Instruments for mental health needs of juvenile justice youths. *J Am Acad Child Adolesc Psychiatry*. 2001;40(5):41-548. doi:10.1097/00004583-200105000-00013

52. Schmidt F, Hoge R, Gomes L. Reliability and validity analyses of the youth level of service/case management inventory. *Crim Just Behav*. 2005;32(3):329. doi:10.1177/0093854804274373

53. Ramirez de Arellano MA, Lyman D, Jobe-Shields L, et al. Trauma-focused cognitive-behavioral therapy: assessing the evidence. *Psychiatr Serv*. 2014;65(5):591-602. doi:10.1176/appi.ps.201300255

54. Wilkinson A, Lantos H, McDaniel T, Winslow H. Disrupting the link between maltreatment and delinquency: how school, family, and community factors can be protective. *BMC Public Health*. 2019;19:588-598. doi:10.1186/s12889-019-6906-y

55. Annie E. Casey Foundation. Youth incarceration in the United States. 2021. https://www.aecf.org/resources/youth-incarceration-in-the-united-states

56. Mendel RA. No place for kids: the case for reducing juvenile incarceration. Annie E. Casey Foundation. 2011. https://files.eric.ed.gov/fulltext/ED527944.pdf

57. Lipsey M, Howell JC, Kelly MR, Chapman G, Carver D. Improving the effectiveness of juvenile justice programs: a new perspective on evidence-based

practice. Center for Juvenile Justice Reform. 2010. https://njjn.org/uploads/digital-library/CJJR_Lipsey_Improving-Effectiveness-of-Juvenile-Justice_2010.pdf

58. Skowyra KR, Cocozza JJ. Mental health screening within juvenile justice: the next frontier. National Center for Mental Health and Juvenile Justice. 2007. https://www.modelsforchange.net/publications/198/Mental_Health_Screening_within_Juvenile_Justice_The_Next_Frontier.pdf

Chapter 20

EATING DISORDERS

Lisa Ann Tauai, RD, MBA, CWP

OBJECTIVES
After reading this chapter, the reader will be able to:

1. *Recognize and differentiate between the different types of eating disorders.*

2. *Comprehend the link between child maltreatment and the manifestation of eating disorders.*

3. *Identify and apply treatment options for patients with eating disorders.*

BACKGROUND AND SIGNIFICANCE

Eating disorders are a debilitating condition that can impact all aspects of an individual's life as well as their family members and friends, who often feel helpless in caring for their loved one. They can affect anyone regardless of their age, ethnicity, or gender, and the results can be emotionally, mentally, and physically devastating if left untreated. There are also immense financial costs associated with eating disorders, with an estimated cost in the United States of 64.7 billion dollars a year.[1] As of the writing of this chapter, the prevalence of eating disorders is increasing. In 2020, there was a 66% increase from the previous year in hospital admissions related to eating disorders.[1] In addition, 9% of Americans (approximately 28 000 000 individuals) will have an eating disorder in their lifetime.[2]

The causes for eating disorders have been well-researched, and studies continue to try to understand the foundational problems that can lead to this condition. Some studies point to genetics as the primary factor in determining if a person will have an eating disorder, while others conclude that the family environment may be the culprit. Although these factors may contribute to the problem, there also appears to be a very strong link between a traumatic event and the later development of an eating disorder. Once the root cause of an eating disorder is identified, the practitioner's goal is to create a personalized treatment plan that involves a multidisciplinary approach.[3]

TYPES OF EATING DISORDERS

Before exploring the link between traumatic stress stemming from maltreatment and the development of an eating disorder, it is important to understand different types of eating disorders. ***Eating disorders*** are behavioral conditions characterized by a severe and persistent disturbance in eating behaviors associated with distressing thoughts and emotions.[4] Without treatment, they can progress into extremely serious conditions, affecting physical, psychological, and social functioning. Eating disorders can fall into a variety of categories, including anorexia nervosa, bulimia nervosa, binge eating disorder, and avoidant restrictive food intake disorder. Although each of these are distinct clinical conditions, the rate of crossing over from one to another is high. Additionally, there are other specified feeding and eating disorders such as pica, which involves a person craving and consuming non-nutritive, non-edible substances[5] and rumination disorder, in which a person inadvertently and repeatedly spits up or regurgitates partially digested food from the stomach.[6]

Anorexia nervosa, or simply "anorexia," is characterized by an abnormally low body weight, an intense fear of gaining weight, and a distorted perception of weight.[7] People with anorexia obsess over controlling their weight and shape and often use extreme efforts such as meticulously controlling calorie intake, exercising excessively, or misusing laxatives, diet aids, or diuretics and enemas.[7] Their biggest fear is weight gain, a fear that controls their daily lives and severely impairs their physical, social, and psychological functioning. Anorexia can potentially lead to a life-threateningly low body weight and is associated with the highest mortality rate of all psychiatric disorders.[1] The average age of anorexia onset is 16 to 17 years old, but, in recent years, there appears to be an increase in the prevalence of this disorder in younger children.[1] Because of the rapid loss of weight, gastrointestinal concerns, and depressed mood, it is often easier for practitioners to identify a patient with anorexia. Some other, more apparent, physical symptoms include thinning hair, absence of menstruation, and soft, downy hair that covers the body. In more severe cases, irregular heart rhythms surface and blood pressure can drop to dangerously low levels.[7]

Bulimia nervosa, or "bulimia," is a serious, potentially life-threatening eating disorder where people secretly binge uncontrollably on large amounts of food and then purge in an attempt to compensate for the extra calories they consumed. One desired effect of purging is to prevent weight gain. Purging can include regular self-induced vomiting or misuse of laxatives, weight loss supplements, diuretics, or enemas. People with bulimia may also use other methods such as fasting, strict dieting, or excessive exercise to rid themselves of calories to prevent weight gain. Like those with anorexia, patients with bulimia are preoccupied with their weight and body shape and often judge themselves severely for any self-perceived flaws.[8] The average age of onset for bulimia is 18 years old, but similar to anorexia, the age of bulimia onset is beginning to be more apparent in younger children across genders.[1]

Binge eating disorder is a serious eating disorder where the individual consumes unusually large amounts of food and feels unable to stop eating. Unlike bulimia, the binge eater does not purge the food or engage in compensatory behaviors. The binge eater often feels embarrassed about their overeating and vows to stop but cannot resist the compulsions and urges to binge eat.[9] Binge eating disorder, if left untreated, often results in one or more comorbidities such as weight gain, type 2 diabetes, cardiovascular disease, and hypertension. There seems to be a strong genetic factor in individuals with binge eating disorder. About 50% of the risk of binge eating disorder is genetic, and the prevalence of binge eating disorder is nearly 2 times greater in obese individuals compared to non-obese individuals.[1] Of all eating disorders, binge eating disorder has the latest average age of onset, estimated at 25 years of age.[1]

IMPACT OF MALTREATMENT ON DISORDERED EATING
There can be several possible reasons for an individual to develop an eating disorder. Some studies suggest that home and family environments (ie, family-related stress or non-abuse situations) are associated with having bulimia and binge eating disorder, and anorexia may be less influenced by psychosocial factors such as family background issues.[10] Other studies point to altered levels of the neurotransmitter dopamine having a strong correlation with binge eating disorder.[11,12] The majority of literature, however, suggests that childhood maltreatment, abuse, and other forms of trauma are the strongest predictors for the development of an eating disorder or other comorbid psychiatric disorders.[3]

Maltreatment, trauma, and stress can take on many forms and can involve emotional, physical, or sexual abuse which leave a lasting impact on the victim's life. These stressors all can lead to the development of post-traumatic stress disorder (PTSD), wherein some people experience flashbacks, nightmares, feelings of numbness, loss of control, fear, and panic that can then impact their eating behavior. *Eating behavior*, as defined by LaCaille,[13] encompasses food choice and motives, feeding practice, dieting, and eating-related problems such as weight gain, eating disorders, and feeding disorders. A disordered eating behavior can later manifest as a result of traumatic events experienced in childhood, adolescence, or even adulthood. These individuals claim to gain short-term relief or suppression from trauma-related thoughts and feelings along with regaining a feeling of control when engaging in a disordered eating behavior.[13]

When someone has experienced trauma, it is common for them to feel stressed. When people become chronically stressed, their brain expresses a strong desire to eat as well as a reduced ability to stop eating. This, in turn, can result in overconsumption of high-fat, high-sugar foods that temporarily improve their mood and help them feel less stressed. This short-lived feeling, however, is often followed by feelings of guilt, depression, and embarrassment that can lead to other disordered eating patterns such as excessive dieting, exercising, use of laxatives, or purging.

For some people, certain foods can provide self-comforting feelings whereas other foods can trigger traumatic memories resulting in feelings of anxiety. Additionally, some people find control and satisfaction in their lives by straying away from any form of unhealthy foods for fear of weight gain or unappealing body image. In the vast majority of cases, however, binge eating or restrictive eating develops in childhood or adolescence as a coping strategy to "survive" painful emotions or forget severe traumatic experiences.[14]

Surviving painful emotions that surface due to past trauma can take on many forms. People who engage in disordered eating often compare their disordered eating to other unhealthy behaviors (eg, alcohol or drug use, tobacco use, or compulsive gambling) that are used to suppress negative feelings. There is a belief that disordered eating may be more of an accepted behavior in society compared to other unhealthy behaviors such as drug or alcohol use. Even though they feel unwell when engaging in disordered eating practices and realize they may develop lasting health consequences, many people report continuing to either severely restrict their food intake or binge eat, as these behaviors feel better than the negative emotions and stress stemming from their traumatic events.[14]

In a study involving 3 focus groups exploring how traumatic stress impacted the participants' eating behavior, it was apparent that changes in eating behavior can appear in people struggling with traumatic stress after experiencing a traumatic event.[14] One common theme among the 3 focus groups was that stress and emotions from traumatic experiences led to impulsive and uncontrolled consumption of fast foods, sweets, and salty snacks.[14] Many of the participants agreed that they had difficulty thinking clearly during these times and were almost on autopilot until they realized what they were doing. Once they realized what they were doing, they would inadvertently throw the food away or punish themselves later by restricting their food intake or purging. The majority of the participants claimed that during times of stress, they resorted to easy food solutions such as fast foods, sweets, and other processed foods and beverages. These foods offered quick energy, were comfort foods that made them feel better, and were extremely convenient. When they felt exhausted or simply wanted to feel less stressed, they believed that preparing a healthier meal would take too much time and effort, resulting in additional stress. On the contrary, on days they felt better and were calmer, they had a better appetite and made time to plan and prepare healthy meals and snacks.

Because traumatic stress often results in feeling overwhelmed or even numb and many people do not have solid coping strategies in place, it is not surprising that the focus group study concluded that eating behaviors were severely affected in various ways by traumatic stress. In situations where prolonged traumatic stress exists, the risk factor for food and sugar addiction rises. In fact, a study involving older veterans found that there was a strong correlation between PTSD and food addiction.[15] Another study determined that children and adolescents who experienced maltreatment had a higher occurrence of social isolation later in adulthood, along with an increased consumption of sugary beverages.[16]

INTERVENTION, TREATMENT, AND PREVENTION

It is important to know that 75% of people with an eating disorder do not seek professional help, and 44% of people with an eating disorder do not know where to seek help.[1] Intervention by family and friends could be the turning point in ensuring a person is receiving the care that they need. Care should include a multidisciplinary approach involving a psychologist or psychiatrist (or both), a dietitian, and a physician. The treatment plan should be centered on the individual with a goal of understanding what motivates the behavior or determining the driving force behind the individual's behavior. According to Hedonistic Motivational Theory,[17] eating disorders may be motivated by a desire for pleasure and avoidance of pain. When an individual binge eats or restricts their eating, they are attempting to avoid their pain, negative emotions, and memories from the trauma. Many individuals are unaware of the connection between their traumatic stress and their eating behaviors. Once their medical team makes them aware of the connection, the individual (if receptive) can begin learning healthier coping methods and skills when stress or negative emotions resurface.[17]

Clinicians treating people with eating disorders must understand the best treatment course to take depending on the type of eating disorder diagnosed. For example, the use of cognitive behavioral therapy (CBT) is the most recommended specific psychotherapy for anorexia patients. However, using an individual-centered approach and a range of different therapies may have merit.[18] Additionally, in family-related non-abuse cases, family separation, or negative parent-child interactions, anorexia patients may be less influenced by psychosocial factors connected to family environment during childhood compared to bulimia or binge eating disorder patients.[18] This knowledge is important for clinicians working from trauma-informed and recovery-oriented approaches in eating disorder treatment.

The dietitian's role in the treatment of eating disorder patients is also individual-centered. The individual must be receiving treatment from other members of the multidisciplinary team for nutrition guidance and treatment to be effective. It is most important for the dietitian to build a good relationship with the patient in which the patient feels comfortable and trusts the dietitian. Because this process may take some time, it is not uncommon for actual nutrition counseling to begin at a later session. Once nutrition counseling does begin, the underlying focus is to help the patient form an improved relationship with food while also helping them normalize their eating behaviors. The dietitian assists in tailoring a patient's eating to promote weight restoration or maintenance, taking into account their eating disorder history. Depending on whether the dietitian is treating the patient in an inpatient or outpatient setting, the number of visits and appointments vary per week and can span from one or two months to upwards of a year. Ultimately, a full medical team approach that includes overall health and lab value monitoring, possible medication prescriptions, and long-term counseling are essential to the patient's healing process and steps toward short and long-term recovery.

CASE STUDY

Case Study 20-1

A 15-year-old female presented to the emergency department with severe dizziness and disorientation. After her evaluation, it was noted that she was extremely underweight and appeared malnourished. The mother expressed concerns that her daughter was overly preoccupied with her appearance and weight, and she noticed that her daughter had been eating very little food. Lab results revealed low albumin and prealbumin levels consistent with being undernourished.

Discussion

It is important to interview the child and parents separately in hopes that the child will reveal more with their health care provider in a private setting. The immediate concern is to treat the acute physical conditions that resulted in the patient being taken to the emergency room. After more is known about the child's condition, a treatment plan that includes a multidisciplinary approach should be initiated. If the diagnosis is determined to be an eating disorder, referrals to a psychologist or psychiatrist (or both) and a dietitian should be generated. Depending on the severity of the symptoms, the patient may be transferred to an inpatient facility that specializes in eating disorders.

KEY POINTS

1. Anorexia nervosa, bulimia nervosa, and binge eating disorder are the 3 most common eating disorders.

2. Traumatic stress and maltreatment are linked to disordered eating, as food temporarily suppresses negative emotions.

3. Effective eating disorder treatment utilizes an interdisciplinary approach with a team including a psychologist or psychiatrist, a dietitian, and a physician, along with familial and community support.

REFERENCES

1. Eating Disorder Statistics. National Association of Anorexia Nervosa and Associated Disorders. https://anad.org/eating-disorders-statistics/

2. Linardon J. 2023 Eating Disorder Statistics: 79+ Unthinkable Facts. March 3, 2023. https://breakbingeeating.com/eating-disorder-statistics/

3. Molendijk ML, Hoek HW, Brewerton TD, Elzinga BM. Childhood maltreatment and eating disorder pathology: a systematic review and dose-response meta analysis. *Psychol Med*. 2017;1-15. doi:10.1017/s0033291716003561

4. Guarda A. What Are Eating Disorders? American Psychiatric Association. March 2021. https://psychiatry.org/patients-families/eating-disorders/what-are-eating-disorders

5. Pica. National Eating Disorders Association. Updated October 18, 2023. https://www.nationaleatingdisorders.org/learn/by-eating-disorder/other/pica?msclkid=68d40cb9cef711ecb864d5f887a380d9

6. Alexandra W. Common Indicators of Rumination Syndrome. Health Prep. https://healthprep.com/stomach-conditions/common-indicators-rumination-syndrome/

7. Anorexia nervosa. Mayo Clinic. February 20, 2018. https://www.mayoclinic.org/diseases-conditions/anorexia-nervosa/symptoms-causes/syc-20353591

8. Bulimia nervosa. Mayo Clinic. May 10, 2018. https://www.mayoclinic.org/diseases-conditions/bulimia/symptoms-causes/syc-20353615

9. Binge-eating disorder. Mayo Clinic. May 5, 2018. https://www.mayoclinic.org/diseases-conditions/binge-eating-disorder/symptoms-causes/syc-20353627

10. Grogan K, MacGarry D, Bramham J, Scriven M, Maher C, Fitzgerald A. Family-related non-abuse adverse life experiences occurring for adults diagnosed with eating disorders: a systematic review. *J Eat Disord*. 2020;8. doi:10.1186/s40337-020-00311-6

11. Yang Y, Miller R, Grow SW. A literature review of dopamine in binge eating. *J Eat Disord*. 2022;10:11. doi:10.1186/s40337-022-00531-y

12. Cristol H. What is Dopamine? WebMD. https://www.webmd.com/mental-health/what-is-dopamine?msclkid=7e4b960acf2311ec90d3daaced34f0de

13. LaCaille L. Eating Behavior. In: Gellman MD, Turn JR, eds. *Encyclopedia of Behavioral Medicine*. Springer; 2013:641-642.

14. Roer GE, Solbakken HH, Abebe DS, Aaseth JO, Bolstad I, Lien L. Inpatients experiences about the impact of traumatic stress on eating behaviors: an exploratory focus group study. *J Eat Disord*. 2021;9:119. doi:10.1186/s40337-021-00480-y

15. Mitchell KS, Wolf EJ. PTSD, food addiction, and disordered eating in a sample of primarily older veterans: the mediating role of emotion regulation. *Psychiatry Res*. 2016;243:23-29. doi:10.1016/j.psychres.2016.06.013

16. Henriksen RE, Torsheim T, Thuen F. Loneliness, social integration and consumption of sugar-containing beverages: testing the social baseline theory. *PLoS One*. 2014;9(8):e104421. doi:10.1371/journal.pone.0104421

17. Williams DM. Psychological hedonism, hedonic motivation, and health behavior in affective determinants of health behavior. In: Williams DM, Rhodes RE, Conner MT, eds. *Affective Determinants of Health Behavior*. Oxford Scholarship Online; 2018.

18. Wade TD, Treasure J, Schmidt U, et al. Comparative efficacy of pharmacological and non-pharmacological interventions for the acute treatment of adult outpatients with anorexia nervosa: study protocol for the systematic review and network meta-analysis of individual data. *J Eat Disord*. 2017;5:24. doi:10.1186/s40337-017-0153-3

Legal Issues in Cases of Child Maltreatment

Eva Klain, JD
Alicia Summers, PhD

Objectives

After reading this chapter, the reader will be able to:

1. *Describe and explain the structure and flow of civil and criminal court cases brought in response to suspected child maltreatment.*

2. *Identify mental health considerations that may arise during each stage or juncture of the court process.*

3. *Identify research findings related to mental health outcomes for court-involved children and families.*

Background and Significance

State intervention in the life of a family is governed by both civil and criminal statutes seeking to protect child victims of abuse or neglect, safeguard the rights of parents to raise their children, and further the interest of the state in preserving the safety of the public and pursuing justice. When parents are unable, unwilling, or unfit to care for their children, the state can intervene to provide the necessary care and safety. The civil child welfare system seeks to preserve family unity whenever possible, ideally only pursuing separation of children and parents when necessary. Criminal prosecution may be pursued whenever a parent or caregiver commits sexual or other serious abuse or neglect of a child, as well as when the offender is someone outside the family. The effects of child abuse and neglect can be traumatic and carry significant implications for physical and mental health into adulthood. At the same time, separation of parents and children, especially when unnecessary, can cause trauma to both the child and parent. Mental health considerations, especially those associated with traumatic stress, arise in both civil and criminal cases addressing any type of abuse or neglect—physical, sexual, educational, emotional, or medical. These mental health challenges may affect children, parents, victims, offenders, and witnesses.

The Civil Child Welfare System

Every state has a child welfare system that provides services to children and families in response to concerns about child maltreatment. The child welfare system is primarily concerned with children who have been abused or neglected, although some states also include truant, runaway, or otherwise ungovernable children within the jurisdiction of their child welfare system.[1]

The child welfare system is governed by both federal and state law. Federal laws set requirements that must be met for the state to receive federal funding for the care and services provided to the child and family (see **Table 21-1**).[2] Since 1980, both federal and state laws require that non-emergency removals of a child from the home must be reviewed by a court, which must regularly review the case of every child who is in out-of-home care. These laws require child protection agencies (also known as child welfare agencies) to preserve families whenever possible, reunite children with parents when safe to do so, or find another permanent home for the child. The term *permanency* in child welfare means a legally permanent (ie, free from court oversight), nurturing family that can provide lifelong connections, support, and stability for every child. Services may be provided to families while children remain in their own homes or after a child has been removed and placed in foster care or another out-of-home placement.

Federal laws governing civil child welfare cases include the Adoption and Safe Families Act (ASFA) of 1997,[3] which was designed to promote permanency for children in foster care and accelerate permanent placements of children but has recently come under increased scrutiny as a family regulation law that unnecessarily separates parents and children.[4]

Table 21-1. Federal Child Welfare Statutes[2]

Child Abuse Prevention and Treatment Act (CAPTA), 1974, amended 1996, reauthorized 2010, amended by Comprehensive Addiction and Recovery Act (CARA), 2016

Indian Child Welfare Act (ICWA), 1978

Adoption Assistance and Child Welfare Act, 1980

Family Preservation and Support Services Program Act, 1993

Multiethnic Placement Act, 1994

ASFA, 1997

Promoting Safe and Stable Families Amendments, 2001

Keeping Children & Families Safe Act (KCFSA), 2003

Fostering Connections to Success and Increasing Adoptions Act, 2008

Child and Family Services Improvement and Innovation Act, 2011

Preventing Sex Trafficking and Strengthening Families Act, 2014

Every Student Succeeds Act (ESSA), 2015

Substance Use-Disorder Prevention that Promotes Opioid Recovery and Treatment for Patients and Communities Act (SUPPORT for Patients and Communities Act), 2018

Family First Prevention Services Act (FFPSA), 2018

ASFA requires specific court findings, including that remaining in the family home would be contrary to the welfare of the child. Such a finding may be that it is contrary to the welfare of an 18-month-old child to remain in the family home because the agency has found severe and frequent bruising resulting from the parents' age-inappropriate attempts to discipline the child. Reasonable efforts to prevent removal findings must also be made by the court within 60 days of the child's removal from the home. Such a finding may be that the agency made reasonable efforts to prevent removal by providing intensive in-home therapy to the family as well as respite child care. If these case-specific and child-specific detailed findings are not made, the agency will not receive federal funds for the length of the child's stay in foster care.

The court must also make reasonable efforts to finalize the permanency plan findings within 12 months of the child's entry into foster care. Such findings can detail the efforts a child welfare agency made to reunify the family, including mental health or substance use treatment for parents, or to find another permanent home for the child, such as locating relatives willing to adopt the child. A negative, late, insufficient, or missing finding makes the agency ineligible for federal dollars until a subsequent finding that reasonable efforts have been made is entered. No reasonable efforts to reunify the parent and child are necessary if a court finds there were aggravated circumstances (eg, abandonment, torture, chronic abuse, sexual abuse, or as otherwise defined in state law), the parent was convicted of one of the enumerated crimes (eg, aided, abetted, or committed murder, involuntary manslaughter, or felony assault causing serious bodily harm to another of the parent's children), or the parent's rights to another child were involuntarily terminated.

If a criminal case is pending against a parent for one of the enumerated crimes, the court has discretion to waive reunification services based on the child's developmental needs and the amount of time until the criminal case will be resolved. If the court decides the agency does not need to make reunification efforts, the court must conduct a permanency hearing within 30 days. ASFA also requires that the child welfare agency file a termination of parental rights (TPR) petition when a court determines a parent has committed certain crimes, the child has been abandoned, or when a child has been in care for 15 of the previous 22 months. The 15 out of 22 months provision is often cited in cases involving parental substance use as ignoring the reality of substance use treatment, the potential for relapse, and the health needs of the parent. All ASFA provisions also relate to delinquency and status offender cases if the agency is receiving federal dollars for the child.

Additional federal statutes establish requirements in civil cases. The Fostering Connections to Success and Increasing Adoptions Act of 2008[5] seeks to ensure permanent relationships with relatives; maintain sibling ties and other family connections; improve outcomes for older children and adolescents in foster care (including extending federal support of those in foster care until they turn 21); address children's health and education needs; and more. Under the Fostering Connections to Success and Increasing Adoptions Act, states must develop a plan for ongoing oversight and coordination of health care services, including mental health. The plans must describe health screening, monitoring, and treatment, as well as how they will ensure oversight of prescription medications, including psychotropic drugs. These provisions, along with other efforts, are significant because children in foster care are overprescribed psychiatric medications at a rate 9 times higher than children not in foster care, with more than 1/4 of foster children prescribed at least one psychiatric drug.[6]

Emphasizing the importance of prevention services and the least restrictive, most family-like placements for children, the Family First Prevention Services Act of 2018[7] allows only 4 types of non-family placements. Among them is a residential placement to meet the therapeutic needs of children and adolescents with serious emotional or behavioral disorders or disturbances, called a qualified residential treatment program (QRTP). The Family First Prevention Services Act details the requirements for this placement type, assessments and treatment planning, and the approval process and timeline.[8] Another of the allowable non-family settings is a high-quality residential care setting for children and adolescents who are victims or at risk of becoming victims of sex trafficking.

The Preventing Sex Trafficking and Strengthening Families Act of 2014[9] includes requirements that states identify, report, and determine services to victims of sex trafficking; encourage developmentally appropriate activities for children in foster care; and strengthen permanency options for older adolescents, among other provisions.

Multiple provisions in these federal statutes address the importance of children's health and wellbeing. One such provision is maintaining sibling relationships and other connections for children, which has been linked to more positive mental health outcomes. A review of sibling research found several articles that linked placement with siblings to better mental health outcomes, including fewer internalizing and externalizing behaviors.[10] Relational permanence (ie, having a person to whom the child feels connected) has been linked to better overall outcomes on a composite measure that included a mental health symptoms checklist.[11] Qualitative research in the form of interviews of former foster children also found a common theme that the most important thing to a foster child is having an authentic relationship,[12] one in which the child feels comfortable sharing their true self with someone else. Child welfare professionals should first focus on preserving families and preventing the need to place children outside of their homes. Clinical research shows that separation from family can lead to children experiencing difficulty sleeping, developmental regression, permanent architectural changes in the brain, depression, higher risk of suicide attempts, and higher risk for addictive behaviors such as alcohol use and gambling later in life.[13] In studies of children facing possible removal by social services, children who were removed were twice as likely to have learning disabilities and developmental delays and 6 times more likely to have behavioral problems than children who remained in their homes.[14] As adults, children who are removed are more likely to have substance-related disorders, psychotic or bipolar disorders, depression, and anxiety disorders.[15]

Mental health needs may affect a parent's ability to care for their child. A study of chronic neglect—defined as 4 or more referrals to the child welfare system for neglect—found that families referred for chronic neglect were more likely to have a parent with mental health concerns than families referred less often.[16] Unfortunately, good data are not available on the rate of mental health concerns among parents involved in the foster care system. National data collects removal reasons, which include parent inability to cope (ie, emotional illness) and substance use as a reason. In the most recent data, 41% of children entering care had a reason of parental drug or alcohol abuse and 13% had a reason of inability to cope.[17] These may be underestimates, as most removal reasons are listed as neglect, which does not address the underlying causes such as mental health concerns or coping mechanisms in response to stressors (eg, poverty, racism, unsafe housing or communities, and other social determinants of health). In one study of mothers involved in child protection proceedings who also self-reported a mental health or substance use disorder (referred to as an "Axis I" in older versions of the *Diagnostic and Statistical Manual of Mental Disorders*), 40% had a diagnosis of polysubstance dependency and 20% had co-occurring mental health and substance use disorders.[18]

When children must be removed to ensure their safety, efforts focus on returning them home as soon as is safely possible or placing them in another permanent placement. These options may include adoptive families, legal guardians, or relatives who obtain legal custody. In many cases, the court will determine that a child may be reunited with their parent if the parent has complied with court-imposed requirements such as mental health or drug and alcohol treatment and otherwise demonstrates their ability to care for the child upon returning home. Reunification with the parent may not be possible when a diagnosable condition makes the parent unable to assume care of the child, such as intractable mental illness, mental deficiency, or in rare cases, extreme physical disability.

For cases in which returning home safely is not possible, the child welfare agency will often move to have parental rights terminated and seek a new permanent home for the child. Often, a permanent home is not found in a timely manner and an individual may age out of the system (ie, transition to adulthood from the child welfare system). Those who age out of the system are frequently ill-prepared to function as self-sufficient adults. Research shows that they are more likely to face homelessness or incarceration and less likely to obtain a high school diploma or GED, attend college, or secure employment. Research following former foster children in several states has shown high degrees of behavioral health needs for adolescents immediately prior to and following aging out of foster care, with 68% reporting some type of behavioral need, 37% reporting depressive symptoms, 25% reporting post-traumatic stress disorder (PTSD) symptoms, and 35% reporting substance dependency symptoms.[19]

FOSTER CARE

Foster care (ie, out-of-home care) is meant to be a temporary service for children who cannot live with their families, whether because of child safety concerns, as a result of serious parent-child conflict, or to treat serious physical or behavioral health conditions that cannot be addressed within the family. Removal from the home and placement in foster care is meant to provide safety for a child while the agency works with the parents to achieve permanency for them.

Whether because of their experiences of maltreatment, their experience of being in foster care, or the correlation between high mental health needs and entry into foster care, children that enter the foster care system have poorer mental health outcomes than those that do not.[20] Approximately 2/3 of children in foster care reported no mental health diagnoses within the last year. However, children in foster care did report a lifetime prevalence of attention-deficit/hyperactivity disorder (ADHD), conduct disorder, major depressive disorder, and PTSD at rates significantly higher than the general population.[21] Overrepresentation of racial and ethnic minority children involved with child protection or placed in foster care, combined with the high risk of serious mental health and social problems for these children, highlights a need for more targeted research for each racial group given the complexities of historical and intergenerational trauma.[22]

Kinship care refers to the care of children by relatives or, in some jurisdictions, close family friends or chosen kin. Relatives are the preferred resource for children who must be removed from their birth parents because kin placement maintains the children's connections with their families. Approximately 1/4 of the children in out-of-home care live with relatives. Kinship placements are typically more stable, providing consistency and a secure attachment to a caring adult. Instability in placements (ie, frequent placement moves) has been shown across multiple studies to be related to child behavior problems.[23] While kinship placement is preferred, research suggests placement with relatives alone is not a sufficient predictor of better mental health outcomes for children or adolescents, even if they are in kinship care the entire length of stay.[24]

REASONABLE EFFORTS TO PREVENT REMOVAL AND ACHIEVE A PERMANENT PLACEMENT

Federal law requires the child welfare agency to make reasonable efforts to keep families together, reunify families when they are separated, and achieve an alternative permanency plan for children who cannot return home. While federal law does not define reasonable efforts, such efforts generally include "accessible, available, and culturally appropriate services that are designed to improve the capacity of families to provide safe and stable homes for their children."[25] The Indian Child Welfare Act (ICWA)[26] requires an even higher level of effort–"active efforts"–in cases involving Indigenous children. Clarifying federal regulations and guidelines issued in 2016 state that active efforts should be "affirmative, active, thorough, and timely" and "must involve assisting the parent or parents or Indian custodian through the steps of a case plan and with accessing or developing the resources necessary to satisfy the case plan."[27]

Courts must approve all decisions to remove children from their homes to ensure reasonable efforts to prevent removal were made. Child welfare agency staff must make reasonable efforts to safely maintain children with their families, including providing necessary supports and services. These services are often called family preservation or in-home services, and are provided by child protective services staff, community agencies, or other service providers.

While in out-of-home care, children and their parents or other family members should receive services specifically tailored to their needs. These are designed to provide support and safety for the child, to remedy the problems leading to the placement, and should be evidence-based and trauma-informed. Out-of-home care is intended to be temporary, and many of the services provided to children in out-of-home care and their families are targeted to achieve the goal of reunification.

Removing a child from their home may be traumatic to both the child and the parent(s). Providers that work with families should consider trauma screenings as part of efforts to effectively address underlying issues and work successfully with the family. Interventions such as Family Centered Treatment (a home-based family trauma and preservation service) have shown positive outcomes related to reduced time in foster care and more timely reunification.[28]

CIVIL CHILD WELFARE COURT HEARING TYPES

In civil child protection cases, the focus is on whether the state can prove that a child is abused or neglected. The cases are usually heard by a judicial officer; jury trials on this issue are used in only a few states. The court's focus is centered on the safety, permanency, and wellbeing of the child. Permanency focuses on having a stable placement and one that can become both safe and permanent as quickly as is practical, and wellbeing focuses on making sure that the child's education, physical and mental health, and other needs are addressed. The parties in civil cases are the parents, the children, and the state. The typical stages of the child protective court process begin with the filing of a petition by or on behalf of a child welfare agency that either removed a child from their home based on emergent circumstances prior to any court hearing or seeks to have the court order that a child be removed from their home and placed in foster care.

The typical hearings in child welfare or dependency court proceedings include an *initial hearing*, which may be called a "shelter care hearing" or "emergency removal hearing" in different jurisdictions, after a child has been removed from the home, usually held within 24 to 72 hours. This hearing is required whenever a child is removed without first giving the child's parent(s) or custodian(s) the opportunity to challenge the decision in court. The *adjudication hearing* is a fact-finding hearing when the judge decides whether the child has been abused or neglected and allows the court to assume jurisdiction over the case. A *disposition hearing* may be held in conjunction with or after the adjudication hearing and entails the court determining whether the child may be placed in foster care, who will be awarded authority to care for and supervise the child (ie, custody), and under what conditions the child is placed, including services to be provided.

After disposition, most state courts conduct periodic *review hearings* to examine case progress and the current wellbeing of the child. Review hearings take place at maximum predetermined intervals, such as once every 6 months, but many judges set earlier times for review hearings, based on the particular circumstances of the case and local practice. The court must conduct *permanency hearings* within 12 months after a child is considered to have entered foster care and then at least once every 12 months thereafter as long as the child remains in care. While the purpose of a review hearing is judicial oversight, a permanency hearing must determine a permanent goal (ie, permanency plan) and the permanent status of the child. When deciding on a permanency plan, the court should place highest priority on reunification, followed by adoption, legal guardianship (often addressed in a separate court hearing), or other permanent placement with relatives. Before approving the placement of a child in some other planned, permanent living arrangement under ASFA, the agency must document and the court must find a compelling reason why the higher priority options are not in the child's best interests.

If adoption is the goal set at the permanency hearing, there may be TPR proceedings to legally free the child for adoption. The TPR decision has significant implications for the child and family because it results in complete and final severance of a parent's legal rights and responsibilities to the child. In most states, TPR requires a new set of legal proceedings.

Children's presence and participation during the various hearings in civil dependency cases depends largely on state law and local court culture. Research on the impact of child attendance at child welfare hearings is limited. However, some research has shown that there were no signs of serious distress prior to or after attending hearings. The same study found nearly all children felt that they should be able to attend court if they so wish.[29]

CRIMINAL CHILD ABUSE PROSECUTION

When there is an allegation of abuse or neglect of a child within the home, a civil child protection or dependency case is far more common than a criminal prosecution of an offending parent. However, with allegations of sexual and serious physical abuse, it is common to simultaneously see both a civil child protection case and a criminal prosecution based on the same parental conduct.

In a criminal prosecution for child abuse or neglect, the parties to the case include the alleged abuser (ie, defendant) and the state (ie, the governmental entity bringing the charges). Most child abuse cases are tried in state courts, although the federal courts have jurisdiction in limited circumstances, such as when the alleged offense takes place on federal land (eg, military bases or other government-owned lands or properties) or involves travel across state lines. Although complex, criminal child abuse cases follow the same process as other criminal cases. After a report of maltreatment is investigated by police, child protective services, or both working together as part of an interprofessional team, child abuse cases are referred to prosecutors for charging decisions. While all child sexual abuse is considered a crime, only serious child physical abuse and neglect are defined as crimes. To decide whether to file criminal charges, prosecutors consider whether there is sufficient evidence that a crime has been committed and whether the probability of obtaining a just result warrants filing charges. These decisions are based on policies and practices that vary across jurisdictions. Prosecutors often take into account the stress that the child victim and family may experience from the prosecution and possible trial. Once charges are filed, prosecutors may enter into a plea bargain with the defendant or proceed to trial. The focus of criminal proceedings is on the defendant—who has certain constitutional protections in criminal cases—and their alleged actions, not on the permanency, safety, or wellbeing of the child as is the case in civil proceedings.

The criminal court does not have the authority to make foster care placements or to terminate parental rights, although it may have authority to order an allegedly abusive parent out of the child's home through a protective or restraining order or to hold the offending parent in custody until the case is resolved. When the alleged criminal conduct occurs within the family, coordination between the civil and criminal proceedings is beneficial. Areas for coordination include synchronizing investigations, scheduling proceedings, keeping judges and parties apprised of orders in other courts (which may include domestic relations or domestic violence), and coordinating dispositional or sentencing options sought in either court.

Children and families involved in criminal proceedings have often been affected by trauma in many forms, including adverse community-based racial or socioeconomic experiences or system-induced trauma. Both civil and criminal child abuse prosecutors should understand the traumatic impact of the proceedings on the child and their ability to participate in the case preparation or trial. The most extreme outcome in these cases, if the criminal abuse or neglect is proved beyond a reasonable doubt, is the sentencing of a parent to incarceration, fines, or restitution (eg, payment for the child victim's treatment expenses).

Children who must testify in court often feel anxiety, stress, and fear. After testifying, they may feel less anxiety, less victimized, and more in control. Children who testified when they were younger and those who had to testify more than once reported more long-term mental health consequences. Those who testified about severe abuse had more trauma-related concerns later. Finally, children who did not testify experienced worse mental health outcomes if the accused got a light sentence.[30]

CASE STUDIES

Case Study 21-1

When Shania was 12, her mother had her hospitalized for extreme behavioral outbursts, aggression, running away, and impulsive behavior. Shania was placed in foster care because her mother was not willing to have her in the home with her 3 younger siblings. She remained in foster care for 3 years, experiencing multiple placement changes when her behaviors became too disruptive for her foster parents to handle. During this time, she was placed on multiple psychiatric medications. Her behavior continued to worsen, and she began using drugs and alcohol and acting out sexually.

At 15, Shania was moved to a therapeutic foster home that made her feel safe. She started treatment with a new therapist who took her off all her medications and started a new treatment modality.

Discussion

As a result of the supports she received, Shania felt safe enough to disclose to her therapist that her uncle had repeatedly raped her while she was living at home and threatened her and her siblings' lives if she told her mother. Once she disclosed the abuse to her therapist, her behavior stabilized, and she continued to improve. Now 18, Shania has graduated high school and has aged out of foster care. She has re-established connections with her mother and siblings but lives on her own, works at a local restaurant, and continues her treatment.

Case Study 21-2

Meaghan, age 25, had 2 children, Tony, age 5, and Nakita, age 4. The family's landlord went to their apartment Saturday afternoon at 2:00 PM to make some repairs and discovered that the children were left home alone. He was surprised because he and his wife had known Meaghan for 6 years. The landlord saw Tony and his sister playing together, using a prescription bottle of pills as a toy. He also noticed dirty dishes in every room, clothes strewn throughout the apartment, empty liquor bottles on the counter, and signs of an insect infestation in the cupboard. After trying to reach Meaghan by phone, the landlord called the child abuse hotline. A child protection services worker came to the apartment and confirmed the condition of the home. Tony said their mother made breakfast for them before she went to work, and they were to eat bread and peanut butter when they got hungry.

Meaghan eventually returned the landlord's call at 6:00 PM. She was not able to access her phone during her shift except during breaks. She was afraid of losing her job but said she would be home as soon as possible. However, the agency worker had already taken the children into custody, citing exigent circumstances and immediate safety concerns in the home, including the condition of the apartment and lack of appropriate supervision of the children.

Discussion

Meaghan acknowledged why the landlord had called the hotline and agreed to cooperate with the agency worker. She explained that she was required to work 10-hour days, 6 days each week. She arranged child care Monday through Friday but on Saturdays sometimes struggled to find someone to watch the children because she had no close family nearby. She stated that she needed to work so she could pay her bills and provide food for her family. On her day off, she cleaned the apartment and spent time with her children. She often felt overwhelmed and sometimes had a drink at night to lessen her stress and anxiety.

An emergency shelter care hearing was held on Monday morning. Meaghan's attorney argued that the child welfare agency had not made reasonable efforts to prevent removal of the children and traumatic separation of the family.

KEY POINTS

1. The focus of civil child protection proceedings is on the safety, permanency, and wellbeing of children. The role of the court in civil proceedings is to ensure children are removed from their parents only when absolutely necessary and are returned as quickly and safely as possible or, when they cannot return home, that another legally permanent placement is found.

2. The effects of child abuse and neglect can be traumatic and carry significant implications for physical and mental health into adulthood. At the same time, separation of parents and children by the state, especially when unnecessary, can cause trauma to both the child and parent.

3. Child welfare agencies are required to make reasonable efforts, and, in the case of Indigenous children, to make active efforts to prevent removal and achieve permanency for the child.

4. Criminal prosecution for child abuse and neglect is mostly under state jurisdiction, although federal jurisdiction exists in certain circumstances. Offenders can be either within or outside the family of the child victim. If the offender is a parent and a simultaneous civil child protection case is open, the criminal and civil cases should be coordinated.

ADDITIONAL RESOURCES

— *Child Welfare Information Gateway*: https://www.childwelfare.gov/pubs/factsheets/cpswork.pdf for general information on how the child welfare system works

— *National Child Traumatic Stress Network*: www.nctsn.org

— *ABA Center on Children and the Law*: www.americanbar.org/child

— *National Council of Juvenile and Family Court Judges*: www.ncjfcj.org including the Enhanced Resource Guidelines, https://www.ncjfcj.org/wp-content/uploads/2016/05/NCJFCJ-Enhanced-Resource-Guidelines-05-2016.pdf

REFERENCES

1. State statutes database. Child Welfare Information Gateway. 2023. https://www.childwelfare.gov/topics/systemwide/laws-policies/state/

2. Child Welfare Information Gateway. Major federal legislation concerned with child protection, child welfare, and adoption. US Department of Health and Human Services, Children's Bureau. 2019. https://www.childwelfare.gov/pub PDFs/majorfedlegis.pdf

3. Adoption and Safe Families Act of 1997, Pub L No. 105-89, 111 Stat 2115 (1997).

4. Trivedi S. The Adoption and Safe Families Act is not worth saving: the case for repeal. *Fam Court Rev*. 2023;61(2):315-340. doi:10.1111/fcre.12711

   Overrepresentation of Black, Indigenous, and other families of color in child welfare affects every decision point in a child welfare case. See: Loe IM, Buysse CA, deBlank M, Kirshbaum M, Augustyn M. Disproportionate representation of children of color and parents with disabilities in the child welfare system: the intersection of race/ethnicity, immigration status, and disability. *J Dev Behav Pediatr*. 2021;42(6):512-514. doi:10.1097/DBP.0000000000000989

5. Fostering Connections to Success and Increasing Adoptions Act of 2008, Pub L No. 110-351, (2008).

6. Foster care: HHS has taken steps to support states' oversight of psychotropic medications, but additional assistance could further collaboration. United States Government Accountability Office. 2017. https://www.gao.gov/assets/gao-17-129.pdf

7. Family First Prevention Services Act, Pub L No. 115-123, (2018).

8. The Family First Prevention Services Act of 2018: a guide for the legal community. ABA Center on Children and the Law. 2020. https://www.americanbar.org/content/dam/aba/administrative/child_law/family-first-legal-guide.pdf

9. Preventing Sex Trafficking and Strengthening Families Act, Pub L No. 113-183, (2014).

10. Washington K. Research review: sibling placement in foster care: a review of the evidence. *Child Fam Soc Work*. 2007;12(4):426-433. doi:10.1111/j.1365-2206.2006.00467.x

11. Cushing G, Samuels GM, Kerman B. Profiles of relational permanence at 22: variability in parental supports and outcomes among young adults with foster care histories. *Child Youth Serv Rev*. 2014;39:73-83. doi:10.1016/j.childyouth.2014.01.001

12. Faulkner M, Belseth T, Adkins T, Perez A. Texas Youth Permanency Project: preliminary findings. The University of Texas at Austin. 2018. https://utyps.socialwork.utexas.edu/2018-pilot-study/

13. Goydarzi S. Separating families may cause lifelong health damage. Scientific American. 2018. https://www.scientificamerican.com/article/separating-families-may-cause-lifelong-health-damage/

14. Lowenstein K. Shutting down the trauma to prison pipeline early, appropriate care for child-welfare involved youth. Citizens for Juvenile Justice. 2018. https://static1.squarespace.com/static/58ea378e414fb5fae5ba06c7/t/5b47615e6d2a733141a2d965/1531404642856/FINAL+TraumaToPrisonReport.pdf

15. Côté SM, Orri M, Marttila M, Ristikari T. Out-of-home placement in early childhood and psychiatric diagnoses and criminal convictions in young adult-hood: a population-based propensity score-matched study. *Lancet Child Adolesc Health*. 2018;2(9):647-653. doi:10.1016/S2352-4642(18)30207-4

16. Logan Greene P, Semanchin Jones A. Predicting chronic neglect: understanding risk and protective factors for CPS involved families. *Child Fam Soc Work*. 2018;23(2):264-272. doi:10.1111/cfs.12414

17. *The AFCARS Report: Preliminary FY 2020 Estimates as of October 4, 2021 – No. 28*. US Department of Health and Human Services, Administration for Children and Families, Administration on Children, Youth and Families, Children's Bureau; 2021. https://www.acf.hhs.gov/sites/default/files/documents/cb/afcarsreport28.pdf

18. Lewin L, Abdrbo A. Mothers with self-reported Axis I Diagnoses and child protection. *Arch Psychiatr Nurs*. 2009;23(3):200-209. doi:10.1016/j.apnu.2008.05.011

19. Brown A, Courtney ME, McMillen JC. Behavioral health needs and service use among those who've aged-out of foster care. *Child Youth Serv Rev*. 2015;58:163-169. doi:10.1016/j.childyouth.2015.09.020

20. Turney K, Wildeman C. Mental and physical health of children in foster care. *Pediatrics*. 2016;138(5):e20161118. doi:10.1542/peds.2016-1118

21. Mental health, ethnicity, sexuality, and spirituality among youth in foster care: findings from the Casey Field Office mental health study. Casey Family Programs. 2007. https://www.casey.org/media/MentalHealthEthnicitySexuality_ FR.pdf

22. Garland AF, Hough RL, Landsverk JA, et al. Racial and ethnic variations in mental health care utilization among children in foster care. *Child Serv.* 2000;3(3):133-146. doi:10.1207/S15326918CS0303_1

23. Konijn C, Admiraal S, Baart J, et al. Foster care placement instability: a meta-analytic review. *Child Youth Serv Rev.* 2019;96:483-499. doi:10.1016/j. childyouth.2018.12.002

24. Fechter-Leggett M, O'Brien K. The effects of kinship care on adult mental health outcomes of alumni of foster care. *Child Youth Serv Rev.* 2010;32:206-213. doi: 10.1016/j.childyouth.2009.08.017

25. *Reasonable Efforts to Preserve or Reunify Families and Achieve Permanency for Children.* US Department of Health and Human Services, Administration for Children and Families, Children's Bureau. September 2019. https://ocfcpacourts. us/wp-content/uploads/2021/09/1.-Reasonable-Efforts-to-Preserve-or-Reunify-Families-and-Achieve-Permanency-for-Children.-new-committee-to-review.pdf

26. Indian Child Welfare Act, Pub L No. 95-608, (1978), upheld in *Haaland v Brackeen,* 599 US ____ (2023).

27. *Guidelines for Implementing the Indian Child Welfare Act.* US Department of the Interior, Bureau of Indian Affairs. December 2016. https://www.bia.gov/sites/ default/files/dup/assets/bia/ois/pdf/idc2-056831.pdf

28. Pierce BJ, Muzzey FK, Bloomquist KR, Imburgia TM. Effectiveness of Family Centered Treatment on reunification and days in care: propensity score matched sample from Indiana child welfare data. *Child Youth Serv Rev.* 2022;136:106395. doi:10.1016/j.childyouth.2022.106395

29. Weisz V, Wingrove T, Beal SJ, Faith-Slaker A. Children's participation in foster care hearings. *Child Abuse Negl.* 2011;35(4):267-272. doi:10.1016/j.chiabu. 2010.12.007

30. Pantell RH; Committee on Psychosocial Aspects of Child And Family Health. The child witness in the courtroom. *Pediatrics.* 2017;139(3):e20164008. doi: 10.1542/peds.2016-4008

ETHICAL ISSUES WHEN WORKING WITH ABUSED CHILDREN

Linda K. Knauss, PhD, ABPP

OBJECTIVES

After reading this chapter, the reader will be able to:

1. *Identify the major ethical issues in working with abused children.*

2. *Describe ethical intervention methods for working with abused children.*

3. *Develop sensitivity to diversity issues when working with abused children.*

BACKGROUND AND SIGNIFICANCE

Research and clinical literature indicate that childhood sexual abuse can result in significant negative short-term and long-term emotional and psychological consequences. Children who have experienced abuse often make extraordinary efforts to cope with and make sense of their experience.[1-3] Effective intervention and assessment with children who have been abused requires competence in working with children as well as competence in working with survivors of abuse. This chapter will focus on practicing ethically with this population in providing both intervention and assessment. The issues of competence, consent, confidentiality, diversity and cultural awareness, mandated reporting, and boundaries will be highlighted.

COMPETENCE

Adequate training is needed to work with children who have been abused. This includes techniques in the assessment of suspected abuse and characteristic indicators of child sexual abuse.[2,4] It is also important to be knowledgeable of the short-term and long-term effects of abuse, the contextual variables associated with abuse,[5] and effective therapeutic interventions for families in which sexual abuse has occurred or is occurring.[6,7] Practitioners working with minors need to be aware of the statutes and regulations in their jurisdictions that apply to minors as well as the Child Protective Services (CPS) procedures.[2,8] These statutes or regulations are subject to change, so it is necessary to remain current.

Another area of competence for mental health practitioners is familiarity with a variety of treatment models, including the efficacy and appropriateness of various interventions. This is also an area where it is necessary to remain current with changing developments in the field.[9] For this reason, the theoretical orientation preferred by the therapist may not be appropriate for sexual abuse treatment. Intervention strategies should be assessed for their usefulness in treating child abuse in both an individual and a family context. Some issues that may arise include the needs of individual family members in contrast to the family system, attributions of responsibility for the abuse, and the value of maintaining an intact family structure.[10] Working with abused children requires skill and practice.

Emotional competence is also very important in working with abused children. It includes the ability to emotionally tolerate clinical material presented in treatment and the skill to recognize and limit personal biases.[11] Another component of emotional competence is acknowledging that not every therapist can work with every type of client or with all kinds of problems.[12,13] If a therapist does not have training in or experience with working with abused children, they may need to refer the child or family elsewhere. This does not constitute a sign of weakness.[11] It is important to help clients understand that the purpose of the referral is to ensure that they receive the best possible treatment. In situations where a referral is not possible due to distance or other factors, consultation or supervision from a mental health professional trained to work with abused children is recommended.[10] Thus, it is important for therapists to maintain an awareness of and sensitivity to the effects of their own emotional needs and reactions, especially when working with children and adolescents who have been abused.

CONSENT TO TREATMENT

The purpose of informed consent is twofold: (1) to provide an adequate basis for making a decision about whether or not to give permission for a child to be seen in therapy or for assessment and (2) enable minors to decide on their level of participation once they are in therapy or being assessed. Establishing a therapeutic alliance and a working relationship of emotional trust is essential to a successful therapeutic outcome, especially when working with abused children. However, this becomes complicated when working with children. In order to give consent for treatment, one needs to be competent, and the law presumes adults to be competent and minors to be incompetent to give consent for treatment.[14] Thus, it is the parent or legal guardian in most cases who is the client of the services, even though the therapist is working with the child. Participation in therapy or assessment may not be voluntary on the part of a minor when consent is given by a parent or guardian. However, the child is always able to make choices about how much and what information to share. This is one reason for including minors in the informed consent process. Minors need to know whether their behavior will be the basis of any decision-making process, such as custody decisions or probation. Children also need to know the limits of confidentiality both to their parents as well as any other parties, such as teachers, school administrators, or probation officers.[15] When children do not have the legal right to consent to or refuse services or hold the right of confidentiality regarding any information they divulge during therapy, the opportunity is present for potentially serious conflicts of interest between the child, parent, and therapist.[16]

It is also important to differentiate between the concepts of consent and assent. To give consent, one must have the ability to understand the facts and consequences relative to a decision and make that decision voluntarily. Informed consent implies that the person has and understands all of the relevant data needed to reach a reasoned decision. Often a person must meet a legal age requirement, usually 18 years old, in order for their decisions to be considered legal or binding. Thus, mental health professionals working with children or adolescents need to know the legal age of consent in their jurisdiction. In addition, some states may have different ages of consent for inpatient or outpatient treatment, or there could be differences related to confidentiality and release of information. Many state professional organizations can be helpful in providing this information.[15]

The assent process recognizes that the minor client cannot legally consent, but nonetheless acknowledges the importance of their active agreement and contributions to the therapy or assessment process. Assent should be obtained using language that the client can be reasonably expected to understand and documented by the therapist. Assent recognizes that although minors may not have the capacity to give fully reasoned consent because of their age and developmental level, they are still able to have and express a preference.[14] Unfortunately, this preference usually can only be expressed by refusing to participate in treatment. However, the point could be made that it sends a mixed message to solicit the assent of a child if refusal would not be honored. Practitioners should be sure that children understand what participation means before asking for assent so the child can make an informed choice. It is both an ethical obligation and sound clinical practice to develop an active and collaborative therapeutic relationship with a child who becomes a client at the request of others.[17] Whether a child has chosen to participate or not, it is important for them to understand the psychological services they will be receiving. In some states, minors may make decisions independently of parental authority in certain circumstances, such as substance abuse treatment or seeking medical care for contraception, treatment for sexually transmitted disease, or termination of pregnancy; however, courts have historically treated children as the property of the parents. It is assumed that the adult is acting in the child's best interest. Even in the best of circumstances, though, not all parental decisions regarding children occur without conflicts of interest.

It is for these reasons that it is the ethical responsibility of professionals to protect the best interest of the child while delivering competent services.[17,18] This is a difficult task, because when providing mental health services to a minor, a therapist always has 2 clients—the minor and their parent(s) or legal guardian(s). As mentioned previously, the best interests of the parents do not necessarily align with those of their children, and different family members may have different goals for the same child. Regarding consent to treatment, services should not be provided to any minor without the knowledge and consent of their parents or guardians, unless it is an emergency, or the child is old enough to give consent on their own. Any treatment plan that is developed should take into consideration the best interest of all parties, although this goal may require assertiveness and strong mediation skills.

CONFIDENTIALITY

Confidentiality when working with children requires special considerations at the start of the treatment relationship. The best time to discuss confidentiality and the limits of confidentiality is during the informed consent process. Mental health professionals were once ethically able to tell clients that everything that was said within the professional relationship was confidential[19]; however, there are now legally mandated limits to confidentiality in all therapy situations. These exceptions to confidentiality include threats of physical harm to oneself or others, mandated reporting of child abuse, and responding to a court order. Thus, therapists should never imply that everything that is shared in the context of therapy is confidential.[19]

The ability to authorize or consent to treatment implies the ability to control confidentiality and the release of information shared in that treatment. Thus, when parental consent is needed to obtain treatment, parents have a right to obtain the information generated from the treatment. Although there are a few exceptions, state and federal laws in the United States generally grant parents full access to the medical and mental health records of their minor children. In addition to learning the content of therapy sessions, this includes signing for release of information and accessing school or hospital records. Thus, it is very important to discuss the limits of confidentiality with both parents and children before beginning treatment because a policy of sharing all information with the parents may discourage a child from being open and honest in therapy. Minors need to know not only the nature and extent of information being shared with others but also the reasons for sharing it. It is good clinical practice to tell the child what information will be disclosed and to whom rather than disclosing without the child's knowledge. This conveys respect for the child and integrity on the part of the therapist.[15,20]

Confidentiality may not often become a significant concern with very young children, but autonomy and privacy issues are very important to adolescents. In places where adolescents do not have confidentiality, therapists can often establish agreements where parents are willing to withhold their requests for information to allow a greater sense of privacy and encourage a stronger therapeutic alliance. The best way to do this is to have a discussion with the adolescent and his or her parent(s) at the beginning of therapy. In addition to assuring the adolescent of confidentiality so that they can talk openly in therapy, it is also important for parents to feel confident about their child's wellbeing and safety.[14] If this agreement is made informally, and parental consent to treatment is legally required, the parents can later insist on obtaining and thus receive the information shared in therapy; however, the Health Insurance Portability and Accountability Act (HIPAA) Privacy Rule[21] elevates the status of private agreements between parents, minors, and therapists. If the parents have signed a written agreement of confidentiality, it can be legally binding and prevents parents from accessing the information covered by the confidentiality agreement.[20] Even with agreements of confidentiality, exceptions to confidentiality include danger to the life or safety of the minor or to a third party, court orders, and the mandated reporting of child abuse. Parents can limit the information they wish to be informed of to only dangers to self and others and child abuse, or they can include sexual activity, substance use, or any other category in which they are interested. Minors should know in advance what information will be shared with parents and make their disclosures accordingly. Agreements of confidentiality require therapists to think carefully about the continuum of adolescent behavior and what information may need to be shared with parents as a result of danger to the adolescent or others. Behaviors such as cigarette smoking, illegal substance use, and sexual activity all present varying degrees of danger. There is no easy answer to when these behaviors cross the line and become dangerous. Therapists need to consider the intensity, frequency, and seriousness of the behavior as well as whether parental involvement would or would not be helpful. These decisions are context-dependent and include the likely response of the parents, the damage to the therapeutic relationship, and the willingness of the client to disclose the information and to work on these behaviors in therapy.[22] It is best when clients recognize through therapy that disclosing the behavior themselves can facilitate growth and communication within the family.[20]

Children who have been abused are sometimes seen in group therapy, which presents another unique set of considerations regarding confidentiality. Group leaders are required to follow the standards of confidentiality set by their profession; however, there are no external mandates requiring confidentiality on the part of group members. Some therapists require a signed confidentiality agreement as a prerequisite for group members. The consequence of breaking such an agreement is usually termination of group membership; however, this is not an effective consequence with children and adolescents, who are often not highly motivated to participate in the group.[23] Thus, it is the group leader's responsibility to establish a climate of confidentiality in which group members agree not to share information discussed in the group context with others outside of the group. Children and adolescents may need to be educated about the importance of maintaining confidentiality and reminded frequently of its necessity. It is also important to stress the importance of maintaining confidentiality after the group ends.

DIVERSITY

As society becomes more diverse, mental health practitioners will be increasingly likely to encounter clients from diverse backgrounds.[22] In order for treatment to be effective, the unique needs of each client must be considered. While each person has their own strengths and concerns, certain themes are commonly found among members of different cultural groups. Ignoring these themes could compromise the quality of treatment.[20]

Clients from diverse backgrounds can express their distress and react to mental health treatment in unique ways. For example, expecting verbalization of thoughts and feelings, confrontations, and conflicts and asking questions to probe feelings can be uncomfortable for members of various cultural groups[24]; however, it is equally important not to stereotype minority clients using broad generalizations.[15]

Mental health professionals will work more effectively with diverse individuals if they recognize the impact of their own cultural heritage and values on their assumptions.[20] There is no definite level of education, awareness, or skill that is needed to be competent to treat an individual from a diverse background. Cultural awareness also means more than memorizing a list of stereotypes about various cultures. According to Knapp et al,[20] "it means being able to think in cultural terms and focus on process as well as content."

MANDATED REPORTING

The reporting of child abuse is mandated by law in every jurisdiction in the United States, although the specific details of reporting vary from state to state. Reporting child abuse is an exception to confidentiality and thus needs to be discussed as part of the informed consent process. Many therapists fear that telling clients, especially children and adolescents, that they are mandated reporters will lead them to avoid discussing abuse. This may be true in certain situations, but it is best that clients know the consequences of their behavior and choose accordingly; however, many minor clients do reveal abuse in therapy with the knowledge that the therapist is a mandated reporter in an effort to obtain protection or assistance.[15] Even when a therapist is working with an abused child, additional incidents of abuse may be revealed.

The decision to report suspected abuse is always difficult because it is not clear when clinical intuition becomes suspicion or belief, which is the legal requirement for reporting abuse in most states. Therapists are often confronted with an ethical dilemma regarding reporting suspected child abuse. It is important to recognize that the threshold of certainty for making reports is low, as most states in the United States only require that mandated reporters suspect that a child was abused; they do not need to have proof.

It is the child welfare agency, not the therapist, that has the responsibility to determine whether abuse actually occurred.[20] Mental health professionals should be aware of important features of the CPS laws in their jurisdiction, such as how abuse is defined, the conditions that activate the duty to report, and the definition of a perpetrator of child abuse. The definition of child abuse also varies from jurisdiction to jurisdiction, but most include nonaccidental injury, neglect, emotional abuse, and sexual abuse.

Privileged communication or confidentiality laws do not excuse professionals from their duty to report suspected abuse. All jurisdictions of the United States grant therapists immunity from civil or criminal liability for good-faith reporting.[25] In fact, because mental health professionals are mandated by law to report abuse, failure to report abuse results in either civil or criminal penalties. Thus, mandated reporting laws are based on the belief that protecting the harmed individual outweighs therapeutic confidentiality.[26]

Concerns about reporting need to be considered in relation to the potential negative consequences of not reporting for children and their families. Failure to report suspected or disclosed abuse is likely to result in the continued victimization of the child(ren) in question and can communicate to the family that the therapist is willing to collude with the perpetrator.

When a report of child abuse must be made, mental health professionals can minimize the negative effect on the child, the family, and the ongoing treatment through proactive efforts. The first step is to thoroughly inform clients of confidentiality limitations at the beginning of treatment. Then, when the therapist learns of abuse, the therapist should remind the client and their parents that it must be reported. From a clinical perspective, it is helpful to discuss with the family the necessity to file a child abuse report and obtain their consent if possible; unfortunately, this step is often neglected. It is best if the family calls the child welfare agency, or the therapist can call with the family present, so they know exactly what was said. The effort to clarify what was done and why may minimize the damage to the therapeutic relationship. It may also be helpful for the therapist to explain that the reporting decision is mandated by law and that criminal or civil penalties can result from failure to report.[20] If the client and legal guardian are not present when the report is made, it is helpful for them to be informed that a report was made. A report of suspected child abuse can be made legally and ethically without the client being present or informed, but this is the least preferable choice from a therapeutic perspective. Although, there may be times when this is the best option.[15] Therapists should carefully document their interactions with families in which child abuse is suspected.

Families also benefit from being kept informed of the procedures that follow the report of abuse, such as the policies and procedures involved in investigating reports of child abuse.[10] Therapists should work as cooperatively as possible with the police and social services personnel investigating these cases. When therapists discuss the limits of confidentiality and report all cases of suspected abuse, they have met both their legal and ethical obligations.

BOUNDARIES

Clinical work with children also presents potential boundary crossings, such as accepting hugs from clients, escorting children to the bathroom, giving food as a reward, buying fundraising items, accepting invitations to significant events, and giving gifts to clients. Clinicians tend to be more flexible with their boundaries when working with younger children. While these things can be beneficial to the therapeutic relationship, it can also be threatening to a child who has been abused. It is essential for therapists to understand their own professional perspective on boundaries and childhood developmental issues in order to maintain a therapeutic relationship with children.[27]

It is more difficult to explain to children the reasons for boundaries. Children may feel rejected if therapists do not allow them to sit on their laps or if they refuse an invitation to a birthday party. Children often bring gifts to their therapists and may expect presents in return. Children are physical and spontaneous, so therapists must decide where to draw the line in terms of physical contact with child clients. Decisions regarding boundaries depend on a variety of factors, such as a child's age, sex, diagnosis, and prior history.[28]

Two boundary considerations that occur frequently when working with children involve gifts and touch. When working with children, gifts may be given by the children or their parents. Accepting small gifts, such as homemade cookies or a child's hand-drawn picture, typically does not pose an ethical problem. As with other boundary issues, the focus should be on client welfare. Turning down small gifts could be seen as rejection. Most therapists accept nominal gifts as courteous social conventions. Gifts should also be considered in the context of the client's culture. Therapists should be aware of their feelings and clinical rationales ahead of time so they can respond appropriately when faced with the issue of gifts.

Touch is especially important to consider with children. Many people, not only therapists, touch children regardless of the child's wishes. It can be therapeutic as well as ethical to help children express their wishes about being touched, both in and outside of the therapeutic relationship. This could include asking clients for their assent to share a "high-five" at the end of a particularly successful session, or redirecting a child who wants to sit on the therapist's lap to sit on a chair or pillow so they can see each other and talk. It can be especially challenging to set and maintain clinically sensitive boundaries when working with children who have been sexually abused and who find a variety of ways to initiate inappropriate touch. While it is not always the therapist who initiates touch, it is important to maintain boundaries of the therapeutic relationship when a client, especially a child client, initiates physical contact.

Boundaries help therapists maintain objectivity, respect for privacy, dignity, and autonomy. They serve as a safety net to minimize the likelihood of exploiting a client for personal gain and they promote trust in the therapeutic process. Maintaining professional boundaries is one-sided, and it is always the responsibility of the clinician. There are many considerations in establishing personal and professional boundaries to make therapy both effective and ethical.

CONCLUSION

There are many ethical challenges that therapists confront when working with abused children. Ethical guidelines and codes aid therapists in making good decisions, but they do not provide solutions to all ethical dilemmas. Ethical dilemmas arise because of the personal and interpersonal nature of the mental health profession. Thus, it is beneficial to discuss ethical issues with colleagues. Consultation helps to ensure that adequate services are being delivered and provides an additional perspective. When working with children who have been abused, it is critical to be sensitive to ethical issues.

KEY POINTS

1. Effective intervention and assessment with children who have been abused requires competence in working with children as well as with survivors of abuse.

2. Numerous ethical and legal issues are unique to working with children and adolescents. Treating children is challenging because there is a range of developmental changes that affect cognitive, emotional, social, and physical abilities. Practitioners cannot effectively provide mental health care to children and adolescents without involving adults who have legal responsibility for them.

3. It is necessary for therapists to be aware of the ethical issues related to competence, consent, confidentiality, diversity, mandated reporting, and boundaries.

REFERENCES

1. Bass E, Davis L. *20th Anniversary Edition: The Courage to Heal: A Guide for Women Survivors of Child Sexual Abuse.* 4th ed. Harper & Row; 2008.

2. Courtois CA. *Healing the Incest Wound: Adult Survivors in Therapy.* 2nd ed. WW Norton & Company; 2010.

3. Herman JL. *Trauma and Recovery: The Aftermath of Violence—From Domestic Abuse to Political Terror.* Basic Books; 2015.

4. What is child abuse and neglect? Recognizing the signs and symptoms. Child Welfare Information Gateway. 2019. https://www.childwelfare.gov/pubpdfs/what iscan.pdf

5. Committee on Child Maltreatment Research, Policy, and Practice for the Next Decade: Phase II; Board on Children, Youth, and Families; Committee on Law and Justice; Institute of Medicine; National Research Council. Consequences of child abuse and neglect. In: Petersen AC, Joseph J, Feit M, eds. *New Directions in Child Abuse and Neglect Research.* National Academies Press (US); 2014.

6. Practice profile: therapeutic appraoches for sexually abused children and adolescents. US Department of Justice. 2015. https://crimesolutions.ojp.gov/ ratedpractices/45

7. Interventions. The National Child Traumatic Stress Network. 2023. https://www.nctsn.org/what-is-child-trauma/trauma-types/sexual-abuse/interventions

8. American Psychological Association. Guidelines for psychological evaluations in child protection matters. *Am Psychologist.* 2013;68(1):20-31. doi:10.1037/a0029891

9. Fairburn CG, Cooper Z. Therapist competence, therapy quality, and therapist training. *Behav Res Ther.* 2011;49(6-7):373-8. doi:10.1016/j.brat.2011.03.005

10. Committee on Child Maltreatment Research, Policy, and Practice for the Next Decade: Phase II; Board on Children, Youth, and Families; Committee on Law and Justice; Institute of Medicine; National Research Council. The child welfare system. In: Petersen AC, Joseph J, Feit M, eds. *New Directions in Child Abuse and Neglect Research.* National Academies Press (US); 2014.

11. Koocher GP, Keith-Spiegel P. *Ethics in Psychology and the Mental Health Professions: Standards and Cases.* 3rd ed. Oxford University Press; 2008. doi:10.1080/10673220600968670

12. Brenner AM. The role of personal psychodynamic psychotherapy in becoming a competent psychiatrist. *Harvard Rev Psychiatry.* 2006;14(5):268-272.

13. Koocher GP. Ethical issues in psychotherapy with adolescents. *J Clin Psych.* 2003;59(11):1247-1256. doi:10.1002/jclp.10215

14. Koocher GP, Daniel JH. Treating children and adolescents. In: Knapp SJ, ed. *APA Handbook of Ethics in Psychology Vol 2; Practice, Teaching, and Research.* American Psychological Association; 2012:3-14.

15. Knauss LK. Legal and ethical issues in providing group therapy to minors. In: Christner RW, Stewart JL, Freeman A, eds. *Cognitive-Behavior Group Therapy with Children and Adolescents.* Routledge; 2007:65-85.

16. Sales BD, DeKraai MB, Hall SR, Duvall JC. Child therapy and the law. In: Morris RJ, Kratochwill TR, eds. *The Practice of Child Therapy.* 4th ed. Lawrence Erlbaum Associates. 2008:519-542.

17. Cotrim H, Granja C, Carvalho AS, Cotrim C, Martins R. Children's understanding of informed assents in research studies. *Healthcare (Basel).* 2021;9(7):871. doi:10.3390/healthcare9070871.

18. Michaud P, Blum R, Benaroyo L, Zermatten J, Baltag V. Assessing an adolescent's capacity for autonomous decision-making in clinical care. *J Adolesc Health.* 2015; 57:361-366. doi:10.1016/j.jadohealth.2015.06.012

19. Fisher MA. Confidentiality and record keeping. In: Knapp SJ, ed. *APA Handbook of Ethics in Psychology, Vol 1: Moral Foundations and Common Themes.* American Psychological Association; 2012:333-375.

20. Knapp S, VandeCreek L, Fingerhut R. *Practical Ethics for Psychologists: A Positive Approach.* 3rd ed. American Psychological Association; 2017.

21. HIPAA Privacy Rules, 45 CFR § 164 (2023). https://www.ecfr.gov/current/title-45/subtitle-A/subchapter-C/part-164

22. Knapp S, Younggren JN, VandeCreek L, Harris E, Martin J. *Assessing and Managing Risk in Psychological Practice: An Individualized Approach.* The Trust; 2013.

23. Brabender V. *Introduction to Group Therapy.* John Wiley & Sons; 2002.

24. Center for Substance Abuse Treatment (US). Understanding the impact of trauma. In: *Trauma-Informed Care in Behavioral Health Services.* Substance Abuse and Mental Health Services Administration (US); 2014.

25. US Department of Health and Human Services; Administration for Children and Families; Administration on Children, Youth and Families; Children's Bureau. Report to congress on immunity from prosecution for professional consultation in suspected and known instances of child abuse and neglect. US Department of Health and Human Services. 2013. https://www.acf.hhs.gov/sites/default/files/documents/cb/capta_immunity_rptcongress.pdf

26. Thomas R, Reeves M. *Mandatory Reporting Laws.* StatPearls Publishing; 2023.

27. Belitz J, Bailey RA. Clinical ethics for the treatment of children and adolescents: a guide for general psychiatrists. *Psychiatr Clin N Am.* 2009;32(2):243-257. doi:10.1016/j.psc.2009.02.001

28. Bhide A, Chakraborty K. General principles for psychotherapeutic interventions in children and adolescents. *Indian J Psychiatry.* 2020;62(Suppl 2):S299-S318. doi:10.4103/psychiatry.IndianJPsychiatry_811_19

Chapter 23

CHILD AND ADOLESCENT MALTREATMENT: *IMPLICATIONS FOR ADULT SURVIVORS*

Matthew A. Myrick, PhD, LSW
Rebecca Vlam, MSS, LCSW

OBJECTIVES

After reading this chapter, the reader will be able to:

1. *Identify the ways in which shame and invalidation experienced during childhood impact those individuals as adults.*

2. *Explain how adult relationships may be impacted by childhood trauma.*

3. *Identify the effects of a provider's childhood experiences and emotional reactions on their clinical practice.*

BACKGROUND AND SIGNIFICANCE

The World Health Organization (WHO) reports that nearly 3 in 4 children (ie, 300 000 000 children) aged 2 to 4 years regularly suffer physical punishment or psychological violence at the hands of their parents or caregivers.[1] Additionally, 1 in 5 women and 1 in 13 men report having been sexually abused as a child aged 0 to 17 years.[1] It should be remembered, however, that these are *reported* statistics, and in many instances, abuse goes unreported, as noted by agencies such as the National Children's Alliance, who state the actual number of children abused is likely under-reported.[2]

Adult survivors of childhood trauma typically experience challenges with interpersonal relationships, emotion regulation, and distress tolerance. Survivors who experience trauma responses "frequently spend their lives experiencing invalidation of their body, experiences, emotions, and sense of self."[3]

Understanding the impact of childhood trauma can become complicated when health and human services and medical professionals pathologize trauma responses through diagnosis and personal reactions.[4] It is important for practitioners working with adult survivors of trauma to see these trauma responses as the coping skills that were used in childhood to ensure "safety." Practitioners should also understand that, while coping skills may be ineffective and even damaging in adulthood, survivors will continue to use these "ineffective behaviors" developed in childhood and experience symptoms until new and effective skills are developed and utilized.

DIAGNOSIS

People are diagnosed in a myriad of ways; most often by social workers, psychologists, psychiatrists, or other licensed mental health professionals. However, it is possible to see diagnoses added to a patient's chart from someone other than the aforementioned. Diagnosis is important for many reasons and may take various lengths of time and visits in order to be obtained correctly; however, the provider is expected to immediately bill the client's insurance company. To do this, providers add a diagnosis to their client's chart so that they may be compensated for the visit, and even though this diagnosis can be changed by the attending psychiatric professional, often the initial diagnosis used for billing purposes remains in a client's chart. This diagnosis and any subsequent changes then create a list of diagnoses that can be very long, confusing, and have the potential to follow clients wherever they go. Clinicians may also add a "rule-out" diagnosis and include any possible diagnoses that may apply to the client. The official diagnosis also allows professionals to identify a cluster of symptoms and have an idea of what may be happening to the person. It is important to note, though, that one size does not fit all, and each person should be asked what they are experiencing and how these experiences impact their lives.

Furthermore, specialists tend to diagnose mental health disorders without looking at the brain itself, which can be problematic, as different parts of the brain can be impacted even within a particular diagnosis. In addition, many assessments categorize trauma as part of the patient's history and not as a factor relevant to what they may be experiencing in the present. "The dominant theory and services provided in American psychiatric hospitals and clinics continues to view mental 'illnesses' as biomedical conditions that can be best addressed with pharmacological treatments."[5] Each diagnosis points toward a medical protocol.

There is evidence to suggest that diagnosis alone can create challenges to trauma recovery, as both the *Diagnostic and Statistical Manual of Mental Disorders* (DSM)[6] and providers can unintentionally perpetuate stigma. Additionally, a misdiagnosis can prevent a client from receiving appropriate treatment. One recorded case notes that for 7 years, in a university mental health clinic, a person was misdiagnosed and had no improvement until the appropriate diagnosis and subsequent treatment was provided.[7] Symptoms from one diagnosis are often seen in another, as noted by Cogan et al,[8] who share that bipolar disorders and post-traumatic stress disorder (PTSD) "have overlapping symptoms, potentially leading to misdiagnosis" and improper care.

We also see stigma around the symptoms and diagnosis of personality disorders.[9] These findings shed light on a particular client's community's attitudes and pre-conceived notions, including the idea that their decisions to not share a borderline personality disorder (BPD) are "attention-seeking and manipulative." This study points out that these and other findings suggest that the mental health care system must change, including in regard to the way providers are educated about and educate others regarding BPD, the way they supervise and receive supervision, and the way they support other organization workers through enhancing "the discourse cultural safety for worker disclosure of mental illness."[9]

BPD and complex post-traumatic stress disorder (CPTSD), also referred to as complex trauma, share many similarities. In 2018, the WHO brought forth the 11th edition of the International Classification of Diseases (IDC) and introduced the distinction between BPD and CPTSD. Some of the common symptoms in this family include re-experiencing trauma by remembering it, experiencing "flight, fight, freeze, fawn" responses, and holding negative beliefs about oneself and others. They are different by the "number and diversity of symptom clusters, and several studies thus far have indicated that they differ by comorbidity and level of impairment."[10] PTSD is considered a response to trauma and BPD has not always been thought of as such; in many circles, the belief that BPD is not a trauma response continues. Proctor et al[11] notes that although stigmas have decreased, "Internationally, individuals diagnosed with BPD still experience increased levels of stigma, are more likely to be viewed as manipulative, and evoke negative responses from health professionals more frequently, compared with individuals with other mental health diagnoses." Hong & Lishner[12] write that those with BPD or PTSD "share a significant number of interpersonal and intrapersonal difficulties, such as the propensity to manipulate others and poor affect and behavioral control." Research has shown that "[1/4] of those with PTSD also meet criteria for BPD and as many as 50% of individuals that meet criteria for BPD have met criteria for lifetime PTSD."[13] A trauma experience is not part of the criteria for BPD, however, a meta-analysis study[14] found that those patients with BPD were more likely to report maltreatment in their childhood than those with other diagnoses.

Health and human service professionals see trauma in their work, yet a diagnosis of trauma or PTSD/CPTSD is not used as often as other diagnoses (eg, depression or anxiety). There is growing attention concerning treatment that addresses the impact of trauma. For example, a 2021 study focusing on college students and the impact of trauma on attention and repetitive negative thinking suggests that childhood trauma increases negative thinking and decreases attention ability, thereby increasing PTSD symptoms.[15] In 2017, Kostaras et al[16] found that major depressive disorder-post-traumatic stress disorder (MDD-PTSD) comorbidity is often overlooked and that, "Prolonged trauma seems to be a major risk factor for MDD-PTSD comorbidity, predisposing subjects to PTSD and later on or simultaneously to comorbidity with MDD." While the recommendation is for further studies, the initial findings suggest that trauma is underdiagnosed. Finally, and perhaps most importantly, it should be remembered that while a diagnosis conveys what a person may be experiencing (eg, grief, sadness, fear, anger, hypervigilance), it conveys nothing about who the client is, their strengths, their ability to survive, or their hopes and dreams.

CONSEQUENCES OF CHILDHOOD TRAUMA

The consequences of childhood trauma can be vast, impacting physical health, self-esteem, and work, among other aspects of a person's life. Consequences also include more nuanced behaviors such as the ability to regulate emotions and the ability to have nurturing relationships. The following section focuses on the developmental consequences of child abuse and neglect, though the list is not exhaustive, and providers should continue to do independent research on the sequelae of childhood trauma.

INVALIDATION AND SHAME

Marsha Linehan is the director of the Behavioral Research and Therapy clinics at the University of Washington, best known for her work in suicide prevention and developing Dialectical Behavior Therapy (DBT). She and her colleagues[17] posit that children coming from an invalidating childhood struggle to identify and regulate emotions without any knowledge or ability of how they will tolerate emotions and distress. Children with this background will often need to act upon extreme emotions to get their needs met, "thus, the social contingencies favor the development of extreme emotional reactions."[17] A study conducted in 2019, based upon Marsha Linehan's biosocial theory of BPD, examined the correlation between childhood history and present-day challenges with emotion regulation and BPD. The study found support for "unique associations between parental magnification of negative emotions, neglect of negative emotions, parental psychological control, and total childhood trauma with BPD features in adulthood."[18] Another study had 127 participants take part in a self-report survey that looked at chronic emotional inhibition and the relationship between childhood emotional invalidation and abuse with psychological distress in adults. The results stated that, "A history of childhood emotional invalidation was associated with chronic emotional inhibition in adulthood," resulting in depression and anxiety.[18] In 2016, Hong & Lishner[12] studied invalidation and the relationship between childhood sexual abuse, finding evidence to support that invalidation predicts depression, anxiety, and symptoms of PTSD. In a recent study, Wasson Simpson et al[19] noted the direct correlation between validation and an acceptance of mental health treatment; it posits that children respond and accept support when they feel validated by both mental health professionals and family members.

A 2022 meta-analysis brought forth the idea that having a definition for shame plays a role in the ability to understand it and approach it.[20] It should be noted, however, that the literature predominately focuses on women, possibly leading to the assumption that women-identifying people experience shame in the same way male-identifying people do, and this may not be true.

Further, shame and guilt are often found hand-in-hand. However, guilt is seen as adaptive and provides a drive to do things differently, thus creating a behavior change. Shame is less about doing and more about being; "shame generates an urgent need to hide and conceal the defective self from exposure."[20]

RELATIONSHIP ISSUES

The impact of trauma on adult relationships has been documented in research. For example, various studies have found that trauma is predictive of antisocial behaviors, problematic peer relationships, sexual promiscuity, and intimate partner violence.[21-23] These maladaptive behaviors are one spectrum of the continuum and can represent an extreme; however, these former coping skills, now "maladaptive" behaviors, do not translate well when attempting to navigate work and healthy adult relationships. It is important to remember that adult survivors of childhood trauma may experience emotion dysregulation that is connected to their trauma experience and interpersonal issues with others.[24] Experiencing childhood trauma, however, does not always result in adverse adult relationships; adult survivors have successfully coped and integrated their trauma prior to or while engaging in relationships.

EMOTION DYSREGULATION

The ability to regulate emotions is connected to the brain and can impact every area of a person's life. People need the ability to regulate in order to work, go to school, have friendships, and navigate the world in a way that allows for an enjoyable life. The brain is impacted in people who have experienced trauma, specifically in responses to negative stimuli and the use of the prefrontal cortex to self-regulate.[25] Trauma experienced in childhood, specifically neglect, is connected to impulsivity, increased reactivity, and challenges with emotion regulation. Studies have shown "depressed neural responsiveness, particularly in the amygdala," symptoms of depression, and challenges with emotion regulation.[26]

According to Miller,[27] trauma responses are often categorized in terms of the 4 Fs: fight, flight, freeze, and fawn/appeasement. "Fawn" is a relatively new concept that is "theorized to be a reaction to childhood exposure to complex trauma."[28] Fawning is frequently seen in survivors who need to "people please" in order to survive (eg, the survivor struggles with maintaining their own boundaries, putting themselves first, or avoiding conflicts).

INTERVENTION AND CARE

It would be remiss to not discuss more common treatment practices, both traditional and nontraditional; however, it is important to note that treatment practices and *available* treatment practices (ie, affordable, accessible, and covered by insurance) are not equally available to everyone in every community.

There is a plethora of evidenced-based, manualized practices that are specific to trauma, including eye movement desensitization and reprocessing therapy (EMDR), cognitive processing therapy (CPT), DBT, and Trauma-focused cognitive behavioral therapy (TF-CBT), among others. For example, one study on EMDR using a linear mixed model approach showed a significant decrease in depressive symptoms, anxiety, other psychiatric disorders, personality disorders, and somatic disorders.[29] Another study specifically looking at brief intensive treatment found "significant decreases" in symptoms of BPD and "32.7% lost their positive screen at post-treatment."[30] Although psychodynamic work is not evidenced-based and is not a "manualized treatment," it is known that this approach aligns with the treatment of trauma and is a trauma-informed approach. Psychodynamic therapy is relationship-focused and "may be especially useful for treating clients with CPTSD because it focuses on establishing a trusting relationship, removing barriers to creating this relationship, and emotion regulation,"[31] all of which are part of a trauma-informed practice and trauma treatment. Nontraditional treatment practices have gained more attention and credibility in recent years. With growing evidence regarding the impact of trauma on the body,[32] activities such as mindfulness, meditation, and yoga are being used in a wide variety of settings and with diverse groups of clients to address stressors and aid in healing. Mindfulness is the practice of directing one's thoughts and emotions to the present moment in order to step away from negative thoughts of self or others that lower emotional reactivity.[33] Meditation has roots in Buddhist and other contemplative traditions and has been practiced for more than 4000 years.[34] Traditionally, yoga unites mind, body, and spirit via techniques such as physical postures, breath work, meditation, or chanting.[35] There is an ongoing movement to decolonize mindfulness, meditation, and yoga so that it is accessible to all people of different races, ethnicities, all bodies, all gender identities, and all socioeconomic statuses.

Summary

Adverse childhood experiences "can produce a sustained, toxic stress response in children that disrupts child development, emotional regulation, interpersonal relationships, and physiologic processes, and ultimately contributes to increased risk for poor outcomes."[36] In addition to topics discussed in this chapter, there are many other factors that can cause trauma in childhood. These include oppression, access to consistent quality care, racism, sexism, heterosexism, classism, access to healthy food, and more. Most importantly, even though providers must remember to leave their own history or trauma out of the office, they must remember to take care of themselves as well.

Case Studies

Case Study 23-1

Penny was a 32-year-old, cisgender, heterosexual woman. She was able-bodied, White, and a non-religious Protestant. She had been in the health care field for many years and loved to work with animals. She volunteered at the American Society for the Prevention of Cruelty to Animals® (ASPCA) on weekends and when she was unable to work. Despite her high intelligence and this involvement, she was persistently sad. When the provider met with her, it was her last try at "traditional therapy," in particular, DBT, before admitting herself for electroconvulsive therapy, which was being prescribed due to the lack of response to any treatment provided. Penny's body was approximately 80% scar tissue as a result of self-harm; the only place she had unharmed skin was her face.

Penny came from a family that placed extreme value on education, behaving perfectly, and acting like an adult. Penny's father was absent most of the time due to work or his own hobbies, and Penny's mother was morbidly depressed. Penny recalled that when she was very young, she thought that her mother was a "witch in disguise." When home, Penny's mother would lock herself in her bedroom, leaving Penny to care for herself and her younger brothers, beginning at the age of 5 or 6 years. Her mother insisted they look like a "perfect family" when in public. Penny was not allowed to be angry or sad, but, in contrast, her mother's moods would go from loving to extreme anger to rejection. Penny reported that she spent her childhood, teens, and early adult years "always doing what I was told." Penny's parents separated when she was approximately 7 years old, and her mother left the state without saying goodbye. Her father began dating immediately, so he hired a full-time, live-in caregiver, Ellis, with whom Penny grew close, even stating that when with Ellis, it was the first and only time in her childhood that she felt safe. Penny shared that she loved Ellis very much and began to experience a healthy attachment. When Penny's mother returned, roughly 6 months after the separation, her parents reconciled, and Ellis was sent away. Ellis was not allowed to say goodbye to Penny, and Penny was not told that Ellis was leaving.

When Penny was 12 years old, she was sexually assaulted by an older cousin, and she began to self-harm shortly after this incident. Penny attempted to tell both parents about her assault, and while her mother was reportedly upset, she did nothing. Her father reportedly responded by saying, "What do you want me to do about it?" When Penny was 13 years old, her parents divorced. Her father remarried in less than a year, and his second wife did not allow Penny to be a part of this new family. Penny's mother also entered into a new relationship and stayed in a different state with her partner on Thursday through Tuesday of each week, leaving Penny home alone. Penny began to use substances and self-soothe with food.

Discussion

Penny shared at her appointment that she wished she had had access to the DBT skills as a child that she had later in life. She described her experience with DBT as "eventually life altering," and shared that it took some time to "buy in" and learn the skills. By learning DBT, she learned about historical trauma, genetics, and the importance of a "healthy" attachment. Penny considered herself a "work in progress," however, she had a fulfilling career as a psychologist working with children, had healthy relationships, and was living a "life worth living."

While Penny had experienced a multitude of traumas in her life, it was not the summation of her character; providers are encouraged to view Penny's trauma as wounds and missed opportunities. Furthermore, Penny was diagnosed as having BPD, a once considered "terminal"[37] diagnosis. However, through a therapeutic relationship, person-centered approaches, and countertransference, Penny began actively healing and navigating her diagnosis.

Case Study 23-2

JC was a 77-year-old, White, able-bodied, gay-identifying male, who met with a family doctor for his dissertation research. JC grew up in a rural area of the southern United States. Growing up, he lived with his father, mother, and older brother, who was 3.5 years older than him. The family identified as Christian, and JC's father was a leader in the church community.

JC was a survivor of incest, whose father would sexually assault him repeatedly from the age of 6 until the age of 14. His mother and father would also physically and psychologically abuse him. His older brother, who was also a victim of his father, sexually experimented with JC during childhood and early adolescence. Upon reflection, JC realized that the experiences with his brother were more confusing because they felt pleasurable. During these years, JC would describe himself as a shy and insecure child who was guilty and angry about what was happening to him. The sexual abuse stopped at 14 years old because JC was then physically able to stop his father from abusing him.

As an adult, JC used alcohol consumption as a coping strategy, and he described himself as a binge drinker before his retirement. After he retired, the start time of his drinking changed from evenings to 11:00 AM. JC described his drinking as a means "to escape his demons." JC did not have any long-lasting romantic relationships in early adulthood.

Discussion

Throughout his life, a protective factor for JC was dance class, as it had a calming effect on him and served as an artistic outlet (important for trauma survivors). This dance interest turned into a professional career and lasted until his retirement from it. JC, with encouragement from his friends, also chose to take part in Alcoholics Anonymous (AA) in his late 50s, after experiencing a blackout post-drinking. This shows the impact of a positive support network in one's healing journey and the benefit of 12-step programs for trauma survivors. In addition to attending AA meetings, JC became involved in therapeutic services for many years. He saw 2 licensed therapists and 1 psychologist. JC did not share with his therapist that he was a survivor of incest until the therapeutic bond had been established, and his therapist was only the second person that he had ever talked to about it. JC noted that his therapists would respect his boundaries and never invade his space. After being sober for 7 years, JC began a long-term relationship with another man, recognizing that he had to address his trauma prior to engaging in a committed relationship. Through dance, AA meetings, a positive support network, and a strong therapeutic relationship, JC was able to begin healing.

KEY POINTS

1. Statistics show that children continue to experience the impacts of their childhood trauma well into adulthood, and it may affect many areas of their lives.

2. Adult survivors of childhood and adolescent maltreatment may experience challenges with emotion regulation, feelings of shame, and interpersonal relationships in adulthood. However, readers should note that additional challenges may arise as well. More education (including research) and exploration of this topic area is needed in the health and human service fields.

3. The diagnoses given to adult survivors of childhood and adolescent maltreatment gives health and human service professionals a means of understanding the person's challenges; however, understanding the whole person and their history gives professionals a wider perspective and allows for a more thorough under-

standing of their trauma and can potentially reduce the risk for ongoing diagnosis-related stigma.

ADDITIONAL RESOURCES

— Information about Trauma-Informed Care: https://store.samhsa.gov/product/SAMHSA-s-Concept-of-Trauma-and-Guidance-for-a-Trauma-Informed-Approach/SMA14-4884

REFERENCES

1. Child maltreatment. World Health Organization. 2020. Accessed 2022. https://www.who.int/news-room/fact-sheets/detail/child-maltreatment/

2. National statistics on child abuse. National Children's Alliance. 2023. Accessed 2023. https://www.nationalchildrensalliance.org/media-room/national-statistics-on-child-abuse/

3. Courtois CA, Ford JD. *Treatment of Complex Trauma: A Sequenced, Relationship-Based Approach.* Guilford Press; 2013.

4. Suhr JA, Johnson EEH. First do no harm: ethical issues in pathologizing normal variations in behavior and functioning. *Psychol Inj and Law.* 2022;15:253-267. doi:10.1007/s12207-022-09455-z

5. Costanzo MS. Ill or injured: shifting the emphasis to trauma in mental health diagnosis and treatment. *Psychiatr Rehabil J.* 2016;39(4):368-370. doi:10.1037/prj0000229

6. American Psychiatric Association. *Diagnostic and Statistical Manual of Mental Disorders: DSM-5-TR.* 8th ed. American Psychiatric Association Publishing; 2022.

7. de Oliveira R, Mendlowicz MV, Berger W, et al. Unnecessarily prolonged suffering: a case of missed diagnosis of post-traumatic stress disorder in a teaching hospital. *J Brasil Psiquiatr.* 2021;70(3):266-270. doi:10.1590/0047-2085000000323

8. Cogan CM, Paquet CB, Lee JY, Miller KE, Crowley MD, Davis JL. Differentiating the symptoms of posttraumatic stress disorder and bipolar disorders in adults: utilizing a trauma informed assessment approach. *Clin Psychol Psychother.* 2021;28(1):251-260. doi:10.1002/cpp.2504

9. Ring D, Lawn S. Stigma perpetuation at the interface of mental health care: a review to compare patient and clinician perspectives of stigma and borderline personality disorder. *J Ment Health.* 2019;1-21. doi:10.1080/09638237.2019.1581337

10. Cloitre M, Hyland P, Bisson JI, et al. ICD-11 Posttraumatic Stress Disorder and Complex Posttraumatic Stress Disorder in the United States: a population-based study. *J Trauma Stress.* 2019;32(6):833-842. doi:10.1002/jts.22454

11. Proctor JM, Lawn S, McMahon J. Consumer perspective from people with a diagnosis of Borderline Personality Disorder (BPD) on BPD management- How are the Australian NHMRC BPD guidelines faring in practice? *J Psychiatr Ment Health Nurs.* 2021;28(4):670-681. doi:10.1111/jpm.12714

12. Hong PY, Lishner DA. General invalidation and trauma-specific invalidation as predictors of personality and subclinical psychopathology. *Pers Individ Differ.* 2016;89:211-216. doi:10.1016/j.paid.2015.10.016

13. Powers A, Petri JM, Sleep C, et al. Distinguishing PTSD, complex PTSD, and borderline personality disorder using exploratory structural equation modeling in a trauma-exposed urban sample. *J Anxiety Disord.* 2022;88:102558. doi:10.1016/j.janxdis.2022.102558

14. Borroni S, Masci E, Franzoni C, Somma A, Fossati A. The co-occurrence of trauma related disorder and borderline personality disorder: AQ study on a clinical sample of patients seeking psychotherapy treatment. *Psychiatry Res.* 2021; 295:113587. doi:10.1016/j.psychres.2020.113587

15. Espeleta HC, Taylor DL, Kraft JD, Grant DM. Child maltreatment and cognitive vulnerabilities: examining the link to posttraumatic stress symptoms. *J Am College Health.* 2021;69(7):759-766.

16. Kostaras P, Bergiannaki JD, Psarros C, Ploumbidis D, Papageorgiou C. Post-traumatic stress disorder in outpatients with depression: still a missed diagnosis. *J Trauma Dissociation.* 2017;18(2):233-247. doi:10.1080/15299732.2016.123 7402

17. Neacsiu AD, Ward-Ciesielski EF, Linehan MM. Emerging approaches to counseling intervention: dialectical behavior therapy. *Couns Psychol.* 2012;40(7): 1003-1032.

18. Hope NH, Chapman AL. Difficulties regulating emotions mediates the associations of parental psychological control and emotion invalidation with borderline personality features. *Personal Disord.* 2019;10(3):267-274. doi:10.1037/per 0000316

19. Wasson Simpson KS, Gallagher A, Ronis ST, Miller DAA, Tilleczek KC. Youths' perceived impact of invalidation and validation on their mental health treatment journeys. *Adm Policy Ment Health.* 2022;49(3):476-489. doi:10.1007/s10488-021-01177-9

20. Plante W, Tufford L, Shute T. Interventions with survivors of interpersonal trauma: addressing the role of shame. *Clin Soc Work.* 2022;50:183-193. doi:10. 1007/s10615-021-00832-w

21. Feiring C, Simon VA, Cleland CM. Childhood sexual abuse, stigmatization, internalizing symptoms, and the development of sexual difficulties and dating aggression. *J Consult Clin Psychol.* 2009;77(1):127-137. doi:10.1037/a0013475

22. Ha T, Kim H, Christopher C, Caruthers A, Dishion TJ. Predicting sexual coercion in early adulthood: the transaction among maltreatment, gang affiliation, and adolescent socialization of coercive relationship norms. *Dev Psychopathol.* 2016;28(3):707-720. doi:10.1017/S0954579416000262

23. Wekerle C, Leung E, Wall AM, et al. The contribution of childhood emotional abuse to teen dating violence among child protective services-involved youth. *Child Abuse Negl.* 2009;33:45-58. doi:10.1016/j.chiabu.2008.12.006

24. Ha T, Otten R, McGill S, Dishion TJ. The family and peer origins of coercion within adult romantic relationships: a longitudinal multimethod study across relationships contexts. *Dev Psychol.* 2019;55(1):207-215. doi:10.1037/dev 0000630

25. Tinajero R, Williams PG, Cribbet MR, et al. Reported history of childhood trauma and stress-related vulnerability: associations with emotion regulation, executive functioning, daily hassles and pre-sleep arousal. *Stress Health.* 2020; 36(4):405-418. doi:10.1002/smi.2938

26. Mccrory EJ, Gerin MI, Viding E. Annual research review: childhood maltreatment, latent vulnerability and the shift to preventative psychiatry - the contribution of functional brain imaging. *J Child Psychol Psychiatry.* 2017;58(4): 338-357. doi:10.1111/jcpp.12713

27. Walker P. *Complex PTSD: From surviving to thriving.* Audiobook. Tantor Audio. 2018.

28. Owca J. The association between a psychotherapist's theoretical orientation and perception of complex trauma and repressed anger in the fawn response. The Chicago School of Professional Psychology ProQuest Dissertations Publishing. July 27, 2020. Accessed 2022. https://www.proquest.com/dissertations-theses/association-between-psychotherapist-s-theoretical/docview/2447256147/se-2

29. Gielkens EMJ, Sobczak S, Rossi G, van Alphen SPJ. The feasibility of eye movement desensitization and reprocessing (EMDR) for older adults with posttraumatic stress disorder (PTSD) and comorbid psychiatric and somatic disorders. *Psychol Trauma.* 2022. doi:10.1037/tra0001402

30. de Jongh A, Groenland GN, Sanches S, Bongaerts H, Voorendonk EM, van Minnen A. The impact of brief intensive trauma-focused treatment for PTSD on symptoms of borderline personality disorder. *Eur J Psychotraumatol.* 2020;11(1): 1721142. doi:10.1080/20008198.2020.1721142

31. Alessi EJ, Kahn S. Using psychodynamic interventions to engage in trauma-informed practice. *J Soc Work Pract.* 2019;33(1):27-39.

32. van der Kolk BA. Clinical implications of neuroscience research in PTSD. *Ann N Y Acad Sci.* 2006:1071;277-293. doi:10.1196/annals.1364.022

33. Salcido-Cibrian L, Ramos N, Jimenez O, Blanca M. Mindfulness to regulate emotions: mindfulness and emotional intelligence program (PINEP) and its adaptation to a virtual learning platform. *Complement Ther Clin Pract.* 2019; 36:176-180. doi:10.1016/j.ctcp. 2019.07.00310.1016/j.ctcp.2019.07.003

34. Nguyen-Feng VN, Clark CJ, Butler ME. Yoga as an intervention for psychological symptoms following trauma: a systematic review and quantitative synthesis. *Psychol Serv.* 2019;16(3):513-523. doi:10.1037/ser0000191

35. Cramer H, Lauche R, Langhorst J, Dobos G. Yoga for depression: a systematic review and meta-analysis. *Depress Anxiety.* 2013;30(11):1068-1083. doi:10.1002/da.22166

36. Choi KR, Stewart T, Fein E, et al. The impact of attachment-disrupting adverse childhood experiences on child behavioral health. *J Pediatr.* 2020;221:224-229. doi:10.1016/j.jpeds.2020.03.006

37. Kwon D. The long shadow of trauma. *Sci Am.* 2022;326(1):48-55.

III

ASSESSMENT

MULTIPLE CHOICE

For questions 1 and 2, read the scenario below and answer the following questions by selecting the best response or responses from those provided.

Sharon is a 14-year-old female high school student. She was referred to a psychiatrist on account of what seemed like recurrent episodes of abnormal behavior. She is often conscious during these episodes but feels like she is watching herself. The episodes are characterized by heavy breathing and feeling very upset about her past. While talking with the psychiatrist, Sharon reveals a history of chronic family dysfunction—which included witnessing frequent fights between her parents—and sexual molestation. She has nightmares and intrusive thoughts about these incidents. On assessment, she reveals that she is unable to sleep well at night, has a low mood, and finds it hard to study, resulting in low grades in school. She has been thinking it might be better if she is dead. Sharon's parents are currently estranged from one another; she is accompanied to the consultation by her mother.

1. What is the possible diagnosis of this girl?

    A. No disorder present

    B. PTSD

    C. Depression

    D. Epilepsy

    E. Complex trauma

2. Appropriate psychopharmacologic agents as adjunctive treatment will include:

    A. Chlorpromazine

    B. Fluoxetine

    C. Escitalopram

    D. Amitriptyline

    E. Olanzapine

For questions 3 and 4, read the scenario below and answer the following questions by selecting the best response or responses from those provided.

Femi is a 17-year-old first year university student. This is his first semester at university, and he has increasingly been struggling throughout the term. He says he has frequent nightmares, has lost interest in his schoolwork, and has started cutting himself. He gives a history of being teased and bullied throughout junior school by his friends. He was often picked on because he wore glasses and at times said things that got his peers into trouble. He currently has no friends, and he believes no one can be trusted. He was diagnosed as having depression, borderline personality traits, and low self-esteem. He commenced TF-CBT but is still unhappy after several weeks. Pharmacotherapy is being considered.

3. Femi does not believe he should take any medication. What do you do?

    A. Explore more sessions of TF-CBT

    B. Prescribe a medication anyway and insist that he take it

    C. Educate the patient and parents on the benefits of the medication but also inform them of the potential side effects

    D. Give the patient and parents time to think about the medication

    E. Provide a referral to see a physiotherapist

4. If he changes his mind, as part of preparing him for medication use, what things must be done?

    A. Consider the pros and cons of available medication options

    B. Say he can use the medication when he feels ready to do so

    C. Explain the need for medication adherence

    D. Plan to review and taper off medication as soon as possible

    E. Educate him on the side effect profile

For questions 5 and 6, read the scenario below and answer the following questions by selecting the best response or responses from those provided.

Kayin is 7 years old. She was adopted by a family in Lagos when she was 18 months of age. The family has 3 other biological children. Kayin had been the product of an unwanted pregnancy, and her birth mother had abandoned her at the orphanage at 3 months of age. The birth mother was known to be abusing multiple psychoactive substances. Kayin's adoptive parents have nurtured her lovingly over the years through nightmares and periods of difficult behavior. They have made an appointment with a psychiatrist because they are worried that she has remained very fidgety, cannot sit still in class, and often acts impulsively, resulting in numerous reports from school and suspension. A diagnosis of ADHD is being considered.

5. What medication options could work for Kayin?

    A. Antidepressants

    B. Amphetamines

    C. Antipsychotics

    D. Antihistamines

    E. Atomoxetine

6. What should you consider when choosing a medication for her?

    A. Her age and weight

    B. Her red blood cell count level

    C. Her height

    D. Her cardiac function

    E. Her gastrointestinal profile

For question 7, read the scenario below and answer the following question by selecting the best response or responses from those provided.

An 8-year-old client is currently participating in TF-CBT with his caregivers after being the sole survivor of a car crash involving his grandparents. In the latest child-oriented session of therapy, the child discussed how he could not be afraid of cars, because "big boys weren't supposed to be afraid of anything." He recalled how his father told him this phrase when he was afraid of the dark. Similarly, in the latest caregiver-oriented session, the client's father considered his own views on masculinity and how these views may have impacted the client's thoughts and feelings surrounding the physiological reactions the client has whenever he is in a car.

7. Based on these discussions, which component of the PRACTICE acronym was prioritized in the most recent TF-CBT sessions?

    A. Psychoeducation

    B. Affective Regulation and Modulation

    C. Cognitive Coping

    D. *In Vivo* exposure

For question 8, read the scenario below and answer the following question by selecting the best response or responses from those provided.

A 14-year-old client has been referred to a clinical psychologist by child protective services after allegations surfaced of physical abuse by her mother and the mother's boyfriend. The client's mother disclosed during a parent interview that she wanted to be involved in the treatment process and wants "to be a better parent." Interviews with the client reveal that the physical abuse has been chronic and most often occurs when her mother engages in substance use. At the end of the multimethod intake assessment, the psychologist discovered that the client meets criteria for both persistent depressive disorder and PTSD. While determining a treatment plan, the psychologist hesitates on whether to use TF-CBT over other therapeutic interventions.

8. Which of the following case details is the primary cause for the psychologist's hesitation to use TF-CBT?

    A. The client is a teenager and is too old for this treatment model

    B. TF-CBT is ill-suited for any comorbid diagnoses

    C. *In vivo* exposure and the trauma narrative revolve around a single event, whereas the client has numerous experiences with physical abuse

    D. TF-CBT is not designed for offending caregivers, regardless of the caregivers' intentions

For questions 9 and 10, read each question carefully and select the best response or responses from those provided.

9. What are the PRIDE skills in PCIT?

    A. Praise (labeled praise), respond, imitate, and be enthusiastic

    B. Praise (labeled praise), reflect, imitate, describe, and enjoy

    C. Praise (labeled praise), reflect, imitate, describe, and be enthusiastic

    D. Prompt, reflect, imitate, describe, and enjoy

10. A 6-year-old girl is a victim of sexual abuse by her biological father. She has a number of aggressive and disruptive behaviors that have been increasing since she disclosed the abuse. Is PCIT appropriate for this child? Why?

    A. No, because she was sexually abused and PCIT is contraindicated with sexual abuse victims

    B. Yes, because she experienced maltreatment and PCIT is effective for child maltreatment

    C. Yes, as long as the parent can be involved in treatment

    D. It depends. If PCIT is done with the nonoffending caregiver, then it may be appropriate. PCIT is contraindicated with an offending caregiver

For questions 11 and 12, read the scenario below and answer the following questions by selecting the best response or responses from those provided.

Billy is a 12-year-old boy who loves to play video games, especially first-person shooter games. When his mother tells him to stop playing video games and prepare for another activity (eg, school, an outing, or bedtime) Billy becomes extremely angry and begins screaming, swearing, throwing things, and striking his mother. Billy's mother ultimately reneges and allows Billy to remain undisturbed, even at the expense of other activities. Billy's excessive gaming has led to reduction in grades and an exceeding number of absences at school.

11. If Billy's family presented to treatment, AF-CBT would not be an appropriate first-line intervention if which of the following is identified as a primary concern?

    A. Aggression (either child or caregiver)

    B. Inappropriate discipline practices (ie, excessive corporal punishment)

    C. Post-Traumatic Stress Disorder

    D. AF-CBT is an appropriate first-line intervention for all of these

12. AF-CBT would likely teach Billy all of the following skills *except*:

    A. Emotion regulation

    B. Thought diffusion

    C. Thought restructuring

    D. Noticing positive behavior

For questions 13-15, read each question carefully and select the best response or responses from those provided.

13. An elementary school teacher would like to incorporate mindful exercises while promoting physical fitness during the recess time block at her school. What are some "golden rule" guidelines she should consider?

    A. Do not be accommodating with yoga poses

    B. Yoga should be ritualistic, and only technical names should be used when practicing various poses

    C. Make yoga fun and enthusiastic

    D. Be very critical of the children if they do not follow directions

14. The same elementary school teacher from the question above would like to incorporate some breathing exercises as a starting point to practicing mindfulness. Which of the following exercises would be an appropriate adaptation?

    A. Calmly and slowly instructing the children when to breath in and out

    B. Rigorous diaphragmatic breathing

    C. Short, shallow, fast breathing

    D. Instructing the children to hold their breath for longer than 1 minute

15. The elementary school teacher from the questions above thought it would be fun to have the children sing as they practice their yoga poses. What body function is stimulated when chanting or singing during yoga?

    A. The cardiovascular system

    B. The endocrine system

    C. The pituitary system

    D. The larynx and brain function

For question 16, read the scenario below and answer the following question by selecting the best response or responses from those provided.

Chris grew up in a home with regular drug abuse, and multiple men were in and out of the house each week depending on their mother's relationship status. Chris was responsible for preparing dinner when the adults were too inebriated, and most nights, the sound of yelling and a loud TV were background noise at bedtime. In school, Chris excelled academically but would often experience verbal and behavioral outbursts "out of the blue." Chris experienced frequent disciplinary action at school for being loud, aggressive, and insubordinate. Chris had very few positive adult interactions and was not involved in camps or community activities. At age 9, Chris was made responsible for contributing financially to the household. When school began in the fall, Chris was not only a student but also responsible for ensuring the other children in the home were fed and put to bed at night. Meanwhile, the adults in the home continued to engage in drug activity into the night. As a result, Chris often went to school tired, unable to focus, and hypervigilant to environmental and educational demands. One day, Chris cussed at a teacher during class after being told to "wake up and pay attention." The teacher sent Chris to the principal's office. Because of the school's zero-tolerance discipline policy, Chris was suspended for disrespect and sent home, back into the exact environment that contributed to their distress.

16. What skills can adults in Chris's life cultivate or learn to help impact a more positive relational template?

    A. Adults can have personal and professional boundaries with Chris so they are not impacted negatively by Chris's bad behavior

    B. Adults can learn about their school's policy on hyperactive children and implement consequences to make Chris learn

    C. Adults can understand how their own sense of self and regulation impact the relational field and cultivate the skills to be present with Chris during hardship, so they can respond, rather than react, to Chris's symptoms of stress

    D. Adults cannot learn any skills to influence positive relational templates

For questions 17-19, read each question carefully and select the best response or responses from those provided.

17. Family strengthening programs are an example of _____ prevention of child maltreatment.

    A. Primary

    B. Secondary

    C. Tertiary

    D. All of the above

18. Trauma can impact which of the following cognitive functions of the brain?

    A. Focus

    B. Focus and aggression

    C. Focus, concentration, and problem solving

    D. Focus, concentration, and aggression

19. _____ consistently emerges as a protective factor that buffers children from experiencing maltreatment.

    A. Access to health care

    B. A supportive family environment

    C. Adequate housing

    D. Parental employment

For questions 20-22, read the scenario below and answer the following questions by selecting the best response or responses from those provided.

Joey was a 16-year-old teenage boy, diagnosed as having ASD and mild ID, who had been in the custody of the office of OCYF for 5 years. After being denied all other residential options, he resided in a hotel room staffed by OCYF workers that served as a temporary shelter. He was listed as being uncooperative, threatening providers, making repeated false allegations of abuse, eloping from placements, hiding and smearing feces where others would come in contact with it, destroying property, and being disrespectful and defiant. He was known to speak in animal-like noises. He was also aggressive with his mother, bordering on sexual assault. He was known for stealing and vandalizing any neighborhood he lived in. He had a list of diagnoses including ADHD, ASD, RAD, mood dysregulation disorder, ODD, intermittent explosive disorder, and depressive disorder.

20. *True or False?* Based on the initial synopsis, you have adequate information to be confident in your assessment, diagnosis, and treatment plan.

    A. True

    B. False

21. Of the following, select the underlying issues that you would like to explore further before recommending treatment options:

    A. Physical health concerns

    B. Developmental trauma

    C. Current lifestyle

    D. Hearing and communication style

    E. Learning style

F. Anxiety level

G. Social history

H. Sexuality and identity

I. Personal likes and goals

J. Status of each relationship in his life

K. Developmental age

L. All of the above

22. What might be the role of the cross-systems collaboration on the behalf of Joey?

A. To figure out which institution to put him in

B. To maximize resources on his behalf

C. To garner the expertise of professionals from a multitude of service systems

D. To work as a team to source more ideas, creativity, and mutual support

E. A & B

F. B, C & D

For questions 23-25, read the scenario below and answer the following questions by selecting the best response or responses from those provided. For this set of questions, you may wish to refer to **Diagnostic Assessment – Structured Interview for Relational Problems – Child Physical Abuse** *found in Chapter 12: Family Maltreatment and Military Families: Prevention and Response Efforts.*

You are interviewing the mother of a 3-year-old child and are told the following: "I grabbed his arm when he would not stay seated at the kitchen table for breakfast. He said it hurt. I saw a dark bruise where I had grabbed him the next morning, and it lasted a few days. He was otherwise okay—going to daycare, playing with his sister, going to bed without a problem."

23. Was this considered a non-accidental use of physical force?

A. Yes—Grabbing or yanking limbs or body

B. Yes—But this was done so the child would stay seated

C. No—This was accidental

D. No—This was done so the child would stay seated

24. Was there a more than inconsequential physical injury?

A. Yes—But this was done so the child would stay seated

B. Yes—Bruising

C. No—A more than inconsequential physical injury was not noted

D. No—The bruising was superficial

25. Was there a more than inconsequential fear reaction?

A. Yes—The child was acting scared

B. Yes—The child said he was scared

C. No—None was reported

D. No—The parent said she did not have a more than inconsequential fear reaction

For question 26, read the scenario below and answer the following question by selecting the best response or responses from those provided.

After experiencing years of maltreatment from within her family while living in her home country of Honduras, Luz Maria, age 13, was kidnapped and beaten by the perpetrators before escaping and coming to the attention of immigration agents at the border. Luz Maria was released to the sponsorship of her mother, from whom she was separated for 10 years of her life. Luz Maria's mother was happy to have her reunited with her but was concerned about how quiet and sullen she was. Their relationship quickly became conflicted, and, in a moment of frustration, Luz Maria's mother slapped her across the face, causing a bruise. The next day, a teacher made a report to child protective services.

26. What are the most important considerations for the CPS worker upon contacting the family?

> A. Provide an assessment worker who speaks Spanish and is familiar with the culture of the family and dynamics of recently reunited parents and children
>
> B. Removal of Luz Maria to prevent further conflict and harm
>
> C. Assess for Luz Maria's psychosocial needs in the context of her migration experience and recent arrival in the United States
>
> D. Ask the mother for her immigration documents to make sure that she is authorized to be in the United States

For question 27, read the scenario below and answer the following question by selecting the best response or responses from those provided.

Orlando had been living in the streets of El Salvador after being abandoned by his parents at 10 years old. He learned how to survive by "hustling" food and other items from passersby in the street, and oftentimes, by stealing. Orlando's freedom became very important to him, so when he was old enough to migrate north to the United States, he did so at age 14, barely surviving the dangerous journey. He was placed with his older brother, who had migrated to the United States before Orlando had been born. Orlando began to run away so he could continue to have his freedom, and his brother became increasingly concerned and frustrated, eventually locking him in a room when he went to work. Orlando became truant from school and the brother was accused of abusing and neglecting Orlando when authorities heard of what the brother was doing to attempt to control Orlando's behavior.

27. When assessing Orlando's needs, what theoretical construct would be useful?

> A. Piaget's theory of moral development
>
> B. Attachment theory
>
> C. Maslow's theory of the hierarchy of needs
>
> D. Herzberg's motivation hygiene theory

For questions 28-31, carefully read and answer each question by selecting the best response or responses from those provided. This set of questions will require you to refer back to Case Studies 17-1 and 17-2, which appear in Chapter 15: The School Environment and the Impacts of Education When the Teacher is the Bully.

28. What are the potential consequences of the bystander effect when an educator does not intervene in a teacher bullying situation, such as in the situation described in Case Study 17-1?

    A. The student victim will often feel revictimized by the teacher who is indifferent to the abuse they witness

    B. The student victim will self-blame and feel they are not worthy of a teacher intervening on their behalf

    C. The student victim may act out in a manner that is considered disruptive to the classroom and school environment

    D. All of the above

29. What are the potential ramifications of teacher indifference as described in Case Study 17-2?

    A. The student is at risk of further isolating and being vulnerable to having mental health issues such as depression or anxiety, which could become lifelong challenges

    B. There are no ramifications; the student will find like-minded friends and will be just fine

    C. The student will feel a sense of shame and embarrassment that she is a cultural-ethnic-religious minority

30. Which of the following can be considered direct teacher-on-student bullying?

    A. A teacher assigning extra homework because they are frustrated

    B. A teacher intentionally embarrassing, shaming, or humiliating a student

    C. Teacher indifference to witnessing the abuse of a student by a peer

31. How can school-based or clinical social workers play a significant role in the identification of teacher-on-student bullying?

    A. Participate in interdisciplinary teams to identify problematic behaviors in teachers

    B. Facilitate trainings on recognizing and addressing abusive behaviors

    C. Identify the offending teacher and have them terminated or transferred to another school

    D. All of the above

    E. A & B only

For questions 32-34, carefully read and answer each question by selecting the best response or responses from those provided.

32. Students report the most frequent location they are bullied is:

    A. Outside on school grounds

    B. The cafeteria

    C. The hallway or stairwell at school

    D. Online or by text

33. What percentage of adolescents reported having experienced at least one type of cyberbullying?

    A. 71.9%

    B. 59%

    C. 19%

    D. 3.9%

34. Revealing and posting someone's personal information (eg, their home address) to enlist others to harass them is known as:

    A. Doxxing

    B. Happy slapping

    C. Swatting

    D. Outing

For questions 35 and 36, read the scenario below and answer the following questions by selecting the best response or responses from those provided.

A 14-year-old girl was referred to you, a dietitian, by her family physician, who suspects the girl has anorexia nervosa. The physician was concerned that her weight was well under what it should be for a girl of her age and stature. He also picked up on a comment she made about being overweight when the medical technician had her step on the scale. The patient was accompanied by her mother, who did all of the talking, not giving her daughter a chance to answer any medical history or other questions asked. The girl appeared sad and standoffish, not making eye contact with the physician or medical technician.

Upon receiving the consultation from the physician, you contact the girl's mother to set up an appointment to see her daughter. At the planned day and time of the appointment, you introduce yourself to the mother and daughter, and ask the mother if it would be alright to see her daughter alone so you can get to know her better. The mother was reluctant at first, but agreed to do this.

35. In this scenario, what is the focus of the first appointment with your new patient?

    A. Asking her if she has an eating disorder

    B. Finding out what she eats and drinks every day

    C. Finding out if she is seeing a psychologist or psychiatrist

    D. Finding out more about her to build a rapport

36. What data should be assessed when treating a patient with an eating disorder?

    A. Weight (using the same scale)

    B. Food intake records

    C. Frequency of disordered eating behaviors and what triggered them

    D. All of the above

For question 37, read the scenario below and answer the following question by selecting the best response or responses from those provided.

Maria Suarez is 8 years old. She has recently been moved into the care of a shelter on an emergency basis, and a dependency petition is being filed by a child protection agency with the goal of placing her in foster care. Prior to the filing of the dependency petition, Maria resided with her mother, Cassie Suarez. The family first became known to the child welfare agency 5 years ago, when the agency received several calls alleging substance use and erratic behavior by Ms. Suarez. The following year, the agency substantiated an allegation when Ms. Suarez admitted to heroin use. Ms. Suarez entered an inpatient substance use program in that same year and successfully completed the program.

During the most recent incident 6 days ago, the Child Protection Hotline received a report from a service provider that Ms. Suarez was observed to be under the influence of an unknown substance. The reporting source and the agency caseworker both observed Ms. Suarez to have slurred speech and an inability to respond appropriately to questions. Ms. Suarez initially stated that she had taken prescription medication but could not produce the medicine bottle or prescription. No father has been identified or located. Maria was removed from her mother's care on an emergency basis.

During the shelter care hearing, the attorney for the agency argued that Ms. Suarez was unable or unwilling to care for Maria, who should be found a dependent child and placed in foster care under the custody and supervision of the agency. The attorney argued the agency made reasonable efforts to prevent the removal and asked the judge to make the appropriate findings.

37. What should the judge consider in finding whether reasonable efforts to prevent removal have been made?

    A. Ms. Suarez's previous successful completion of the inpatient substance use program

    B. The agency's conclusion that the substances Ms. Suarez was using were illicit because she could not provide the prescription or bottle

    C. The agency's previous involvement 5 years ago

    D. Whether the agency provided any in-home support or services after the most recent report was received and prior to Maria's removal from her home

For question 38, read the scenario below and answer the following question by selecting the best response or responses from those provided.

A therapist has been seeing a 16-year-old male for several months for his anxiety and mood dysregulation. At the most recent therapy session, the therapist noticed a large bruise and a cut on the client's face. When asked about the injury, the client said that his mother slapped him and the cut resulted from the ring she was wearing. The client admitted that he had been arguing with his mother and was giving her a "hard time." The therapist reminded the client about the discussion they had at the beginning of therapy regarding mandated reporting of child abuse, and told the client that this incident met the reporting requirements.

The therapist then invited the mother to join her son in the session and told her of the obligation to report the incident. She expressed remorse about what happened and said it would never happen again, asking the therapist not to make a report. The therapist repeated the need to report the incident and made the report with the mother and her son present.

38. In which of the following ways did the therapist meet the highest clinical, ethical, and legal expectations for a professional in her position?

    A. Reminding the client of the discussion of mandated reporting that took place at the beginning of treatment

    B. Making a report of suspected child abuse

    C. Making the report with both the mother and client present

    D. All of the above

For question 39, read the scenario below and answer the following question by selecting the best response or responses from those provided.

A mother brought her adolescent daughter for therapy. The daughter requested therapy regarding peer and romantic relationships. As part of the informed consent process, the therapist told the mother and her daughter about the limits of confidentiality. Because the legal age to consent to treatment in this area was 18 and the client was 16, in addition to consent to treatment, the mother owned confidentiality (the client's father was deceased). The client then did not want to participate in treatment until the therapist mentioned that the three of them could make and sign an agreement detailing what information would be shared with her mother.

39. What would you call the solution proposed by the therapist?

     A. Emotional competence

     B. Assent to treatment

     C. Agreement of confidentiality

     D. Good boundaries

For question 40, read the scenario below and answer the following question by selecting the best response or responses from those provided.

A couple brought their 8-year-old foster son to a psychologist for an assessment. The parents were concerned that their son may have ADHD because he was struggling in school and having difficulty following directions at home. The parents signed the consent to treatment form for the assessment. The psychologist explained to their son the purpose of the assessment, the measures she would be using, who would see the results, and possible outcomes. The psychologist then asked for the son's active agreement to the assessment process and a commitment to do his best work.

40. In this scenario, the therapist asked for the son's ____:

     A. Cooperation

     B. Assent

     C. Agreement

     D. Consent

CONSTRUCTED RESPONSE
For questions 41-43, read each question carefully and formulate a response.

41. What challenges might be faced in coordinating care when using telehealth?

42. What risk factors and warning signs should a provider be aware of or watch for during a telehealth visit?

43. How would you measure the success of telehealth?

For question 44, read the scenario below, then formulate a response to the following question.

A 6-year-old client just finished the intake process to receive psychotherapy. The multimethod assessment process led to a diagnosis of PTSD and a recommendation of TF-CBT as treatment. During the parent interview, the client's mother inferred that symptomology began to emerge after the client witnessed gun violence while walking home from school. The client's mother also disclosed that the community has high rates of violence, but that she had no plans or means to move. Given the client's ongoing risk of further exposure to community violence, the clinician assigned to the case was concerned about the Enhancing Safety and Future Development component being at the end of the TF-CBT treatment model.

44. How might the therapist address this client's safety concerns while still maintaining fidelity to the TF-CBT treatment model?

For question 45, refer back to the scenario provided for questions 11 and 12, then formulate a response to the following question.

45. Complete the functional analysis below as it applies to Billy's negative behavior.

   Antecedent:_____

   Behavior:_____

   Consequence:_____

For questions 46 and 47, refer back to the scenario provided for question 16, then formulate a response to the following questions.

46. How were Chris's relational templates impacted by their early life experiences?

47. What systemic barriers are in place that prevent the adults in Chris's life from meeting their needs and cultivating relational resilience?

For questions 48-50, read the scenario below, then formulate a response to the following questions.

You are completing an intake for a client, Kelly. Kelly is a 16-year-old transgender girl who is currently in foster care after being physically and emotional abused by her biological parents. Because she is currently in the custody of CPS, you first meet with Kelly's caseworker to complete the intake paperwork and informed consent. You notice that the caseworker continuously uses Kelly's deadname as well as masculine pronouns when referring to her.

48. Describe 2 of the trauma-informed care principles and how they may be implemented with Kelly.

49. How might you address the caseworker's use of deadnaming and incorrect pronouns? What other considerations might you have related to Kelly's gender identity when working with the caseworker or CPS more generally?

50. Thinking about clients like Kelly, what affirmative and trauma-informed care practices do you, your practicum/internship site, organization, or educational institution currently implement with clients, and what are some ways these practices could be improved as they apply to work with LGBTQIA+ clients who have experienced child maltreatment or other traumas?

For questions 51-53, read the scenario below, then formulate a response to the following questions.

It is the holiday season, and a local preschool wants to be inclusive to all the faiths and cultural beliefs that make up their school's demographic population.

51. What would be some examples of age-appropriate activities that the children and their respected families can participate in?

52. How can the educators ensure that the children participating in the events feel safe, respected, and seen during such a rich cultural experience?

53. Do you recall an event in your primary or secondary schooling years that invited you to learn about someone else's cultural, ethnic, or religious practices? Was it a pleasant memory? How important was that experience to you, now understanding diversity?

For question 54, read the scenario below, then formulate a response to the following question.

Jeffrey, who is 12 years of age, and Anna, who is 7 years of age, are siblings who live in the same household with their biological parents. Anna reported to her parents that she and Jeffrey "played house." When their parents inquired about this further, Anna reported that this was "acting like a Mommy and Daddy" and involved touching each other's "private parts" while "cuddling" in their parents' bed. At the time of the incident, the parents were out and Jeffrey was watching his sister. Jeffrey reports that they were just playing, and he had heard about this type of fondling from peers and wanted to know what it was like.

54. What further questions would you have about this scenario before making an assessment?

For question 55, read the scenario below, then formulate a response to the following question.

Daniel, who is 10 years of age, and Eric, who is 6 years of age, are siblings in a household with their single mother. Their parents divorced 1 year ago, and the boys see their father most weekends. While the mother works full time, she has noticed an increase in bullying behavior by Daniel towards Eric. Daniel often orders his brother around, makes fun of him for the way he talks and plays, refuses to engage with him in games they used to share, and has banned him from entering his bedroom. In addition, Eric has shown evidence of physical altercations (ie, bruises) after fights with Daniel. Daniel insists that they were "wrestling," but Eric now clearly avoids Daniel and has had bruises on his arms and back on a few different occasions. Eric's first grade teacher reports that Eric has had difficulties with his classmates and is increasingly aggressive in interactions. He also has difficulty focusing in class and needs consistent redirection to stay on task.

55. How would you educate the parents about what is happening with Daniel and Eric?

For question 56, read the scenario below, then formulate a response to the following question.

Joelle, who is 14 years of age, and Samantha, who is 8 years of age, are siblings in a household with their biological mother and stepfather of 4 years. Their biological father died 5 years ago in a car accident. The girls share a bedroom and reportedly argue constantly. Recently, their mother has noticed that Samantha has regressed in her behavior, playing with toys from earlier in her childhood, talking to a make-believe friend, and engaging in baby talk and clingy behavior. Their mother also reports that she has heard Joelle constantly berate Samantha, calling her "ugly," "fat," and a "baby." Joelle has been preoccupied with her own appearance and a group of girls at school who seem to readily judge and ostracize others.

56. What might be causing Joelle to act this way toward her sister?

For question 57, read the scenario below, then formulate a response to the following question.

Oliver is a 17-year-old male who lives with his grandparents. His grandparents put him into therapy for support after his parents' rights were terminated. While he was at basketball practice, his grandmother found a vaping device used for nicotine in his bedroom. At his next therapy appointment, Oliver told his therapist about the incident and how he felt violated that his grandmother was going through his things. His therapist screened for other substance use and assessed his patterns of nicotine use. Oliver denied the use of other substances. He reported using nicotine when he feels stressed and when he hangs out with friends. There has been no change in Oliver's grades or social life.

57. What services and interventions would Oliver benefit from?

For question 58, read the scenario below, then formulate a response to the following question.

Shannon is a 13-year-old female who lives with her father and stepmother. She does not feel supported by them, but lives in a safe environment. At her annual physical, Shannon's physician screened for substance use. Shannon shared that she has been hanging out with an older group of peers who use marijuana and alcohol regularly. She has tried these substances and only liked alcohol. She reported bingeing patterns of alcohol use on Fridays and Saturdays and other risk-taking behavior, such as getting into the car with intoxicated teenage drivers. Her physician also administered a depression screening in which Shannon disclosed suicidal thoughts. Upon talking to her father, the physician learned that Shannon has been refusing to attend school since transitioning to seventh grade.

58. What services and interventions would Shannon benefit from?

For question 59, read the scenario below, then formulate a response to the following question.

Lily is a 16-year-old female who lives with her mother. She has a good relationship with her mom, an active social life, and is involved in a variety of school clubs. Since Lily entered high school, however, her mother has noticed a change in Lily's behavior, as she seems to have a low mood, her grades have been declining, and she has expressed a desire to quit some of her extracurricular activities. Lily agreed to see a therapist, who assessed for mental health concerns and screened for substance use. Lily disclosed that she has been using marijuana 3 to 5 times weekly to cope with her low mood and socially on the weekends. Lily's therapist noted symptoms of depression without suicidal ideation.

59. What services and interventions would Lily benefit from?

For questions 60 and 61, read each question carefully and formulate a response.

60. Why are so many detained and incarcerated child and adolescent offenders also victims of maltreatment?

61. What are some of the most common mental health difficulties found for adolescents involved in the juvenile justice system? What are some of the possible reasons for this?

For question 62, read the scenario below, then formulate a response to the following question.

Malia is a 13-year-old girl sent from abroad to live with her maternal uncle for the purpose of attending school in the United States and helping her uncle's family with their new baby. 6 months after her arrival, Malia's uncle began to sexually abuse her, and she became withdrawn and depressed. Her counselor at school noticed her mental health struggles, and Malia disclosed the abuse during a counseling session. The school reported the abuse to the police and CPS; both investigated the allegation as part of a multidisciplinary team approach. The child welfare agency filed a petition to remove Malia from her uncle's home and place her into foster care. The prosecutor's office filed criminal charges.

62. Name 3 ways in which Malia's civil and criminal cases can be coordinated.

For questions 63-65, read the scenario below, then formulate a response to the following questions. You may wish to refer back to Chapter 23: Child and Adolescent Maltreatment: Implications for Adult Survivors for this set of questions.

Elijah is a 30-year-old heterosexual, able-bodied Latino male who presents with depression. He struggles with maintaining employment and is fearful of losing his longtime partner with whom he lives. Elijah reports having a "short temper," "going from 0 to 60," and feeling both anxious and depressed most of the time. Elijah shares that he grew up with both parents, his mother and father. He also shares that there was interpersonal violence in the home between his parents, and that both parents physically abused him. He says that he was often told he was "no good" and would "never amount to anything." His mother would tell him throughout his childhood that she wished she had an abortion.

63. Given what Elijah has shared about his past experiences, list 3 trauma responses that Elijah appears to be experiencing.

64. Are there issues not discussed in Chapter 23 that would be helpful in understanding and working with Elijah? What other information would you want to know about Elijah?

65. Applying this scenario to your own career, are there any strategies that you use in your discipline that would assist you in collaborating with Elijah to address his areas of concern? What do you need to know more about? How might you collaborate with other disciplines to learn more?

ANSWER KEY

1. B, C, or E	15. D	28. D
2. B or C	16. C	29. A
3. A, C, or D	17. A	30. B
4. A, C, D, or E	18. C	31. E
5. B or E	19. B	32. C
6. A, C, or D	20. B	33. B
7. C	21. L	34. A
8. D	22. F	35. C & D
9. C	23. A	36. D
10. D	24. B	37. D
11. C	25. C	38. D
12. B	26. A & C	39. C
13. C	27. B	40. B
14. A		

41. Some of the challenges nurses often face when using telehealth include:

> **Technology Barriers**—Patients in rural and low-income areas, along with older adults, may not have access to reliable internet, wireless service, or computers or smartphones.

> **Educational Barriers**—This might stem from a lack of training related to telehealth practice. Telehealth was not a standard inclusion in interdisciplinary health care curricula before COVID-19. Clinicians need to be educated early, especially while training as health care students. The early exposure through dedicated training will help build confidence and comfort in using telehealth in their future practice. On the other hand, the literacy of the client (both traditional and digital) and their education level may pose a barrier due to the nature of telehealth. This may necessitate designing telehealth applications based on simplicity and ease-of-use, keeping in mind such limitations.

> **Insurance Coverage Issues**—Some insurance companies require in-person assessments for specific health conditions, even when this is difficult for the patient to do so based on their physical or mental condition, or geographic location.

Regulatory Obstacles—Telehealth services have proven to be indispensable to health care practitioners and patients during COVID-19, allowing for greater accessibility and alignment with technological innovation. Still, after the expiration of the Public Health Emergency Declaration, many factors will need to be addressed to ensure an adequate telehealth infrastructure. The potential for fraud is a key concern. Telehealth's accelerated growth and fast-tracked implementation raise many concerns, including provider licensure compliance and fraudulent behavior by health care providers.

Ethical Barriers—Due to widespread social media usage, there is generally a great awareness of data privacy and confidentiality issues associated with being online. These issues are critical since it concerns health records and other private information related to treatment. These fears might discourage some from accepting telehealth as an alternative mode of availing health care services. Telehealth systems that incorporate data encryption and similar cyber-security measures must be employed. Clinicians must seek informed consent from their clients before each telehealth consultation and in a specific format.

42. During child telehealth visits, risk and warning factors are assessed via **verbal**, **behavioral**, **interactional**, and **environmental** assessment. Below are examples of indicators and related assessment categories (this list is not exhaustive):

    — Observe and consider family/child interactions. (verbal, behavioral, interactional)

    — Does the child seem fearful of the caregiver? (behavioral, interactional)

    — Does the caregiver speak for the child directly without allowing the child the opportunity to share? (verbal, interactional)

    — Observe any nonverbal cues that may be indicative of potential abuse and neglect. (verbal, behavioral, interactional)

    — Does the child demonstrate expressions of pain despite any visible marks or bruises? (behavioral)

    — Does the child seem shutdown? (verbal [ie, nonverbal], behavioral, interactional)

    — Do members of the home engage in traumatic play? (behavioral, interactional, environmental)

    — Pay attention to the background. Are there any safety hazards, either physical or environmental? Can yelling or screaming be overheard? How does the child appear in the environment? (verbal, behavioral, interactional, environmental)

    — Be mindful of who may be listening in the background. (behavioral, interactional, environmental)

    — Ask probing questions such as, "What does a day look like at home for you right now?" (verbal, behavioral, interactional, environmental)

43. If IPV is disclosed in a telehealth context, clinicians are able support to their patients' circumstances (ie, the child or the nonoffending parent) by establishing a referral to a social worker within the clinical care team, online support services, local community-based organizations that specialize in IPV, or support groups with text/chat options. In addition to providing such resources to all patients, an in-person health care visit may be needed due to the inextricable links between IPV and physical ailments.

44. The therapist would engage in general safety planning with the child and the caregiver at the beginning of treatment and engage in safety checks throughout the course of the therapy. The therapist would be cognizant, however, that the components of the PRACTICE acronym are ordered with the concept that the introduction of each new component builds on previous components. One reason why the Enhancing Safety and Future Development component is at the end of the therapeutic process is due to the possibility that teaching safety skills specifically related to a trauma could serve as a reminder of the traumatic event and elicit negative reactions. This possibility is minimized when introduced towards the end of the therapeutic process, as coping skills, affective regulation, and relaxation skills will have been practiced, and the trauma will have been processed by now for both the child and their caregiver. Therefore, the therapist is recommended to teach general safety skills at the beginning of treatment and emphasize trauma-specific safety skills in the last third of treatment.

45. Antecedent: Billy's mother interrupts him playing video games; Behavior: Billy throws a tantrum; Consequence: Billy is allowed to continue playing video games, thus reinforcing the tantrums.

46. It does not seem like Chris had predictable, safe, or reliable experiences with adults. Chris was surrounded by drug abuse and a revolving door of relationships in addition to taking on the responsibilities of caring for young children. Chris's teachers had little to no understanding, tolerance, or curiosity about the contributing factors to the behaviors they saw in the classroom. These experiences have set a relational template for Chris that adults are not to be trusted or turned to for support, care, or validation of difficult circumstances. It is probable that Chris developed a relational template that set them up to be distrustful or protective/defensive towards adults as a way to survive the environment.

47. The school's zero-tolerance policy for "disrespect" is short sighted and harmful not only for children but adults alike. No one thrives in an environment where they are reduced to the sum of their survival strategies. The zero-tolerance policy is an example of a systemic barrier that does not allow for a teacher to tap into their own humanity to meet a child in need of warm, responsive, and safe interactions.

48. One principle of trauma-informed care is safety, which involves helping the client feel both physically and emotionally safe. For example, making arrangements to have a gender-neutral restroom, particularly one with a lock, may help Kelly feel both physically and emotionally safe. Using affirmative language as well as Kelly's correct pronouns (ie, the ones that match her gender identity as opposed to her sex assigned at birth) are other ways to increase a sense of safety. Another principle is trustworthiness, which involves being transparent and making sure the client is informed about the services they will receive and any policies they should be aware of. For example, for LGBTQIA+ children who have experienced maltreatment, they should be informed about the rules related to confidentiality as it relates to their identities, the trauma they have experienced, and any other relevant factors. In this situation, Kelly is in CPS custody, so information about her progress will be periodically shared with her caseworker and the agency. Prior to meeting with Kelly, it would be helpful to discuss with her caseworker what information will need to be shared in any therapist reports.

49. It may be helpful to provide the caseworker with information on the importance of using the client's proper name and pronouns. For example, exposure to deadnaming is a type of minority stress, and minority stress has been found to be predictive of distress in LGBTQIA+ children and adolescents. As the caseworker may be unaware of inclusive language and up-to-date terminology, it may be helpful to provide them with some information resources developed by

an LGBTQIA+ child and adolescent advocacy organization. Since working with children in CPS custody often requires periodic reports on the client's progress to be made, additional information on the required content and format (eg, verbal or written) of progress updates should be ascertained. This information should be shared with the client as well. When written reports are required, efforts should be made to only include the client's deadname to the absolute minimum required. For example, if the client's legal name is required to be included in any written report, determine if is it sufficient to only include the client's legal name at the start of the document, clarify their current name, and then use the current name for the remainder of the report. Finally, it may also be helpful to determine the current visitation and permanency plan (ie, the long-term goal for ending CPS involvement) for the client. For example, is reunification with Kelly's biological parents the current goal? This information could inform the content of treatment with Kelly and determine the need and ability to potentially involve caregivers in treatment.

50. Personal reflection – responses vary

51. **Oral History**: Children can ask their parents about any fairy tale that may have originated within their cultural, ethnic, and religious upbringing. The children can participate in a show and tell.

    Food: Children and parents can bring in their favorite foods to share with the class, and write down a short description of the dish and why it is important to their family unit. If engaging in this exercise, the recommendation is to write down all the ingredients so there is consideration for those individuals with food allergies or food restrictions.

    Music: Children and parents can participate in making a short music playlist with songs that are traditional to their cultural, ethnic, or religious customs. They can play these songs during the multicultural event.

    Regalia: Invite both children and parents to participate in showcasing their traditional regalia if they would like.

    Arts: Allow children to color, make, or craft various ideas that represent different culture, ethnic, or religious customs of the population within the preschool.

52. Educators should constantly check in with the children to gauge if they are enjoying the festivities. The educators should also create an area that is quieter and less stimulating in case any child feels overwhelmed by the activities and would like to step away as needed with supervision and age-appropriateness. Parents and volunteers should be open and gentle when introducing new language and customs to the children. Finally, educators should create an assignment the next day that mimics a debriefing for the children so they may share how they felt about the multicultural festival.

53. Personal reflection – responses vary

54. Further questions should include how often this has occurred, whether this behavior developed from sexual curiosity or exploitation, the effects of the incident(s) on either child, family dynamics, the parents' responses to the situation, and a plan for safety as well as who to call as a mandated reporter. Such a comprehensive assessment is needed to contextualize the family dynamics and the propensity of the 12-year-old to be a perpetrator. The following list is intended to guide an assessment of this nature.

    A. The number of times such incidents occurred can help distinguish between "curiosity" and an ongoing threat/pattern.

B. The degree of exploitation that was involved in those incidents can help identify the dynamics of abuse. For instance, asking the younger child how she was approached, what was said, and how she responded and felt can help determine the power exerted by the older sibling.

C. Dysfunctions in the family dynamics, such as substance abuse, lack of parental supervision, and other experiences of sexual abuse (with these children, others, or the parents themselves) would lead to more concern about risks.

D. Exploring the interest of the 12-year-old and distinguishing between curiosity versus desire/attraction would help identify risks for him as a perpetrator. For example, helpful questions may include: What did you hear from your friends? What part were you curious about? What did you think might happen? How did this affect you?

55. Parents should be educated about the signs and symptoms of sibling abuse, the need for mandated reporting, resources available to them, and ways to develop safety in the house.

56. Joelle may be exerting control over her younger sister because she is feeling disempowered and insecure in her peer relations. She also may have less tolerance for her sister due to developmental differences, and may be acting out as a result of family dynamics which are unknown.

57. Though Oliver is using substances, the severity is low. Oliver is almost of legal age to buy nicotine himself, and his use has not interfered with his academic or social functioning. Oliver would benefit from a continuation of individual therapy with a focus on emotion regulation and concept of self. Oliver's therapist should monitor for progression of substance use. Basketball may be a potential coping skill for stress to replace the use of nicotine. Oliver may benefit from a family session with his grandparents. Oliver may also benefit from some education on nicotine use and the risk of using other substances.

58. Shannon's presentation is high risk. Due to the suicidal ideation in combination with the substance use, Shannon would benefit from Multisystemic Family Therapy as this is an in-home service that offers 24/7 crisis support. If this level of care does not facilitate improvement after a trial period, Shannon may benefit from residential care. Therapy should focus on how Shannon can feel supported by her father and stepmother, development of coping skills for depression, and an increase in community support by increasing school engagement.

59. Lily's presentation is high risk as she is using marijuana frequently, and it has begun to interfere with her functioning at school. Lily would benefit from a continuation of individual therapy with a combination of CBT and MI. CBT would allow her to develop self-regulation tools and coping skills to replace marijuana use, as well as explore thoughts, feelings, and behaviors that are contributing to low mood and substance use. The use of MI may help Lily explore her values and future goals, and how participation in extracurriculars, school performance, and substance use could influence her goals. It may be beneficial to encourage Lily to stay engaged in extracurriculars, or to try new activities that provide similar community support benefits. Lily would also benefit from psychoeducation and involving her mother in the treatment process.

60. Being a victim of any of the maltreatment types increases the risk for other delinquency-related troubles. Some of these may be related directly to the maltreatment (eg, trauma from sexual abuse that causes serious mental health troubles and functioning), while other experiences may be cumulative in building delinquency risks (eg, neglect that is experienced by a parent/guardian

and living in unsafe neighborhoods). It is often this accumulation of difficulties and experiences as a younger person that gravely increases school difficulties and involvement with the juvenile courts.

61. The most common mental health difficulties are disruptive behavioral disorders, substance use/abuse, anxiety, and depressive problems. These mental health difficulties all have trauma symptoms as part of the possible diagnosis/history. This is not surprising, since many of the adolescents involved with the juvenile justice system have trauma/maltreatment histories.

62. The multidisciplinary team can continue to synchronize the investigation for both the civil dependency and criminal cases. Scheduling of hearings can be coordinated. Judges and parties to the proceedings can be apprised of orders in the other court. Dispositional or sentencing options sought in either court can be coordinated. Both civil and criminal child abuse prosecutors should understand the traumatic impact of the proceedings on the child and her ability to participate in case preparation or testify at trial.

63. Elijah is experiencing all the trauma responses described in this chapter. He is having emotion regulation issues due to his temper going from 0 to 60 when activated. Elijah may be experiencing feelings of shame surrounding his history of witnessing violence from his caregivers and experiencing abuse from his caregivers. Additionally, Elijah's memory of not being wanted (his mother saying: "I wish I had an abortion") may also make him feel unwanted. Finally, he has challenges with interpersonal relationships as evidenced by the loss of a longtime partner and issues maintaining employment.

64. Having biopsychosocial knowledge of a client and understanding the whole person and their history gives professionals a wider perspective of the person and allows for a thorough understanding of their trauma. Elijah's age, gender, culture, environment, social supports, coping strategies, strengths, and socioeconomic status, both when the abuse occurred and now, all impact how he navigates the world.

65. Personal reflection – responses vary